P9-DMJ-305

The Healing Powers of Chocolate

"The powerful polyphenols in dark chocolate are a 21st-century health food—your Rx for longevity."

—Karlis Ullis, M.D, Santa Monica, California

"Chocolate is a taste of divine ecstasy on Earth. It is our sensual communion. Orey's journalistic style and efforts share this insight with readers around the world."

—Jim Walsh, founder of Intentional Chocolate

PRAISE FOR CAL OREY'S CLASSIC HEALTH BOOKS

The Healing Powers of Vinegar

"A practical, health-oriented book that everyone who wants to stay healthy and live longer should read."
  —Patricia Bragg, N.D., Ph.D., author of *Apple Cider Vinegar*

"Deserves to be included in everybody's kitchen and medicine chest."
  —Ann Louise Gittleman, Ph.D., author of *The Fat Flush Plan*

"Wonderfully useful for everyone interested in health."
  —Elson M. Haas, M.D., author of *Staying Healthy with Nutrition, 21st Century Edition*

The Healing Powers of Olive Oil

"One of the most healing foods on the planet. A fascinating read—olive oil is not only delicious, it is good medicine!"
  —Ann Louise Gittleman, Ph.D.

"Orey gives kudos to olive oil—and people of all ages will benefit from her words of wisdom."
  —Dr. Will Clower, CEO, Mediterranean Wellness

"Olive oil has been known for centuries to have healing powers and now we know why. It is rich in monounsaturated fats similar to avocado and macadamia nut oils. The information in this book will help you understand the healing powers of oils."
  —Fred Pescatore, M.D., M.P.H., author of *The Hamptons Diet*

The Healing Powers of Coffee

"A cup or two of joe every day is a good way to boost mood, energy, and overall health."
—Julian Whitaker, M.D., Founder of the Whitaker Wellness Institute

"For heart, mind, and body, Cal Orey shows us why coffee is the most comforting health food on the planet."
—Will Clower, Ph.D., founder and president of Mediterranean Wellness, Inc.

"All of the Healing Powers books have been widely popular on our network of thousands of food bloggers. Her latest book on coffee is no exception!"
—Jenn Campus, Foodie Blogroll

The Healing Powers of Honey

"Cal Orey has done a wonderful job of thoroughly explaining the great value of honey. *The Healing Powers of Honey* is an easy-to-read book that's an invaluable addition to anyone's library. It's full of practical tips and applications for medical conditions that everyone should know about."
—Allan Magaziner, D.O., Magaziner Center for Wellness, Cherry Hill, New Jersey

"Cal Orey scores again with *The Healing Powers of Honey*, a continuation of her widely praised Healing Powers series. Orey's honey book is well researched in a manner that makes it both entertaining and informative. This book will make you look at honey in a new way—as a bona fide health food, as well as a gastronomic treat."
—Joe Traynor, author of *Honey: The Gourmet Medicine*

"Not everyone can be a beekeeper, but Cal Orey shares the secrets that honey bees and their keepers have always known. Honey is good for body and soul."
—Kim Flottum, editor of *Bee Culture* magazine and author of several honey bee books

The **HEALING POWERS** of **VINEGAR**

Books by Cal Orey*

The Healing Powers Series

The Healing Powers of Vinegar
The Healing Powers of Olive Oil
The Healing Powers of Chocolate
The Healing Powers of Honey
The Healing Powers of Coffee

Doctors' Orders
202 Pets' Peeves

*Available from Kensington Publishing Corporation

The HEALING POWERS of VINEGAR

A COMPLETE GUIDE TO NATURE'S MOST REMARKABLE REMEDY

REVISED AND UPDATED THIRD EDITION

CAL OREY

KENSINGTON BOOKS
www.kensingtonbooks.com

Permission to reproduce The Mediterranean Diet Pyramid
granted by Oldways Preservation & Exchange Trust, www.oldwayspt.org.

KENSINGTON BOOKS are published by

Kensington Publishing Corp.
119 West 40th Street
New York, NY 10018

Copyright © 2000, 2006, 2016 by Cal Orey

All rights reserved. No part of this book may be reproduced in any form or by any means without the prior written consent of the Publisher, excepting brief quotes used in reviews.

All Kensington titles, imprints and distributed lines are available at special quantity discounts for bulk purchases for sales promotion, premiums, fundraising, educational or institutional use.

Special book excerpts or customized printings can also be created to fit specific needs. For details, write or phone the office of the Kensington Special Sales Manager: Kensington Publishing Corp., 119 West 40th Street, New York, NY 10018. Attn: Special Sales Department. Phone: 1-800-221-2647.

Kensington and the K logo Reg. U.S. Pat & TM Off.

eISBN-13: 978-1-4967-0381-1
eISBN-10: 1-4967-0381-2
Kensington Electronic Edition: September 2016

ISBN-13: 978-1-4967-0380-4
ISBN-10: 1-4967-0380-4
First Kensington Trade Paperback Edition: October 2000
Revised and Updated Edition: September 2006
First Kensington Mass Market Edition: January 2009
Revised and Updated, Third Edition: September 2016

10 9 8 7

Printed in the United States of America

I dedicate this book to tea, for keeping me balanced during the bumps in the road while revisiting changes in Vinegar World.

CONTENTS

PART 6 Vinegar Remedies

PART 7 Future Vinegar

PART 8 Vinegar Recipes 267

PART 9 Vinegar Resources 343

Foreword

Vinegar is a most lovely contradiction. Born of bacteria, it helps prevent bacterial infection. The flavor of its acetic acid may seem overly sharp, and yet it acts as a natural flavor enhancer to bring out all the delicious notes in any savory food preparation. Its medical roots extend as deep as the ancient Greek and Islamic physicians Hypocrites and Ibn Sina, who prescribed apple cider vinegar remedies, and yet new discoveries of its medical benefits are being unearthed every year. Vinegar is so common, and yet uncommonly healthy, for a laundry list of health issues.

A perfect example is the everyday role it assumes in one of the healthiest diets on Earth, the Mediterranean diet. Along with extra virgin olive oil, this culture regularly uses a rich and varied array of vinegars such as balsamic, cider, and a range of infused vinegars limited only by the imagination.

The use of vinegar is an expression of their culture, and much of it driven by their love of good food. For example, I was speaking at an event in Berkeley, California, on the health properties of the traditional Mediterranean diet. Afterward, one of the audience members approached me to talk about the vital importance of the salad to this diet. Although small in stature, he nevertheless strode up to me to make what he and his waving hands certainly considered to be an over-size point.

"Why is the salad so important to this diet?"

Oh no, a rhetorical question! Certainly a trap I was not to escape from, there was no way I was going to venture a guess. "Wow," I floundered. "Yes, so, I mean . . . so why do YOU think it is?" When in doubt, always answer a question with a question.

"Ha," he responded triumphantly, "it is the chemistry of the vinegar!"

Okay, I didn't see that coming, but his point turned out to be quite thoughtful. He enthused on, in words and gestures, to explain that the acetic acid found in vinegar acts as a palate cleanser, allowing you to better appreciate the flavors of your next course of food. The salad is important on its own, but also to reset your tastes to better appreciate the next round of the meal. And for a culture famous for the love of food flavors, combinations, and interactions, this made perfect sense.

As Cal Orey details throughout *The Healing Powers of Vinegar*, the dramatic flavor added to the meal by vinegar confers an equally broad net of health benefits. The third edition is an ideal resource for this, showing the new findings in a way that makes them accessible to everyone. Expect to learn about the many kinds of vinegar, and how they can be used to help control weight, blood sugar for diabetics, and help protect your heart.

And now is a perfect time for *The Healing Powers of Vinegar*, too, as more people look for natural alternatives to older chemical solutions. Rather than using bleach or other harsh chemicals to clean counters, vinegar-based solutions provide the antibiotic cleaning power without worry. Rather than monosodium glutamate (MSG) as a flavor enhancer, vinegar brings out the flavor without the health problems MSG produces. And the idea of incorporating vinegar to help control weight, stabilize blood sugar, and improve heart health is such a delicious addition.

Taste this work and enjoy.

—Dr. Will Clower, CEO, Mediterranean Wellness
and award-winning author of *The Fat Fallacy*,
and *Eat Chocolate, Lose Weight*

Acknowledgments

At the edge of the new millennium, I was asked by the late Lee Heiman, my former editorial consultant, to write the bible on vinegar, focusing on red wine vinegar—not apple cider vinegar. At first, I was anything but enthusiastic. However, it was either create a book about the "new" ancient cure-all or ghostwrite a book for a cardiologist. After flip-flopping, I chose the different vinegar book. And oddly enough, today I am glad I did.

I admit that when I wrote the first edition, I had no clue how versatile vinegar was, so it was a big learning experience for me. Plus, Heiman wanted me to tout the health benefits of red wine vinegar and its potential link to disease-fighting red wine, which I did. However, I realized during my interviews with nutritionists, scientists, and medical doctors that while red wine vinegar certainly has perks (even though you'd have to drink gallons of it to get the exact same benefits as from red wine), it isn't the only healthful vinegar on the shelves.

The second time around, I decided to explore the wide world of vinegar and weight loss, heart health, and longevity; and the ignored health benefits of other vinegars, too. Also, I recall receiving a fan letter from the United Kingdom that was written by a woman who was disgruntled with the first edition of *The Healing Powers of Vinegar*. She noted that while it was a popular book in her country, she felt let down when she saw that it had only 30 home cures. That honest comment hit home. I realized she was right on the money.

So to prepare the second edition, I went to work again. I decided to discover (and to try) some additional home cures using vinegar. I confess: That time I really was amazed by the healing powers of the wide world of vinegars.

Fast-forward to the present and future. I am now one more aging human who is fighting to keep lean, control my cholesterol levels and blood pressure numbers, and stave off type 2 diabetes. And I realize that the new information I bring to this book, the third edition, is a gentle reminder that while I was on the right track, it's vital to my good health that I practice what I preach.

Thus, I am thankful to Heiman, who gave me this original assignment, because I have learned that he was right after all. Perhaps red wine vinegar by *itself* doesn't prevent heart disease. However, the touted Mediterranean diet—which does indeed include vegetables, fruits, grains, fish, olive oil, and vinegar—does keep you healthy, as do other vinegars used internally and externally. Heiman told me this book would have a long shelf life—like vinegar. And I will be forever thankful to him because it just may help me, and you, stay healthier, be happier, and live longer, too.

But the third time is a charm. I want to acknowledge all of the apple cider vinegar followers in the world of vinegar. I ignored this vinegar because my interest took me to the Mediterranean countries, a place where vineyards are plentiful as are balsamic and red wine vinegars. This time, however, I took another look at apple cider vinegar; but since I do things differently, I teamed this timeless vinegar with other healing foods to give you "vinegar trios" and three times the health benefits.

I cannot forget the "Vinegar People" who gave me a nod of approval when I told them I baked and cooked with vinegars—all kinds. We know like an exclusive club that vinegar is not only good for you, offering benefits from weight loss to heart health, but it also opens up a whole new world of flavors.

Also, it's not just the folks who cook for a living whom I thank, but it's vinegar companies that explained to me why vinegar works the way it does, whether it's in a food recipe, for beauty, household cleaning, or other versatile uses.

I want to dish thanks to my editors and publisher, who have faith in me and my research and writing efforts. This timeless topic—ideal for any book—and the first and second edition have received a lot of attention. They've been featured in major book clubs, including Good Cook and One Spirit, have been published in more than a dozen foreign languages, and they ignited the Healing Powers series.

A genuine sense of gratitude is felt toward the people who assisted me this time around as I look back at working through this project. It was challenging because people come and go, as do companies, so many recipes and go-to people in the Vinegar Resources section have been replaced. But change is a good thing because, this time, the Vinegar World has expanded for you and your health.

Credit goes to my comforting and demanding companion animals (who forced me to take breaks and provided unconditional love) and my social media network, who kept me company during the time I was at the computer—busy researching and writing. After all, being an author is a lonely job, but the rewards are worth the efforts.

Overall, I thank each and every person behind the scenes of *The Healing Powers of Vinegar* (all editions and formats). I promise you that this time you will discover even more amazing secrets about the remarkable remedy in Vinegar World. Enjoy.

How to Use This Book

When I was a little girl, my mother's dog-eared *Joy of Cooking* amused me. I can close my eyes and go back in time to the kitchen floor. I'd lie on my stomach and skim through the pages, one after another. So many terms and methods were foreign to me. Often when I'd try one of the recipes, I'd leave out an ingredient or would dump a step and my dish flopped. I'd blame it on the complicated recipe that could have been dumbed down for impatient kids like me.

If you have read the first and second editions of *The Healing Powers of Vinegar*, you know the drill. But if this is your first visit to Vinegar World with me, let me introduce you to some things that could be helpful so you won't get lost like I did when I was a kid.

At the end of each chapter, I include a related recipe (in case you want to take a mini break or are eager to try your hand at using vinegar), a nice introduction to the next chapter, and bullet-point recaps that repeat the highlights of the most important vinegary healing hints to preserve.

PART 1: Welcome to the basic vinegars: apple cider and red wine. These are the two vinegars I used, and chances are, this is why you are reading this book. I take you to the present-day and show you how two household superfoods are still popular in your world and mine. Then, we go back centuries to show you how vinegar isn't anything new, but its shelf life is amazing in the medical world.

PART 2: Next up, I focus on apple cider vinegar—and explain why it's still "in" after centuries. I also scrutinize cider vinegar and show you the ingredients and the real deal as to why it may prove healthful. And that's so not all. I go further into why this vinegar is getting new kudos as a disease fighter as well as fighting pesky ailments—yes, more home cures from the start for you.

PART 3: Then, I go where many vinegar authors don't: into the world of red wine vinegar.

Delving into the past of this vinegar, analyzing its healthful ingredients is what makes this superfood interesting. Also, I take you to the Mediterranean world—and an update of the diet and lifestyle that may be what keeps French women slim, especially if they don't adopt the Western diet of fast, processed food. And, of course, I scrutinize why red wine vinegar may stave off diseases.

PART 4: I don't stop at two vinegars—a place where other vinegar book authors stop. Think of Vinegar World as an amusement park and we are not done. I take you into the land of other healing vinegars: rice, balsamic, herbal, and fruit-flavored varieties. Indeed, since the second edition I wrote a decade ago, some of these vinegars have new information to share—and I'm the hands-on author to take you there.

PART 5: Moving onward, I don't forget olive oil—an important superfood of the Mediterranean diet—and why combining it with other superfoods and vinegar(s) can lead to heart health, losing weight forever, and stalling Father Time.

PART 6: I know I teased you with apple cider vinegar home cures (something readers love), but in this section, I go into mixing and matching vinegars and include new home remedies, tried and true— but no frills and hype. I am not the author to tell you vinegar is going to make you a famous celeb, land you a million dollars, or give you eternal life like a vampire. It's real.

PART 7: Here you'll find how the craze for vinegar—all kinds, not just apple cider—is not a trend but a mainstay around the world because of its versatility and health virtues.

PART 8: Enter one of my favorite places—recipes! This time, dozens of recipes are replaced because the vinegar products are defunct. The exciting news is that I share some of the classic recipes by seasoned chefs and my own easy-to-follow rustic recipes with vinegars that are readily available. An extra bonus: In this fresh edition I have included new recipes using healing foods paired with healing vinegars at the end of each chapter. The ACV Smoothie full of fruit and honey may boost energy, the Peasant Salad with Red Wine Vinegar with its fiber-rich vegetables is pound-paring, and the calcium-rich Mac and Cheese with an Herbal Vinegar Twist helps strengthen bones. Each recipe with its different health benefits deserves to be a stand-out in your diet repertoire.

PART 9: Last but not least, I provide a reader-friendly Resource section—it's not long and boring—and this time I've cut to the chase with the contact information and my take on products.

So, here it is in a vinegar bottle: everything you need to know before you flip through the pages. What's more, I love stories, past and present, so enjoy the different people and places I share with you. Grab a cup of tea spiked with apple cider vinegar or a fruit-flavored vinegar drink and sit down, lie down—get cozy and cuddle up, as I am your guide and here we go into the exciting Vinegar World. No dinosaurs— just unforgettable, enlightening information you and yours can savor. Enjoy!

Author's Note

This book is intended as a reference tool only. It does not give medical advice. Be sure to consult your doctor or the appropriate health-care professional before starting any new diet or exercise program.

Real recipes, tried and true: The recipes in this book have been tested by me, my family and friends, and/or veteran chefs, bakers, and vinegar experts. Changing ingredients or using different vinegar brands or kitchen methods may alter taste, texture, and presentation of a dish. Plus, culinary palates vary. So use your own judgment and follow your instincts and personal tastes when you create a vinegar dish.

In many vinegar home cures and recipes, honey, nature's remarkable nectar, is used.

NOTE: The American Dietetic Association changed its name to Academy of Nutrition and Dietetics.

WARNING: *To avoid infant botulism, do not feed honey to a baby who is younger than one year.*

PART 1

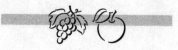

A Time for Vinegar

The Power of Vinegar

Vinegar, the son of wine.

—Babylonian Talmud:
Baba Metzia[1]

More than half a century ago, a vineyard in Sicily, Italy, was the place of my home and heart and unforgettable meals—many complete with vinegar. At the age of six, I was a nature-loving tomboy living a life full of home and family. My grandfather, a big, jovial man, tended to the grapes for winemaking, but he also doted on his homemade red wine vinegar kept in the wine cellar. He used old wooden casks. With child-like fascination I watched him at work providing tender loving care to his vinegars. The liquid with a robust odor bonded us—grandfather and granddaughter—into a sweet underground secret world of making a wonderful thing.

One summer afternoon my mother and father were busy preparing for dinner at our small but quaint family Italian restaurant. It was tourist season and my role was mother's little helper. Sicilian Caponata—one of our signature appetizers—was lacking a special ingredient. "It's empty," she said, holding up a red wine vinegar bottle. I shouted, "It's in Grandpa's barrels!"

I fled outdoors on a vinegar mission to save the dish on the stove-top. I was acquainted with the vats. I filled a large bottle with the robust red liquid produced worldwide. A strong red wine aroma permeated the air. I ran back to the morning sun–lit kitchen, smiled, and delivered the red vinegar. Out of breath, I sat on a bar stool, dangled my legs, and watched as my mother diced vegetables and herbs from the outdoor garden.

Our eyes met. I connected with the woman I admired: She worked hard to feed hungry people looking for authentic, countryside Mediterranean fare, including red pasta sauce and marinated dark meats, like quail and duck. I still can smell the garlic and onions of yesteryear, and see the vintage vinegar bottle on the granite countertop. This vivid memory is my fantasy.

I don't have roots in Italy, where vinegars play a role, but I do feel an uncanny tie to the diet and lifestyle of the European world.

In the real world, more than half a decade ago, I was born and raised in San Jose, California, a region once touted for its fruit orchards and suburbs. Back in the twentieth century my mother did cook Italian dishes (and some recipes included vinegar). I wasn't brought up by an extended family in Italy by the sea, but we did go on picnics to the Pacific Ocean, thirty miles away, and vinegary foods, whether it was salads or sandwiches, were real. And I did imagine living in a European country. In our family room, framed posters of France, Spain, and Italy greeted me every day and night. True, the Sicilian childhood is fabricated, but I was fortunate to taste exotic dishes from the Mediterranean, thanks to my mother, who had traveled abroad and used her talents in the food world.

Those days seem like light-years ago. I can look back at my wonder years and see how the poor man's wine (vinegar) paved the way for me as a woman, author, and health nut who enjoys creating rustic food that is noble and doesn't have to look perfect. I wasn't surrounded by a winery that produced vinegar worth a billion dollars and I didn't grow up in Europe. But I got a taste of vinegar(s) throughout the awkward years of blossoming and embracing different passages as a woman lured by wholesome food.

HELLO, VINEGAR! NATURE'S HELPER

More than 25 years ago, I had a weight problem. One night, I stepped on the scale in my bathroom. It was a shock! At 5 feet 5 inches, I weighed 150 pounds. I blamed it on typical American fast food and a slow sofa-spud lifestyle.

Things changed when I went to college. I wanted to be a dietitian. In basic nutrition class, I was smitten by the fact that food and health were linked. I'd spend time riding my bike to health food stores around town. My diet awareness soared, and my eating habits changed once again, like when I was a teenager. I ate natural, whole foods and plenty of raw green salads splashed with red wine vinegar and olive oil.

My body took on a new shape. Within months, I weighed 120 pounds, and my attitude toward food changed. Food was my friend, not my enemy. I gave all the credit to learning about eating the right amount of the right stuff the way slim and healthy European women and men do.

Kris Cercio* tried just about everything to prevent heart disease—a major killer of women and men in the United States—but nothing worked.

Then she normalized her cholesterol levels by turning to the age-old remedy of apple cider vinegar. As an active 55-year-old woman, she is thin, but she faces the scourge of hereditary high cholesterol. "My doctor couldn't believe I got my numbers down in three short months," she says proudly.

Angelo Salcia* was a 95-year-old man who used his Italian family's old-fashioned remedies for good health. Every day, he took one tablespoon of raw, unfiltered apple cider vinegar in a glass of warm water. After years of using this apple cider vinegar "cocktail," this man stayed active in body and spirit. He vowed the golden liquid kept his blood thin and prevents arthritis.

For countless other people—and perhaps for you, too—the healing powers of vinegar are well known. Like me, people use vinegar not only as a versatile home remedy but also as an integral part of the renowned slimming, heart-healthy, and age-defying Mediterranean diet, where it provides a health boost by teaming up with fruits, vegetables, grains, fish, olive oil, and regular exercise.

If you haven't heard by now, listen up. Your health may depend on

---

*Names of individuals have been changed to protect their privacy.

it. Chances are, you already have two great folk remedies in your kitchen cupboards. It's time to start using them more.

Medical doctors and even scientists are now saying just what folk herbalists in Europe have been saying for years, that *both* apple cider vinegar and red wine vinegar may have a host of amazing healing powers.

I remember as a teenager my mother made sure that I ate my "good for you" dinner. She used both apple cider vinegar and red wine vinegar in her dishes. On Sunday nights I enjoyed eating a fresh cucumber salad: sliced cucumbers, tomatoes, and onions smothered in red wine vinegar. And for dessert, a homemade apple pie was our treat. Real apples were always used for their wholesome goodness and apple cider vinegar for that extra tang. Well, it turns out Mom knew best.

Today, we know even more about the natural goodness behind these two vinegars. Both apple cider vinegar and red wine vinegar are good folk medicine. And this healthful duo promises to be a major home remedy in the new millennium, when alternative medicine will be widespread.

Health Fact!

A survey published in *Journal of the American Medical Association* shows that Americans paid more office visits to alternative medicine practitioners than to primary care physicians.[2]

Medical researchers believe some known trace elements and even the new health-promoting "nutraceuticals" (nutrient supplements that act like pharmaceuticals, which are currently being researched for their potential to treat cancer and heart disease) may be in apple cider vinegar and red wine vinegar.

In addition, foods that are nutritious and prevent diseases are called "functional foods," according to the American Dietetic Association. Scientists have linked functional foods with the prevention or treatment of cancer, diabetes, and heart disease. And studies are ongoing.

Well-known health gurus continue to praise "cure-all" apple cider vinegar, a timeless superfood, as others have done in the past. I watched Dr. Mehmet Oz, for one, on *The Dr. Oz Show*, taste the vinegar and say (not unlike other doctors) this ancient remedy may help to curb the appetite before eating (a good thing during holidays, when we are tempted to overindulge and pack on unwanted pounds). Food Network chefs use apple cider and red wine vinegars (as well as balsamic, wine, fruit-flavored, and herbal varieties) in an array of dishes for the flavor of it. Emeril Lagasse's Seared Quail with Cranberry Vinegar Reduction and Guy Fieri's Vinegar Brined Baby Back Ribs are just a few vinegary dishes and their creative masters at work. And other well-liked food leaders have praised the perks of vinegars too.

The Greenbrier luxury spa in West Virginia is no stranger to the world of vinegars, either. Chef Bryan Skelding uses three basic vinegars I grew up with that are still popular staples in kitchens around the world: apple cider vinegar in his North Carolina BBQ Sauce and red wine vinegar in his Mignonette Sauce. But the seasoned cook also uses champagne vinegar in Pickled Carrots and Vinegar Chips; not to forget balsamic for a dressing recipe made in a large quantity for the luxury spa-goers.

THE APPLE AND THE GRAPE YIELD TWO POWERFUL VINEGARS

Apple cider vinegar has been touted by vinegar gurus as one of nature's most healthful foods, especially if made from fresh, organically grown apples, then allowed to age. And now, red wine vinegar, the ignored condiment, may be its new sidekick, thanks to the grape known as "the vine healer."

People from all walks of life—as well as some vinegar pioneers and contemporary medical experts—believe apple-rich apple cider vinegar aids digestion, helps maintain weight, and keeps blood pressure down. Apple cider vinegar is also known to relieve congestion and maintain healthy skin.

One of the earliest doctors to praise apple cider vinegar was D. C. Jarvis, M.D. Dr. Jarvis strongly recommends its use in his book *Folk Medicine: A New England Almanac of Natural Health Care from a Noted Vermont Country Doctor*, a book that promotes alternative medicine. It's the potassium content, says Jarvis, that makes apple cider vinegar work. "It is so essential to the life of every living thing that without it there would be no life."[3]

Potassium Plus in Apple Cider Vinegar

It's unanimous. As you learn more about apple cider vinegar, you'll continue to hear about the wonders of its high potassium content. Potassium in apple cider vinegar promotes cell, tissue, and organism growth.

In addition to potassium, apple cider vinegar contains these and other health boosters:

Enzymes: chemical substances your body produces to help boost chemical reactions in your body.

Calcium: necessary for transmitting nerve impulses, regulating muscle contraction, and maintaining healthy bones.

Iron: an essential mineral that is important for your blood.

Magnesium: a mineral that has many beneficial effects on you body, most important its impact on heart health.

Two of America's popular antiaging health authorities, the immortalized Dr. Paul Bragg and Dr. Patricia Bragg, spread the good word about potassium-rich apple cider vinegar's health benefits, too. This health-minded team gives credit to apple cider vinegar as being one of the best aids to health and long life known to mankind. They give kudos to its natural substance produced by powerful enzymes—living chemicals.[4]

And now, New Age doctors claim red grapes yield another amazing vinegar. *Red wine vinegar*, claim medical experts, contains healthful nutrients that are part of the "neutraceutical revolution," too. While it's apples that make apple cider vinegar what it is, it is the grape that may be the core of red wine vinegar's nutrients.

For example, one of the nation's leading authorities in preventive, nutritional, and environmental medicine, Allan Magaziner, D.O., founder and director of the Magaziner Center for Wellness and Anti-Aging Medicine in Cherry Hill, New Jersey, says red wine vinegar may have some disease-fighting antioxidant vitamins which are not listed on its label—and yet can be beneficial to our health and well-being.

Andrew Waterhouse, Ph.D., a wine chemist at the University of

California at Davis agrees. Like in wine, red wine vinegar may contain a "new class" of antioxidants or polyphenolics—quercetin, catechins, tannins—which may lower the risk of heart disease and cancer.

Both vinegars have been noted for their folklore remedies in ancient history to modern times, and have gained the respect of countless people, past and present. Before I provide a guide to the health virtues of vinegar, here's what you need to know.

Polyphenols in Red Wine Vinegar

Like apple cider vinegar, red wine vinegar contains polyphenols, naturally occurring compounds that act as powerful antioxidants (enzymes that protect your body by trapping the free-radical molecules and getting rid of them before damage occurs).

Science continues to find new "cutting edge" health-promoting nutrients in grapes and red wine, and these may be in red wine vinegar:

Catechin: a flavonoid believed to prevent cancer.

Flavonoids: antioxidants that belong to the phytochemical family. They are the substances found in fruit and vegetables that give them their colors and flavors.

Quercetin: belongs to the class of nutrients known as bioflavonoids, which provides allergy relief and has been shown to protect from stomach disorders.

Resveratrol: a compound that may have anticancer properties; and may have substances that can also protect against heart disease.

VINEGAR BASICS 101

Vinegar is one of the oldest fermented food products known to man—except for wine and perhaps certain foods made from milk. The word "vinegar" comes from the French *vin aigre* which means "sour wine," a definition that is a no-brainer to anyone who has left a bottle of Chardonnay exposed to the air too long. And someone did just that about 10,000 years ago.

So what exactly is vinegar, anyhow? Simply put, when air is exposed to a fermented liquid, like wine or ale, bacterial activity occurs. This process helps combine oxygen with the alcohol. The end result: acetic acid or sour vinegar.

> **Vinegar:** 1. an impure dilute solution of acetic acid obtained by fermentation beyond alcohol stage and used as a condiment and preservative. 2. Sourness of speech or mood; ill temper. 3. Liveliness and enthusiasm; vim.
>
> —*The American Heritage Dictionary*

Vinegar can be made from any fruit, such as apples or grapes, or any material containing sugar. The following kinds of vinegar are categorized according to material from which they are made and method of production.

VINEGAR POTPOURRI

Kind	Materials Made From	Method of Making
Apple cider vinegar	Apples, apple juice	Twofold fermentation
Wine vinegar	Grapes, peaches, and berries	Twofold fermentation
Malt vinegar	Barley malt or other cereals where starch has been converted into maltose	Twofold fermentation
Sugar vinegar	Solutions of sugar, syrup, or molasses	Twofold fermentation
Spirit or distilled vinegar	Alcohol which comes from whole grain products	Acetic fermentation of dilute distilled alcohol

(*Source:* The Vinegar Institute.)

High-tech manufacturing companies speed up the vinegar-making process. Their method is to circulate fermented liquid through large vats, incorporating lots of air and quickly producing a product. Better-quality vinegars, however, are often left unfiltered and unpasteurized, in which case the bacteria or "mother" will form at the top.

Mother or "mother-of-vinegar" is a term used to describe the excess liquid that accumulates on top of cider or other juice, which turns them into the most nutritious vinegars for health. As the fermentation progresses, mother forms a floating clump or filmy substance, like a coffee latte with the foam on top. Mother, the latte-like foam, is a living mixture of "good" bacteria and enzymes.

All-Natural Orleans Process

The slower the conversion from wine to vinegar, the better the vinegar will be. If you're looking for good vinegar, you want one that's been made using the traditional, all-natural Orleans process, which takes weeks, not hours, to make vinegar. Early vinegar experts fine-tuned this method during the Middle Ages in Orleans, France.[5]

The best vinegars are made from whole apples ground into pulp, cold-pressed to extract the cider, fermented in wooden barrels, and aged for at least six months. Organic cider vinegars are available at health-food stores and usually unfiltered. Other kinds are made from apple cores and peelings, then quickly processed. Some companies, such as Heinz, follow the traditional process of pressing whole apples for their juice.

Naturally Organic

Organic vinegars are made from fruits and grains that are not sprayed with chemical insecticides or pesticides. Natural types of repellents and fertilizers without chemical pesticides and fewer sulfites (a food additive) are used instead. Also the vinegars are free of chemicals or additives. In addition, natural vinegars are free of artificial colorings, flavorings, dyes, and preservatives.

Though the acidity and nutrient content of vinegars may vary, legal standards in America require vinegar to be at least 4 percent acidity, or 4 grams of acetic acid per 100 cubic centimeters. Most are 5 percent acidity. The acidity is defined by the word "grain," which refers to the amount of water dilution. For instance, a 40-grain vinegar is 4 percent acetic acid.[6]

Despite vinegar's acidity strength, health experts are now discovering what the old country folks knew all along: both apple cider vinegar and red wine vinegar have amazing healing powers.

ACV Super Smoothie

❖ ❖ ❖

So what exactly is a smoothie, anyhow? It's a blended beverage created with fruit and other ingredients such as ice cream, milk, and other good-for-you add-ins for health nuts, including honey, wheat germ, and even vinegar(s) for wholesome goodness. I know from personal experience smoothies in the seventies were big and today they thrive, especially in coastal towns up and down our Golden State.

¾ cup fresh strawberries or peaches, sliced and frozen
⅓ cup 2 percent organic low-fat milk
1 cup all-natural organic strawberry ice cream or gelato
1 teaspoon wheat germ (optional)
1 capful pure vanilla extract
2 tablespoons organic strawberry preserve

1 teaspoon honey
1 teaspoon Bragg Organic Raw Apple Cider Vinegar
whipped cream (Optional. I prefer the real thing that you whip up rather than store-bought in a can.)
fresh mint leaves

In a blender, mix the fruit, milk, ice cream, and wheat germ. Add vanilla, and strawberry preserve, honey, and vinegar. Pour into a glass. Top with whipped cream and mint leaf. Serves two.

VINEGARY HEALING HINTS TO PRESERVE

New evidence shows that *both* apple cider and red wine vinegars, which are made from whole apples and red grapes—as well as other healthful vinegars—may help you to:

✓ Fight fat.
✓ Enhance your immune system.
✓ Lower blood pressure.
✓ Lower risk of heart disease.
✓ Prevent cancer.
✓ Slow the aging process.

In this book, I will show you how using both vinegars can be one of the best things you do for yourself—and your health. But note, many people will not want to reap the benefits of vinegar by drinking the healthy brew solo. While vinegar is great for salad, it also is a great seasoning for many foods. Vinegar has a vast number of uses in cooking, and I've included more than 100 recipes to help heal your body, mind, and spirit.

But first, let's go way, way back into the past. Take a close-up look at why and how vinegar is one of the world's first—and most prized—natural medicines.

A Genesis of Sour Wine

*Pour vinegar and oil into the same cruse and thou
wilt say that, as foes, they keep asunder.*
—Aeschylus, *Agamemnon* (458 B.C.)[1]

My real-life first vinegary memory is when I was a curious five-year-old kindergartener who spent lingering afternoons at a semi-rural nursery school. It was at this two-story white house with a big backyard boasting a playhouse, swing set, and sandpile that I learned about the world of food and vinegar.

One cold, rainy fall morning I was recovering from a bout of strep throat. As a little girl with a stubborn streak, swallowing a bitter-tasting antibiotic pill was a bad dream. Ida, a stern, but savvy, salt-and-pepper-haired, heavyset woman who wore glasses, didn't force me to take the titanic tablet when I sat down at the big, oval-shaped wooden kitchen table. I watched her like I do the Food Network chefs as she shaped pie dough with a rolling pin on a cutting board. She added a golden liquid from a bottle (like in my Sicily fantasy) to the raw dough.

I asked my domestic caretaker, "What's that?" She answered, "Vinegar. It helps make the crust flaky." I asked: "Like magic?" She laughed, and our eyes connected. Once the pastry dough was put in several pie pans, the leftover pieces captivated me. Ida rolled them into one large rectangle like our neighbor's swimming pool next door.

I helped her brush the dough with melted butter; sprinkle it with raisins, cinnamon, and sugar. We rolled it up like a snake. She cut it into pinwheel-shaped pieces and plopped them, one by one, on a cookie sheet.

Once in the oven the wonderful aroma made me forget the medicine; out of the oven, the cinnamon cookies cooled on a rack. She gave me two with a glass of orange juice. "What about the pill?" I asked Ida. "You took it," she answered, and smiled. "I put it in the cookie." I sighed with relief. So, the introduction of versatile vinegar in the twentieth century played a role in my life, as it was recognized in other people's lives around the globe for centuries long ago.

As early as 400 B.C., Hippocrates used vinegar to treat his patients. In the era of the Romans and Egyptians, there were many potent vinegars on meal tables. During the nineteenth century, vinegar was used as a healing dressing, and in the twentieth century, people drank vinegar cocktails of all kinds.

Today, nutritionists, doctors, chefs, and researchers around the world continue to utilize other powerful uses of this universal liquid. And history shows that people of yesteryear took advantage not only of the internal benefits of vinegar, but of its external virtues as well. It's no secret.

Vinegar's great power is timeless. The earliest historical record of vinegar may be the Babylonians. In 5000 B.C. they made vinegar as an end product of a wine from the date palm. Since that time, vinegar has been used as a food preservative, a medicinal agent, an antibiotic, and even as a household cleaner. Then and now it's known for its "good" antimicrobial properties—it kills "bad" microorganisms—and healers of the past observed this vinegar power.

Hippocrates, for one, known as "the father of medicine," treated his patients with vinegar as an antibiotic. It was one of our first medicines. Hippocrates used vinegar to treat a variety of illnesses. For instance, he told his patients that oxymel (a honey and vinegar combination) was a good remedy for getting rid of phlegm and breathing easy. It is believed that strong acid, such as in the honey and vinegar, helps to clear up congestion.[2]

Hippocrates also prescribed this potent honey-vinegar combo for other ailments. Not only was oxymel to aid in regularity, but it also treated respiratory disorders such as peripneumonia and pleurisy, too. Vinegar was used to treat inflammations and swellings and even burns.

Also, the ancient medicine man used vinegar for disinfecting ulcerations.[3]

Vinegar is mentioned eight times in the Bible: four times in the Old Testament and four in the New Testament. In fact, there is even a Vinegar Bible. In the sixteenth century the Clarendon Press in Oxford, England, typeset the word "vinegar" instead of "vineyard" in the top-of-the-page running headline of the twenty-second chapter of Luke. And soon, the edition was coined the "Vinegar Bible."[4]

Since biblical times, vinegar, known as "the poor man's wine," has played a major role in the lives of both the rich, such as in royalty, and in the poor. Laborers, for instance, would add a splash of wine vinegar to water, perhaps with a pinch of salt. This ancient version of an energizing drink was teamed with bread to help people persevere as they worked under the hot sun. Even in the eighteenth and nineteenth centuries, this age-old vinegar tradition was used by laborers. For example, a fruit-flavored vinegar known as "shrubs" or "switches" was used by workers during harvesting.[5]

The Royal Power of Vinegar

Remember Cleopatra, the legendary Queen of Egypt? The strong-willed woman led her husband, Mark Antony, into an ironic, no-win wager. She put her vinegar smarts to work. According to Pliny, a Roman scholar, the savvy queen claimed that she could eat one meal that would cost a million sisteries (an old Roman coin). The bet seemed absurd, since one human can only consume so much at one sitting, right? Not exactly.

The queen simply dropped a million sisteries' worth of pearls into a glass of vinegar. Meanwhile, the "meal" was put aside while food preparations were made. At mealtime, the queen just swallowed the dissolved pearls. Thanks to her vinegar knowledge—she knew the acidic strength of sour wine—the "liquid meal" was not only an expensive one, but a surefire way to win the bet.

During the Middle Ages, vinegar made its mark, too. Four robbers in the French town of Marseilles preyed upon the homes and belongings left behind by the people who fell victim to the bubonic plague,

OTHER PAST MEDICAL USES OF VINEGAR

Historical Vinegar User	Method	Ailment
Assyrian tablets[7]	Vinegar	For ear diseases
Ancient Persian physicians[8]	Mixture of lime juice, the sour juice of certain fruits, and vinegar	To prevent fat accumulation in the body
Greek, Roman, and Asian doctors[9]	Vinegar	Aiding digestion, preventing scurvy, lowering bile levels
Spartianus, historian[10]	Mixture of vinegar and water	Helped soldiers survive rigors of battle
Medieval people[11]	Herbal vinegar with lavender and rosemary	Unease of stomach and brain
Galen, doctor in the second century A.D.[12]	Honey and vinegar	Coughs
B. Boyles, fellow of Royal Society of London[13]	Vinegar	Used as a gargle
Genteel people of the 17th/18th centuries[14]	Vinegar-soaked sponges	To ward off the noxious odors of raw sewage and garbage
Hippocrates[15]	Vinegar, honey, and pepper	Feminine disorders
Egyptians[16]	Vinegar	Mushroom poisoning, worms in the ears, bleeding wounds, severe loss of appetite, and gangrene
Theophrastus, a Greek[17]	Mixture of vinegar with pepper	Revives a victim of suffocation

VINEGAR MILESTONES

Year	What Happened	What It Did
794–1185	Japan's Samurai warriors used vinegar tonic.[18]	They believed it gave them strength and power.
1735–1826	Our second president, John Adams, drank apple cider every morning for breakfast.[19]	Showed how the components of ACV may support longer life.
1909	Dr. Jarvis began studying herbal medicines and folk remedies after he began practicing medicine.	Helped treat people with ACV for a variety of ailments.
1912	Dr. Alexis Carrel began an experiment that successfully kept the cells of an embryo chicken heart alive for 30 years.	Showed the importance of ACV in health and longevity.
1920s	During the "Roaring Twenties," apple cider was made and drunk more than any other fruit juices in America.[20]	Implied that ACV provides vim and vigor.
1958	*Folk Medicine: A Vermont Doctor's Guide to Good Health* was published.	Chronicled the ACV remedies Dr. D.C. Jarvis studied to treat many diseases.
1968	On January 17, the Vinegar Institute began.	Helped vinegar producers to protect their rights.
1973	Marcella Hazan, a cooking teacher and author, introduced America to balsamic vinegar from the provinces of Modena and Reggio Emilia.[21]	
1990s	The Braggs provided self-help books: such as *Apple Cider Vinegar: Miracle Health System*.	Helped teach people to live healthier lives.
1999	On June 4, in Roslyn, South Dakota, the international Vinegar Museum was opened.	It will inform you about the wonderful power of vinegar.

or "Black Death" of Europe. Eventually they were caught and brought before French judges, who wondered how these four thieves had protected themselves from the deadly plague while looting plague-ridden possessions.

The legend is that the four thieves bargained and exchanged the famous Four Thieves Vinegar formula for their freedom, explaining that they washed themselves with the infection-fighting liquid every few hours. Upon learning about these immunity-boosting qualities, the formula was used by priests and doctors who treated the ill.

No one seems to know who wrote the formula, which differs from recipe to recipe, but it is basically the same and it works in various ways. It can be used to disinfect sick rooms. If diluted with water, it can be used as a body wash. Taken by the teaspoonful (consult with your doctor for the safe amount), it can be used as a preventive measure to stave off viral infections, such as the flu.

> **Therapeutic Formula of the Four Thieves**
>
> Basic ingredients: Combine 3 quarts apple cider vinegar; 3 tablespoons *each* of rosemary, lavender, sage, mint, rue, and plantain; and 6 cloves of garlic. Let it sit in a covered container for at least 24 hours.

In the American Civil War, vinegar is believed to have prevented scurvy—the disease caused by a vitamin C deficiency. It was also used as a disinfectant and healing agent to treat wounds in both the American Civil War and World War I.

Favorite Tender Crust

❖ ❖ ❖

The following crust, a hybrid between short-flake and medium-flake, combines the best attributes of both: short-flake's melt-in-the-mouth texture, and medium-flake's tender flakiness. Baking powder enhances the flakiness, vinegar makes it tender, and the buttermilk adds flavor.

Note that this is a single, rather than double crust, making it ideal for open-faced pies (pumpkin, pecan, custard), pies with a streusel or meringue topping, or quiches.

1½ cups (6¼ ounces) unbleached all-purpose flour or a combination of all-purpose and pastry flours

1 tablespoon (⅛ ounce) buttermilk powder (optional, though it will help make the crust tender)

1 teaspoon salt

¼ teaspoon baking powder

4 tablespoons (½ stick, or 2 ounces) butter

¼ cup (1⅝ ounces) vegetable shortening

1 teaspoon white or cider vinegar

3 to 5 tablespoons (1½ to 2½ ounces)

ice water

In a medium-sized mixing bowl, combine the flour, buttermilk powder, salt, and baking powder. Using a pastry fork, pastry blender, your fingers, or a mixer, cut in the butter and vegetable shortening, leaving some baby pea–sized lumps.

Mix the vinegar with 3 tablespoons of the water. Sprinkle this mixture over the flour and fat and toss with a fork. Squeeze the dough together; if it's not cohesive, add an additional 1 to 2 tablespoons water (just enough to make the dough stick together comfortably). Shape the dough into a flattened disk, wrap it in plastic wrap, and refrigerate it for 30 minutes before rolling.

Note: At King Arthur Flour, the bakers believe measuring ingredients by weight (ounces) is more accurate than measuring by volume (cups and spoons). But since the volume system is still standard, they use it along with weight measurements. You may use either in the recipe included in this book.

(Courtesy: The King Arthur Flour Baker's Companion: The All-Purpose Baking Cookbook.)

VINEGARY HEALING HINTS TO PRESERVE

As you can see, versatile vinegar has been praised for centuries—in the United States and around the world—as a healing medicine. Vinegar devotees, past and present, believe that vinegar—both ACV and RWV—can fight disease and add years to your life by:

✓ Acting as a safe and effective natural preservative in food.
✓ Fighting deadly food bacteria.
✓ Aiding in digestion.
✓ Preventing infection.
✓ Enhancing immune system function.
✓ Fighting viruses.

No doubt, vinegar back then had a wide variety of powerful health benefits. And it's managed to hold up to its good name. Now it's time to get the lowdown on one of the nation's most popular kinds of vinegar—apple cider vinegar—then . . . and now.

PART 2

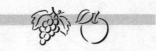

APPLE CIDER VINEGAR

A Historical Testimony

Sour makes sweet happen.
—The Vinegar Man[1]

My second encounter with vinegar was when I was a seven-year-old, spellbound by the great outdoors and indoors if it was linked to eating. Sometimes kids, like me, discover their favorite foods by accident, as was the case when I was in Santa Cruz, a popular beach town in California. One summer afternoon, I sat cross-legged on a red-and-white-checkered blanket on top of the sand next to a picnic basket full of cold cuts, olive oil, vinegar, and cold potato salad with a vinegary taste.

In search of adventure, I wandered off looking for seashells, and played in the ebb and flow of the cold, salty ocean water. When I looked up at my whereabouts—my two siblings and parents had vanished. Strange faces were everywhere. I was disoriented. My eyes were drawn to sand crabs on the wet sand; they were the size of sand dollars. I ran up to two elderly fishermen. I cried, "I'm lost!" They took me on a search. By dusk I was cold and hungry. At last, I saw my mother folding the checkered blanket. After the reunion we went to the boardwalk and ate hot fish and chips. The crispy fried fare with a paper cup of coleslaw had a tang to its taste. My mom said it was vinegar. As time passed, I learned that, like my lost-at-the-beach day, there was more than just apple cider vinegar in the bold land of vinegars.

One health leader, Paul Bragg, fell into the world of vinegar at an early age, but even more so than I did. He reminisces about his father in his book *Apple Cider Vinegar: Miracle Health System*. He recalls his early youth when he enjoyed "robust health" on an apple farm. He wrote, "I was a great apple eater. Each year my father made natural Apple cider vinegar and stored it in wooden barrels. On our table we used this natural Apple cider vinegar and our large family loved it."[2]

Bragg was impressed by his hardworking father. Often he would watch him add apple cider vinegar to the feed and water of sick farm animals and watched it restore health to cattle, horses, sheep, dogs, and cats. The apple cider vinegar worked like a magical potion. Because the farm family lived out in the country, they turned to self-health remedies like vinegar.[3]

The apple cider vinegar advocate remembers his father working long hours during harvest time. His father would be up before dawn and work without rest until late at night. Bragg observed him come into the kitchen and fix a honey and apple cider vinegar cocktail. "I would say, 'Father, why do you drink vinegar, honey and water?' And father would reply, 'Son, farm work is long hard work, it can produce chronic fatigue in the body.'" Bragg learned about a powerful ingredient in that drink that renewed his father's vitality and relieved him of fatigue and stiffness. That ingredient was potassium, which along with healthful enzymes, minerals, and trace elements, are all found in apple cider vinegar[4] (as noted in Chapter 1).

Apple cider vinegar gurus of the 1900s such as Dr. Paul C. Bragg and Dr. Patricia Bragg will not be forgotten. This father-and-daughter health-minded team believe apple cider vinegar has internal and external benefits that include: helping to control and normalize weight, improve digestion, promote a youthful, healthy body, and even prevent dandruff.

Paul and Patricia Bragg: ACV Pioneers

Paul Bragg: World Health Crusader. Bragg, N.D., Ph.D., life extension specialist, originated, named, and opened the first "Health Food Store" in America. He introduced juice therapy in America by bringing the first hand-operated vegetable-fruit juicer from Germany. He was the first to introduce and distribute honey nationwide. He inspired millions to "go organic" in their gardening.

Patricia Bragg: Paul Bragg's daughter, N.D., Ph.D., a doctor of naturopathy, and health and fitness expert, carries on the family name. She lectures on health via radio and TV, and is co-author of *Apple Cider Vinegar.*

(*Source:* Live Food Products: C. S. Lewis & Co. Publicists.)

THE VERMONT COUNTRY DOCTOR

These two vinegar advocates shared the same path that great folk medicine doctor D. C. Jarvis traveled, too. This family doctor noticed that many of his patients—down-to-earth country people—used folk remedies to prevent and treat most illnesses.

Dr. Jarvis offers many uses for apple cider vinegar. Apple cider vinegar is used for many ailments, from poison ivy, burns (including sunburn), varicose veins, impetigo, and bacterial infections, to more serious problems—such as high blood pressure in one of his patients. (See Chapter 18: "Home Cures.")

Acid-Alkaline = Better Blood. A Vermont woman showed a whopping blood pressure reading of nearly 300 when it was taken at a clinic, reports Dr. Jarvis. "However, by controlling the alkalinity of her blood in the manner taught by Vermont folk medicine, she was able to live to the age of 84 years," he says. How? In a nutshell: She upped her daily intake of acid in organic form. That can be in the form of apples or two teaspoons of apple cider vinegar in a glass of water.[5]

A high-protein, high-fat diet increases the alkalinity in the blood, causing it to thicken as in this Vermont patient. It is believed by Dr. Jarvis that apple cider vinegar affects the acid-alkali balance. It thins the blood, which may help lower blood pressure and improve blood circulation.

Today, the American diet high in meat and lower in alkalizing fruits and vegetables leaves an acid residue in the body. The acid residue, in turn, imbalances our biochemistry or pH blood levels in a direction where we are out of acid-alkaline balance. And that can lead to high blood pressure and other heart ailments, say vinegar experts.

"Thus, it is necessary for you to eat as much vegetables as possible to prevent acidity in your body fluid, which may result from taking too much animal protein," reports Togo Kuroiwa in his book *Rice Vinegar:*

An Oriental Home Remedy.[6] The organic acids found in fruits, vegetables, and apple cider vinegar provide the body with important minerals such as potassium, calcium, sodium, and magnesium. These and other minerals form compounds in the body that turn acid body fluids alkaline. Because of this, they are called alkalizing minerals, and the food that supply them—such as apple cider vinegar—are called alkalizing foods. Animal proteins and other acidifying foods cause the body fluids to be more acid, which favors bacterial growth and leads to disease. That's why to stay healthy, our bodies need a constant fresh supply of the alkalizing minerals that are found in fruits, vegetables, and apple cider vinegar.

Food Poison Prevention. Another one of the Vermont doctor's patients experienced the quick healing power of apple cider vinegar. At a Shriner's summer picnic in Vermont, lobster salad was the main course. The salad was spoiled and nineteen people suffered the consequences: food poisoning. One of the diners had taken preventive measures. Dr. Jarvis advised him whenever there was any chance that food might be spoiled, use apple cider vinegar. "At the onset of dinner he poured a generous amount into his glass of water. It happened that he was particularly fond of lobster salad and he had two extra helpings. Whereas many of his table companions suffered bad effects from the spoiled lobster, the apple cider vinegar had so sterilized it in his digestive tract that nothing disagreeable happened to him."[7]

Lameness Rx. One day a farmer at Dr. Jarvis's office reported his bothersome arthritis. He told the doctor that before taking 10 teaspoonfuls of apple cider vinegar in a glass of water with each meal, he had lameness in all the joints of his body. The first day after he started taking apple cider vinegar, he reported his lameness was 20 percent better. The second day he said he was 50 percent better. By the end of a month 75 percent improvement. Not only did the lameness clear up, but so did the pain.[8]

Dr. Carrel's Famous Longevity Experiment

Dr. Alexis Carrel, a New York City doctor back in 1912, administered apple cider vinegar daily to the cells of an embryo chicken heart. That was to ensure that it got a full quota of potassium. The normal life span of a chicken is 7½ to 8 years. Amazingly, Dr. Carrel kept the chicken heart alive and healthy for over three decades—thanks to potassium.

"Dr. Carrel definitely proved to the entire world that the body has a seed of eternal life that man kills himself by wrong habits of eating and living," the Braggs report. The conclusion: Apple cider vinegar is vital to good health and longevity. The question is, can it apply to human beings, too?[9]

CONTEMPORARY DOCTORS: THE ACV LATE BLOOMERS

"Do as I do—drink vinegar," said best-selling author Julian Whitaker, M.D., who has practiced medicine for over 20 years at the Whitaker Wellness Institute in Newport Beach, California. He is the author of *Reversing Hypertension: A Vital New Program to Prevent, Treat, and Reduce High Blood Pressure* (Warner Books, 2000) and other health books about the prevention of diabetes and heart disease. Dr. Whitaker admitted in May 1997 that for a few months he'd been drinking a glass of warm water with a teaspoon each of raw honey and apple cider vinegar once a day. "I'm not ready to commit to it as a ritual but there's enough anecdotal evidence for me to add it to my daily routine."[10]

He is hardly alone. John, an elderly man, had a variety of stomach woes all his life, reports Dr. Whitaker. "After countless GI workups, most recently a series of tests costing $2,000, he was told by his doctor that they could find nothing to explain these problems and recommended he take Zantac every day." But John took an alternative route. For one week he drank one teaspoon of raw, unfiltered, organic apple cider vinegar and one teaspoon of raw honey in warm water once a day. Afterward, his heartburn and stomach problems were no longer a problem.[11]

Dr. Whitaker recalls another man who gives a lot of credit to his "vinegar cocktails" which help remedy angina pain. At 66, Bob was being treated for heart disease. He mixed a shot glass of vinegar with molasses and grapefruit juice and downed it twice a day. "Of course," says Dr. Whitaker, "he was pursuing several other therapies for his chest pain at the same time, but he feels that the vinegar had a decided effect."[12]

Adds Dr. Whitaker: "This is pretty strong testimony for an unglamorous and inexpensive product like vinegar, but stories like this abound. Although it has little mention in the medical literature, apple cider vinegar has a solid and respected place in folk medicine."[13]

Perhaps its best known application is for indigestion, as John experienced so dramatically. Other conditions vinegar reportedly improves include arthritis, leg cramps, swimmer's ear (rinse with equal parts vinegar and water), urinary problems, and excess weight. When applied topically, it can relieve athlete's foot and dandruff, and it makes a good hair rinse, as thousands will attest.[14]

"Daily I drink two ounces of ACV because it's a great source of potassium, good for blood pressure and muscles since I run/walk every day," says Jan McBarron, M.D., a Columbus, Georgia, weight-loss specialist. Dr. McBarron lost 65 pounds—and she's kept it off for over 10 years. She also believes apple cider vinegar helps digestion and aids in staying regular.

YOU CAN'T ARGUE WITH SUCCESS

Plenty of people have reaped the health benefits of apple cider vinegar. Take a look at these success stories:

Longevity Booster. My dear late friend, Virginia,* an elderly, young-at-heart musician who lived in Redwood City, California, believed apple cider vinegar is healthful. She believed in home remedies for good health. No unnatural drugs for her. She lived to be ninety-nine.

She recalls, "As a child I would daily drink apple cider vinegar straight from its container. I liked the tart taste." She continued to use vinegar and remained mentally and physically energized, driving, dining, and attending the opera. Just one more of Mother Nature's miracles.

A *Healthier Life.* Bonnie Raley,* a middle-aged-woman, has been using (and selling) apple cider vinegar with herbs (see Chapter 12: "Healing Herbal Vinegars"). "I have found that I have fewer colds, and if I do seem to be catching a cold, I can fight them off much better than before. I also have no more pain and stiffness in my ankles. I used to awaken with such stiffness that I had pain for several minutes of walking. I no longer have any pain or stiffness.

"My husband and I began taking it after our daughter was able to get her blood sugar in control after just 2 weeks. We have been so pleased with our level of energy and the way our bodies have been able to fight off colds and other viruses that other people seem to have.

"I also am going through menopause. I was having periods during the night in which I experienced 'hot flashes.' I no longer have this problem, however, it does recur if I forget to take the product for more than three or four days."

Digestion Protection. For 20 years Pat Gilmore,* a psychologist in Burlingame, California, has turned to apple cider vinegar as an antibacteria protectant before going to a potluck dinner. "I have no control over who puts what into what food or how clean their hands were. I want to eat their food—I don't want to be all picky and weird. So about a half hour before I go, I just take a tablespoon of vinegar and put it in a glass of cool water and drink it."

Apple Honey Slaw

❖ ❖ ❖

2 teaspoons lemon juice	*dash of crushed red pepper flakes*
2 teaspoons honey	*1 medium red onion, sliced thin*
2 teaspoons balsamic honey	*3 cups of shaved brussels sprouts*
vinegar	*2 Granny Smith or Gala apples*
1 tablespoon olive oil	*salt and pepper to taste (optional)*

In large bowl whisk lemon juice, honey, vinegar, olive oil, and crushed red pepper flakes; add sliced onion. Peel outer layer of brussels sprouts, chop off roots and slice very thin. Core and halve apples, then slice very thin. Add sprouts and apples to bowl, and gently toss until all pieces are coated. Refrigerate 1 hour before serving. Sprinkle with salt and pepper. Makes 6–8 servings.

(*Courtesy:* Honey Ridge Farms.)

So, what exactly makes apple cider vinegar a superfood—or is it just hype when fools rush in hoping it will work wonders? I go face-to-face with this controversial nutrition subject in the next chapter. It's time to scrutinize what's in the vinegar that you have used and may be pondering using even more.

APPLE CIDER VINEGAR IS TIMELESS

In short, apple cider vinegar was healthy in the twentieth century and is healthy in the twenty-first century, too. While its uses are plentiful—both inside and outside your body—its healing powers are due to its healthful ingredients. And now, research reveals more about apple cider vinegar nutrients (which may be missing from our daily food intake) more than ever before.

VINEGARY HEALING HINTS TO PRESERVE

✓ Potassium in apple cider vinegar may renew vitality and relieve fatigue.

✓ Apple cider vinegar has external and internal benefits—from dandruff to digestion.

✓ Apple cider vinegar may help lameness and heartburn.

✓ Apple cider vinegar may boost your immune system and add years to your life.

Where Are the Secret Ingredients?

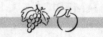

Natural apple cider vinegar
can really be called
one of nature's most perfect foods.[1]
—Drs. Bragg and Bragg

I did have a few more experiences with apple cider vinegar as a child (in my adult years my vinegar palate is more cultured). Still, sweet versatile memories of cider vinegar are part of my growing-up years. My multitasking mom kept baking products in the kitchen cabinets and used frozen foods for the weekday nights, but one weekend she ignored convenient chow in a box or bag. It was a cool, autumn Sunday afternoon—a perfect time for baking pie with our neighbor's fruit from their apple tree.

On the kitchen table, a white-lattice, round, European-style piece, Granny Smith apples were piled high in a wooden bowl. I observed my mother wash the fruit, remove the skins, quarter, core, and slice each one. The apple wedges were plunged into a large ceramic bowl filled with ice water and apple cider vinegar. "The liquid keeps the fresh fruit from turning brown," she explained as I watched the process of making a traditional apple pie.

As I munched on a tart green apple, I watched my mother as I did one of the first classic cooking shows, *The Galloping Gourmet,* a charming man who concocted rich and decadent recipes and knew all the cookery tricks. She fascinated me, so I wasn't paying attention to our type-A dalmatian, Casey. He put his black-and-white-spotted paws on the kitchen table and half of the perfect pie dough filled with apples fell onto the floor. The mishap was messy, but not unfixable. My mom showed me how to piece a piecrust, giving it a rustic look. An hour later, two deep-dish pies were baked and cooling on the rack and we were laughing at the canine faux pas. It was an unforgettable moment that taught me accidents can happen in the kitchen, but they are not always beyond repair and can give food a countryside appeal.

PORE OVER AMERICA'S CIDER VINEGAR

In the twenty-first century, after distilled white vinegar, apple cider vinegar is America's favorite. As far as vinegars go, cider vinegar is a front-runner for both internal and external use. And these days, I am personally beginning to use it along with the other types of vinegar that I favor.

People believe that apple cider vinegar, which is found in most of our homes, stores, and restaurants—and costs just pennies—can stave off arthritis, fight body fat, regulate blood pressure, and even maintain healthy bones. Sound silly? It's not, according to medical experts who believe in the power of home remedies.

The problem is, mainstream nutritionists, doctors, and apple cider vinegar makers play down the good-for-you nutrients in this liquid "cure-all." Even the vinegar trade associations will not link themselves to health or nutritional claims. As for alternative health experts, even though they aren't exactly sure what accounts for vinegar's health benefits—owing to a lack of conclusive scientific data—they do agree that there is an enormous amount of anecdotal evidence of its healing powers. Here's what I discovered:

When you look at apple cider vinegar's product label, it appears to be a dieter's dream: no calories, fat, or sodium, right? But where are the potent nutrients, I pondered.

Dazed and confused, I went straight to the vinegar makers, and obtained a nutritional breakdown of the golden liquid. The nutrition facts seem to be a bit different, and the measurements a bit bigger.

Nutrition Facts

Serving Size 1 Tablespoon (14)
Amount per serving

Calories 0

Calories from fat 0

Total Fat 0 g

Sodium 0 mg

Total Carbohydrate 0

Sugars 0 g

(*Source:* Eden Organic Apple Cider Vinegar.)

More Apple Cider Vinegar, Anyone?

100 grams (three-and-one-half ounces) contains:

95% water
14 calories
0 protein
0 dietary fiber
0 fat
5 grams of carbohydrates
6 milligrams of calcium
9 milligrams of phosphorus
0.6 milligrams of iron
1 milligram of sodium
100 milligrams of potassium
22 milligrams of magnesium
0.04 milligrams of copper[2]

Apparently, more cider equals more nutrients. One cup contains:

98% water
34 calories
a trace of protein
0 fat
14.2 grams of carbohydrates

14 milligrams of calcium
22 milligrams of phosphorus
1.4 milligrams of iron
2 milligrams of sodium
240 milligrams of potassium[3]

People who have written about vinegar claim that apple cider vinegar contains more than thirty important nutrients, a dozen minerals, over half a dozen vitamins and essential acids, several enzymes, and pectin. The bottom line is that more research will be needed before more doctors—conventional and holistic alike—truly understand what accounts for vinegar's healing powers.

QUALITY COUNTS

Not all vinegar is nutritionally equal, natural, organic apple cider vinegar and made using the slow Orleans method. Some producers speed up the process so that vinegar can be bottled within three days.

"For medicinal purposes the apple cider vinegar should be made from the crushed whole apples," says Dr. Jarvis. "Following the line of changes when the whole apple is crushed to make apple cider vinegar," adds Dr. Jarvis, "it is found that the healthful properties in the original apple are passed down to the apple cider vinegar."[4]

The fact is, the best cider vinegars are made from whole apples ground into pulp, cold-pressed to extract the cider, fermented in wooden barrels, and aged for at least six months for rich full flavor. This is the ideal way.

Apple cider vinegar contains the same important nutrients as nature's apples—pectin, beta-carotene, and potassium—plus it contains enzymes and amino acids which are formed during the fermentation process.

"Vinegar possesses the same essential nutrients as the ingredients originally used to make it, but gains nutrients during the fermentation process, notably enzymes and amino acids. Many believe it is the natural fermentation process which endows the final product with its diverse healing properties," explains co-author Earl L. Mindell in his book *Amazing Apple Cider Vinegar* (Keats Publishing, February 1, 1996).

Apple Nutrition

One apple contains 100 calories, mainly from carbohydrate; 2 grams of fiber; 10 mg vitamin C; 150 IUs vitamin A; modest amounts of B vitamins—B_1, B_2, B_3, B_6, and biotin; 159 mg of potassium; over 15 mg each of calcium, magnesium, and phosphorus; about 0.5 mg of iron; traces of maganese, copper, selenium, and zinc; some vitamin E (mostly in the seeds).

(*Source: Staying Healthy with Nutrition: The Complete Guide to Diet and Nutritional Medicine*, Elson Haas, M.D., Celestial Arts, 1992.)

AN APPLE A DAY MEANS FEWER DOCTORS TO PAY

Eighty percent of the fiber found in an apple is soluble fiber—or pectin, which may be of help in lowering blood cholesterol levels. Also, apples are a good source of potassium, which helps provide protection against strokes. And like most other fruits, they're also lower in sodium (for better blood pressure), calories (for staying slim), and unhealthy fat.

Research suggests naturally occurring chemicals found in apples, called flavonoids, may reduce the risk of heart disease and inhibit the development of certain cancers, too. And that makes sense. Because the remaining fiber in apples is known as insoluble fiber. This type of fiber is thought to prevent certain types of cancer. A *health bonus*: health-boosting apples are a good source of the mineral boron, which may help prevent the calcium loss from bone that may lead to brittle bone disease.

POTASSIUM: THE MIRACLE WORKER OF ACV

Apple cider vinegar, again, which is made from healthful apples, contains 240 milligrams of potassium per cup. And medical experts emphasize the importance of regulating the sodium-potassium balance in our nervous and muscular systems. Potassium counteracts the damaging effects of too much sodium and can help prevent high blood pressure. This powerful mineral inhibits fluid retention, too, which is caused by an accumulation of sodium in the body. As a result, this also helps ward off high blood pressure.

Healing apple cider vinegar is also believed to help prevent energy diseases. Folk medicine doctors claim that preventable diseases or conditions such as high blood pressure, impaired memory, and even fatigue can be helped by apple cider vinegar because of its energizing potassium.

While a well-balanced diet is essential for staying power, loading up on complex carbohydrates, protein, iron, and potassium-rich foods (paired with apple cider vinegar) can help you perk up *and* slim down. "Nutrient-dense foods maintain your energy levels, which helps stave off fatigue," says Jeffrey Blumberg, Ph.D., an antioxidant researcher at Tufts University.

Eight Potassium-Rich Foods

Try teaming apple cider vinegar with these potassium-rich foods:

- 4 oz broiled chicken = 350–500 mg of potassium
- 1 cup dried apples = 350–500 mg of potassium
- ½ cup dried apricots = 500–750 mg of potassium
- 1 potato = 500–750 mg of potassium
- 1 cup broccoli = 350–500 mg of potassium
- 1 cup collard greens = 500–750 mg of potassium
- 1 cup low-fat yogurt with fruit = 350–500 mg of potassium
- 1 cup canned tomatoes = 500–750 mg of potassium

(Source: The Healing Foods: The Ultimate Authority of the Curative Power of Nutrition by Patricia Hausman and Judith Benn Hurley [Rodale Press, 1989].)

It's the potassium that helps energize you. Low potassium levels bring on fatigue. You need a daily minimum of 1,875 milligrams of potassium, and apple cider vinegar can help you get that.

Doctors Paul and Patricia Bragg note in their book that potassium-rich apple cider vinegar is the key to good health and longevity, too. One of the best ways to prevent age-related illnesses is by eating a healthy diet, one that is chock-full of those foods that are potassium-rich. And apple cider vinegar is one of the best—and cheapest—sources of potassium.

The Braggs describe potassium as "the mineral of youthfulness." And, they add, potassium is so important that without it there would be no life on Earth. Yet today millions of people struggle without realizing that their quality of health would be better by alleviating their potassium deficiency.[5]

I remember what it was like to watch my mother suffer. She was an alcoholic. The doctor prescribed high blood pressure medication *and* a potassium liquid to take daily. Every morning my father would fix a cranberry juice and potassium cocktail for my mom to drink. Evidently, the taste of the medicine was so bad she refused to drink it. I can't help but wonder if a well-balanced diet, less alcohol, and more exercise—plus taking potassium-rich apple cider vinegar—could have helped my mother live a longer life. She died at age 52.

Potassium helps if you are malnourished. If a disease, such as alcoholism, has progressed to where it has damaged the body's metabolism (as in the case of my mother), you would need extra potassium to keep the potassium-sodium ratio in balance for proper bodily functioning, explains Connie Diekman, R.D., a former American Dietetic Association (see Author's Note) spokesperson. "The biggest reason potassium and sodium need to be in direct balance in the body is to ensure that muscles can contract and relax. The heart is the major muscle in the body, so when these two minerals are out of sync, the heart muscle can beat irregularly, which can result in heart failure."

Since Dr. Jarvis began celebrating the benefits of potassium-rich apple cider vinegar, medical experts have confirmed that it is vital for good health to maintain the proper ratio of potassium to sodium in your diet. The perfect potassium to sodium ratio is 5:1; but unfortunately most Americans have a ratio of 1:2. That means we consume twice as much sodium as we do potassium. Thanks to a modern, fast-

Do You Have a Potassium Deficiency?

When there is a deficiency of potassium, these symptoms can occur: muscle weakness, fatigue, mental confusion, heart rhythm disturbances, and problems with nerve conduction. And note, potassium deficiency occurs when the body is losing more potassium than it is taking in and usually through loss in the urine, excessive perspiration, or with severe vomiting or diarrhea.

paced society, we eat more processed foods today, so our salt intake is higher, and potassium consumption is shrinking. And more Americans are growing unhealthier. Apple cider vinegar is a great way to bring back potassium, the way it used to be when we ate whole, natural foods such as vegetables and fruits, which are naturally potassium-rich.

This ratio can be imbalanced by excessive consumption of sodium, along with a low intake of potassium. Caution ahead: An out-of-whack potassium-sodium ratio can lead to high blood pressure, heart disease, and even strokes.

Health Fact!

Attention Coffee Drinkers: Alcohol, coffee, tea, and sugar are diuretics and therefore potassium drainers. If you drink too much coffee, you might find yourself feeling fatigued. The cause: It depletes your body's required potassium.

"Only five percent of Americans' sodium intake comes from the salt shaker. Ninety-five percent of Americans' sodium intake comes from hidden sodium from the packaged foods," says Georgia-based diet doctor Jan McBarron, M.D. Apple cider vinegar gives you more potassium so that you maintain your sodium-potassium ratio levels for better health and well-being.

Vinegar Is Sodium-Free

While vinegar is high in potassium, it is low in sodium! After sampling a number of vinegar products, the United States Department of Agriculture reports that an average serving size, a tablespoon of vinegar, contains just a trace of sodium. That means, according to labeling guidelines for sodium in foods, vinegar is a "sodium-free" product.

SIX SUPER HEALTH-PROMOTING
ACV COMPONENTS

A friend of Angelo (the elderly man who drinks his daily apple cider vinegar cocktails), Erminia Marcini* who lives in San Jose, California, is starting to worry about age-related diseases, from arthritis to cancer. Erminia says she is eating a healthy diet—but what else can she do?

All women and men need an adequate amount of many other essential minerals and vitamins to help the body maintain good health. Experts urge people of all ages to get plenty of nutrients. Apple cider vinegar contains some of them:

1 **Beta-carotene for Healthier Cells:** Beta-carotene, a carotenoid, and trace element found in apple cider vinegar, is a potent antioxidant. This vitamin will help neutralize the free radical molecules that cause normal cells to become cancerous.

   Foods rich in beta-carotene are sweet potatoes, carrots, and spinach. Team apple cider vinegar (see Part 8, Vinegar Recipes), with baby carrots and seasoned apple cider vinegar, and you get beta-carotene in a one-two punch.

2 **Get Your Boron:** This important trace element, which is found in apple cider vinegar, is essential for good health and strong bones. Boron plays a major role in utilizing calcium and magnesium, which are necessary for beating bone loss, too. Still, most Americans are probably not getting enough of this bone-building buddy.

   You can get more boron by eating boron-rich foods such as apples. Just make up a batch of Apple Chutney (see Part 8, Vinegar Recipes), which is brimming with red tart apples and apple cider vinegar.

3 **Bone Up with Calcium:** As noted before, apple cider vinegar contains a trace of needed calcium. This mineral is necessary for transmitting nerve impulses and regulating muscle contraction. If your diet is deficient in calcium, the body will steal it out of your bones. This, in turn, weakens your skeleton and can lead to brittle bone disease.

"Calcium is the primary mineral in your bones. That is what keeps them strong," says Georgia Kostas, former director of nutrition at the Cooper Clinic in Dallas. "It is critical to the physical structure as well as functioning of the human body."

Note these important calcium facts:

- Ninety-nine percent of the body's calcium is stored in your bones and teeth.
- One percent is in blood and tissues.
- It is necessary for transmitting nerve impulses and regulating muscle contraction.
- The need for calcium starts in infancy and continues throughout life. If your diet is deficient in calcium, the body will steal it out of your bones. This weakens your skeleton and can lead to brittle bone disease.

While apple cider vinegar may only contain a trace element of bone-building calcium, you can add it to calcium-rich dishes. Try cheese or broccoli dishes (in Part 8, Vinegar Recipes) and apple cider vinegar. That way, you are adding extra tangy flavor to calcium-boosting sources and keeping your bones healthy, too.

4 **Enzymes for Good Digestion:** "They're protein molecules and they're what actually digest the food you eat. You can only get enzymes by eating plant foods—live food such as apples, and apple cider vinegar," explains Dr. McBarron.

What better way to get enzymes than eating plenty of fresh fruits and vegetables tossed in enzyme-rich apple cider vinegar. May I suggest indulging in main-dish salads. Not only are they one of my personal favorites, they're packed with live foods such as cabbage, carrots, red peppers, and apple cider vinegar.

5 **Boost Your Fiber:** When vinegar is made from fresh apples, it contains pectin or soluble fiber. Soluble fiber blocks fat absorption, which lowers blood cholesterol and reduces risk of heart disease and high blood pressure.

Naturally, foods that are fiber-plentiful will help you reach your daily fiber intake. Our vegetables/vegetarian recipes in

Chapter 8 will help take you there. They're full of fiber-rich goodness tossed in apple cider vinegar.

6 **Pump Up Your Iron:** Your body needs iron. Apple cider vinegar delivers iron in an easy to digest and absorbable form. Iron deficiency anemia is a common problem and can easily be avoided.

ACV's Nutrient Source Chart

While apple cider vinegar contains these nutrients, so do these nutrient-dense foods, which can be enhanced even more by using natural apple cider vinegar or herbal apple cider vinegar in our tasty recipes at the end of this book.

Beta-carotene: carrots, asparagus, broccoli, red pepper, and green leafy vegetables.

Boron: apples.

Calcium: broccoli and green leafy vegetables, tofu.

Enzymes: carrots, apples, red peppers.

Fiber: beans, potatoes.

Iron: raisins, asparagus, leafy green vegetables, spinach, kale.

Potassium: apples, onion, garlic, green leafy vegetables.

Rather than only thinking of eating liver, you can enjoy recipes that contain iron-rich raisins and apple cider vinegar to help you boost your iron intake with a smile.

OTHER ACV INGREDIENTS

Not only does apple cider vinegar contain plenty of vitamins, minerals, and potassium—it contain carbohydrates and amino acids, which are essential to boost brain power and other important healthful components.

Carbohydrates Supply Mental Energy. Simply put, the brain needs many different kinds of nutrients—vitamins, minerals, and carbohydrates. We know that carbohydrates, which are found in apples and apple cider vinegar, are broken down by the body into the brain's most important food—glucose, a basic sugar.

Carbohydrates enhance a boost of mind fuel (like you get from a cup of coffee) because your brain requires glucose all of the time. It provides your brain with the energy it requires to think. A daily intake of complex carbohydrates from a host of foods (vegetables, fruits, whole grains) and apple cider vinegar are important for mental performance.

Amino Acids and Brain Chemistry. Welcome to the world of amino acids, the building blocks of all protein molecules. There are 22 amino acids—14 of these can be made by the body; thus they're considered "nonessential." The remaining 8 amino acids must be obtained from our diets; thus they're considered "essential."

Is the concept of "brain food" just wishful thinking? If an apple a day keeps the doctor away, can a cup of apple cider make us rocket scientists? Although that may sound far-fetched, scientists now say that we can indeed refuel our brain power with certain nutrients that promote clearer thinking and mental energy.

The brain, like any part of the body, depends on fuel to ensure peak performance. Your brain cells communicate by releasing neurotransmitters or "smart" nutrients that relay a message to other cells in the brain and your body. Thus, essential compounds in foods contribute to the brain's own "smart" chemicals.

Studies show that when people become deficient in one or more of these nutrients, cognitive functioning becomes impaired. Correcting these deficiencies helps us feel better and function optimally. And that's where good nutrition—including apple cider vinegar, a source of brain food—comes into play.

Apple cider vinegar is believed to contain amino acids; however, it is unknown how many and which ones. Scientists are constantly finding new amino acids that the body needs to stay healthy. Although it is not put on the label, it does indeed contain trace elements of amino acids—which are essential to brain chemistry and emotion. (See Chapter 10: "Healthy Rice Vinegar.")

Acid/Alkaline Balance. In addition, natural vinegar can affect your body's pH, or acid/alkaline balance, according to Dr. Jarvis. His urinalysis research conducted in the 1950s showed that pH levels in the body (like in a fish aquarium) become alkaline just before and during illness.

For example, he noted that when a common cold was imminent,

the urine changed to alkaline, staying this way for several days before the cold hit. "During recovery from the cold, the urine reaction shifted back to acid and continued so. It was possible to induce recovery from the common cold by shifting the urine reaction to the acid side," he explained.[6]

Also, Dr. Jarvis discovered that the urine reaction shifted from acid to alkaline before the onset of childhood diseases such as measles and chicken pox, as well as asthma, hay fever, sinusitis, and even a drop in weather temperature. Dr. Jarvis says that you can shift the reaction to acid, relieving sinus problems as well as these other ailments, by taking 1 teaspoon of apple cider vinegar in a glass of water several times a day.[7]

Today, twenty-first-century vinegar remedies can affect your body's pH, or acid/alkaline balance, in a number of ways:

- You can change the pH of the vaginal environment at the first sign of a pesky yeast infection by turning to a natural vinegar-and-water douche. (See Chapter 18, "Home Cures.")
- In folk medicine natural healers often prescribe lemon juice and cider vinegar for detoxification and purification of the body. They have been recommended as alkalinizing agents because of their purported high content of alkaline minerals, reports Susan Lark, M.D., a preventive health doctor in Los Altos, California.[8]
- Apple cider vinegar is used to treat skin ailments such as acne and warts. Its pH (the number that indicates how much acid or alkaline is present in a solution) is identical to normal, healthy skin. It's believed that applying apple cider vinegar to skin areas will help normalize the pH on skin and speed up healing.

Hydrochloric Acid. Apple cider vinegar also helps the stomach to produce hydrochloric acid, which aids digestion. We lose acid as we age, a big reason to take apple cider vinegar to prevent digestion disorders as we get older.

"As we get older, the symptoms of lack of acid are the same as too much acid," explains Dr. Earl Mindell. For instance, indigestion may arise from either excess acid or insufficient acid in the stomach (which leads to poor digestion). "You want to have a balance. That's why a little apple cider vinegar before a meal or with a meal can help produce enough acidity that will help the normal digestion."

Dr. Jan McBarron, a dedicated diet doctor, agrees. "Vinegar is an acid—acid helps dissolve things. In order for our food to be truly digested it has to be broken down 100 percent to a pure liquid. That's the only way the small intestine can absorb the nutrients—it has to be in total liquid form," she explains. And vinegar does the trick.

I can personally attest to that. A while ago, for dinner I ordered a cobb salad. Instead of a high-fat blue cheese dressing, I opted for a red wine vinegar. The result? After my meal, rather than feeling bogged down as I have in the past with blue cheese, I felt light and energized. It was like switching from whole milk to low-fat milk. You can't go back. And I won't.

Purifying Apple Cider Vinegar. The acetic acid in apple cider vinegar is believed to help detoxify the body from foreign substances such as drugs and alcohol. And many medical doctors and folk remedy users believe vinegar—internally and externally—helps to purify your body's system.

Here is a brief recap of how apple cider vinegar can work for you, from head to toe.

ACV Health Boosters

What It Is and Does	Diseases It Prevents
ACID: aids in proper digestion of food.	Digestive disorders such as heartburn and gas.
AMINO ACIDS	Impaired memory.
BETA-CAROTENE: contains carotenoids, which the liver converts into vitamin A, a cancer-fighting antioxidant.	Cancer: When your body doesn't get adequate beta-carotene, you are more likely to develop cancer of the lung, stomach, or mouth. Smokers are at a higher risk for lung and mouth cancers.
BORON: works like estrogen to prevent loss of mineral from bone; aids in utilization of vitamin D.	Osteoporosis.

CALCIUM: maintains strong, healthy bones and teeth, which store 99% of the body's calcium; helps enzymes in fat and protein digestion and energy production; helps regulate contraction of muscles, including the heart; aids absorption of other nutrients.	Osteoporosis.
ENZYMES: aid food digestion.	Digestive disorders such as poor metabolism.
FIBER	Heart disease, cancer (colon, breast).
GLUCOSE	Impaired brain power.
IRON: plays a role in immune system functioning and is important to cognition.	Anemia, fatigue.
MAGANESE: necessary for maintaining normal cholesterol levels.	Heart disorders, high cholesterol.
POTASSIUM	Fatigue, high blood pressure, heart disease, strokes, and fatigue.

Mile-High Apple Vinegary Pie

❖ ❖ ❖

This old-fashioned pie recipe of mine is sweet and tart (thanks to vinegar) and doesn't look like a cookie-cutter packaged one in the store. It's good to savor both warm and cold for Thanksgiving, Christmas, Valentine's Day, and Fourth of July. The berries add a festive color combo to the green apples. And the raw sugar gives it a super crunch.

While you can overindulge in cookies and candies, a slice of fresh fruit pie paired with hot herbal tea or gourmet coffee will give you a nice holiday fix and has some health perks, too. Whether you're alone or with friends and family, this holiday apple pie will feed your sweet tooth, fill you up, not out, and boost your spirit.

5–8 *Granny Smith apples, peeled, cored, sliced thin*

½ *cup premium fresh berries (blueberries or cranberries or strawberries), chopped*

2 *tablespoons European-style butter, cold, cubed*

¼ *cup granulated white sugar*

½ *teaspoon cinnamon*

½ *teaspoon nutmeg*

1 *teaspoon orange rind (optional)*

1 *teaspoon fresh lemon juice (optional)*

1 *tablespoon Bragg Organic Raw Apple Cider Vinegar*

2 *store-bought premium piecrusts*

4 *tablespoons half-and-half (½ for apple mixture; ½ for crust)*

2 *tablespoons each, raw sugar and cinnamon (for crust)*

walnuts for garnish (optional)

In a large bowl, combine sliced apples, cranberries, butter, sugar, spices, citrus, and vinegar. Place in one piecrust. Put other piecrust on top. Flute edges with thumb to give it a homemade, imperfect rustic look. (If pieces break, use warm water to mend.) Brush top with half-and-half. Sprinkle sugar-cinnamon mixture. Cover with foil (so edges of piecrust don't burn). Bake at 375 degrees for 15 minutes, then bake for another 45 minutes. Cool for one hour before cutting. Sprinkle top with chopped walnuts and serve with a small scoop of all-natural vanilla ice cream, or put in the oven with a piece of cheese on top, and then the cheese melts as the pie warms up. Serves approximately 10.

VINEGARY HEALING HINTS TO PRESERVE

✓ Apple cider vinegar contains plenty of healthful nutrients.
✓ The quality of vinegar counts. Natural, organic, and made the slow Orleans method are recommended by folk medicine doctors.
✓ Apples, a component of apple cider vinegar, are fiber-rich and potassium-plentiful.
✓ Potassium, the miracle worker of apple cider vinegar, helps keep the body's sodium-potassium levels in balance.
✓ Apple cider vinegar contains beta-carotene, boron, calcium, enzymes, fiber, and iron.
✓ Other good stuff is in apple cider vinegar such as carbohydrates and amino acids.
✓ Apple cider vinegar can aid in maintaining your body's acid/alkaline balance.
✓ Hydrochloric acid in apple cider vinegar can help aid digestion.
✓ Apple cider vinegar can help your body to excrete toxins, which purifies your system.
✓ The total ingredients of apple cider vinegar can help prevent health ailments such as fatigue and poor digestion and ward off heart disease and cancer.

Researchers and real people will show you how this nutritional wonder can help you—without ill side effects or a high cost. Read on and discover how apple cider vinegar can be healthful for your heart, weight, bones, and so much more!

It's clear that ACV has a powerhouse of health-promoting nutrients. But how exactly does this golden liquid help your body to prevent disease? Researchers and real people will show you how this nutritional wonder can help you—without ill side effects or a high cost.

Why Is Apple Cider Vinegar So Healthy?

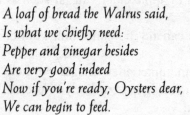

A loaf of bread the Walrus said,
Is what we chiefly need:
Pepper and vinegar besides
Are very good indeed
Now if you're ready, Oysters dear,
We can begin to feed.

—Lewis Carroll[1]

My mom wasn't the only one who used apple cider vinegar in baking and cooking in the mid-twentieth century. In the fifth grade, at ten, I loved testing recipes at home more than school classes. Often I'd play hooky just so I could play with the dog and cook up a recipe or two I'd find in my mother's well-used cookbooks (which were often too difficult to understand, so I'd revise and concoct my own version).

One school day I invited a classmate to join me as my guest for an American main-dish salad with vinaigrette. There was a problem, though. I broke the rules (twice). Students were not allowed to leave the premises. But my desire to flaunt my budding culinary skills was worth the risk. Time wasn't on my side, but putting together a Cobb salad (as ordered in an *I Love Lucy* episode when the comedienne was at the Hollywood Brown Derby restaurant) was almost foolproof. The protein—bacon and chicken—was leftovers in the fridge. I had to boil eggs, prepare the iceberg lettuce, tomatoes, avocado, chives, and crumbled blue cheese. It was easy for a kid to do.

The glitch was, my dad came home unexpectedly; so per my request, my visitor hid in the bedroom closet while I made up a story. "I came home to get my homework. Do you want a salad?" Surprisingly, my dad was happy to eat my lunch; he asked for dressing. The red wine vinegar bottle was almost empty, so I turned to apple cider vinegar, inspired by the basic vinaigrette recipe of the twentieth century. The salad was a winner, but I didn't win any feel-good compliments from my friend who left hungry and with a rain check to have a luncheon salad with a tasty vinaigrette that I put together all by myself.

Years later, I did cross paths with a food-savvy doctor who gets vinegar and its virtues. She told me the story about how the superfood entered her life—and how she made a big life change for the better.

Five years ago, Jan McBarron woke up at her regular time. Rather than pouring herself a cup of coffee, she had 2 tablespoons of vinegar in a glass of water. Then, while clad in leotards and a T-shirt, she ran three miles for her A.M. exercise routine.

Today, Dr. McBarron, a weight-loss specialist in the Deep South, a region called the "Stroke Belt," uses this same energizing ritual every other day before she goes to work. It's the perfect stay-slim, keep-healthy therapy for the doctor who specializes in overweight disorders.

So, do you want to be energized? Do you feel like your weight is out of control? Do you have skyrocketing cholesterol levels? Are you suffering from high blood pressure? If you answered "yes" to any of these questions, apple cider vinegar may be the solution to help you cope, too.

FIGHTING FAT WITH APPLE CIDER VINEGAR

"If I could do it, anyone can." That's what Dr. McBarron assures the patients who come to her with seemingly hopeless weight problems. And they believe her, because they know she's speaking from experience. Years ago, Dr. McBarron dropped 70 pounds from her 5 foot 10 frame—and she's kept the weight off.

For a decade, Dr. McBarron fought a battle with her weight. "I lost 50 pounds—five times!" she says. "I tried every diet you can name. I'd finally attained my dream of becoming a doctor, but I was miserable because I weighed over 200 pounds! It was time to get off the roller coaster," Dr. McBarron says. And vinegar—both apple cider vinegar and red wine vinegar—is part of her meal plan that has helped her and her patients lose weight and keep it off.

Staying lean is a big health concern for Americans today. And it should be. Excess body fat is linked to killer diseases—such as high blood pressure, diabetes, stroke, and heart attack. Despite the danger of fat, losing weight is not easy. Americans are losing the battle of the bulge.

TRANS FATS AND VINEGAR

Have you noticed those three little words, "No trans fats," on a variety of food products? Nutritionists will tell you that trans fats are partially hydrogenated vegetable oils found in unhealthy, high-fat foods such as fried foods, baked pastries, cookies, cakes, muffins, commercial breads (not all of them), margarine, and vegetable shortening. Research shows that people who eat these bad-for-you, artery-clogging goodies chock-full of trans fats are more likely to up the odds of developing heart disease.

The good news is, most vinegars have less than 3 calories per tablespoon and no fat, according to the experts at the Vinegar Institute. But note, they recommend checking the label of your favorite vinegar products (especially the seasoned varieties) to find out the nutrition information for those specific products. And if those products include trans fats, you need to beware.

Keep in mind that labels for vinaigrettes may note "0 trans fats," but don't be fooled. The sodium content can be high, as can the amount of saturated fat. I just looked at a bottle in the fridge. The lesson: If you're watching your sodium intake because you're prone to hypertension, stay clear of the fancy flavored vinegars.

The Academy of Nutrition and Dietetics recommends that you limit your intake of trans fats to 2 grams per day. That way, you're more likely to keep a trim, healthy body.

THE SKINNY ON ACV

But apple cider vinegar comes to the rescue. Doctors can vouch for this. People from coast to coast in America will tell you that they know about the weight loss–apple cider vinegar connection. Folks will religiously drink a tablespoon of apple cider vinegar, especially raw (unpasturized) and organic in a glass of warm water every morning because they believe it will help them to lose pounds, boost energy, and aid digestion.

Meanwhile, I have not heard of any groundbreaking, controlled weight-loss studies in this country that document apple cider vinegar as a weight-loss aid. However, research does show how apple cider vinegar's fat-fighting ingredients—such as fiber—can indeed help pare excess pounds.

Furthermore, the fiber and nutrients in apple cider vinegar can help keep you healthy if you are watching your caloric intake. Both apples and apple cider vinegar contain pectin, a type of fiber found mostly in fruits. It can help suppress a runaway appetite.

Here's proof: Scientists at the University of Southern California found that adding 15 grams of concentrated pectin to the meals of nine overweight people delayed the time required for food to leave their stomachs by 45 minutes. The reason: Pectin plumps up food as it's processed by the stomach, boosting feelings of fullness and suppressing the appetite. The pectin-rich meals helped the people in the study to eat less and shed more than 6½ pounds in one month.[2]

And some people, who mix 1 tablespoon of vinegar in a glass of water and drink the solution a half hour before meals, vow that it curbs the appetite. Could it be possible that the fiber in apple cider vinegar, like apples, fills you up?

Another boon to apple cider vinegar's slimming power is how it can keep the body's sodium-potassium levels in check. According to Dr. McBarron, when the ratio of sodium-potassium is balanced, you'll eat less, because you're not going to be as hungry.

Potassium-rich foods can help decrease unwanted water retention—and flatten the tummy, too. "Potassium works on the body to counterbalance sodium. And sodium is another factor that may cause you to retain water and feel bloated," says Terri Brownlee, R.D., M.P.H., in Durham, North Carolina. ACV and potassium-rich foods like watermelon, bananas, cantaloupe, dried apricots, and vegetables can act as natural diuretics, which may reduce bloating.

Not only is apple cider vinegar rich in pectin and potassium, it's got another fat fighter that you should know about. Acetic acid, the primary ingredient in vinegar, has long been believed to boost metabolism and to dissolve fats.

Bloat-Busting Meal Plan

This slimming, healthy meal plan—designed by New Jersey–based nutritionist Toni Gerbino—can flatten your tummy fast! Give it a try for two days before a special occasion. I tried it, and even though I am a slim 120 pounds at 5-5, it worked wonders. My tummy was flatter and I felt energized!

Breakfast: Fresh berries (no limit)

Lunch: 4 ounces fresh white meat turkey
greens with dressing made of fresh parsley, 1 tablespoon each virgin olive oil and apple cider vinegar, and spices to taste
1 cup fresh berries

Dinner: 6–8 ounces fresh flounder, sole, or salmon
asparagus with lemon, apple cider vinegar, and parsley
1 cup fresh berries

• Drink a minimum of six 8-ounce glasses of water with fresh lemon throughout the day.

• Check with your doctor before starting this or any diet.

Switch to Apple Cider Vinegar

In addition to vinegar cocktails, easy menu changes can help to melt pounds away as easy as 1-2-3. Here, take a look:

1 Change to fat-free vinegar for salad dressing. One of the biggest sources of fat and calories in the average woman's diet is salad dressing. When you toss a salad of mixed greens, substitute 2 tablespoons vinegar for the 2 tablespoons of regular dressing you normally use three times a week.

2 You'll whittle your waistline faster when you trim your sandwich, even just a little. Once a week, build a more slimming sandwich just by leaving out one slice of meat and the cheese, and replacing mayonnaise with vinegar. Then add flavorful, filling layers of fiber- and water-rich dark, leafy greens and tomatoes.

3 Eliminate 1 teaspoon of margarine a day. Giving up just 1 teaspoon of margarine a day will make a big difference. Instead of sautéing your vegetables in the yellow stuff that clogs your arteries, try a splash of vinegar to avoid adding extra calories from fat.

ACV Fat-Fighters' Factoids

Tangy apple cider vinegar is delicious. But with its other fat-fighting qualities, it is not just for salads. It's a refreshing and tasty addition to sandwiches, main dishes, and more.

- It has only 15 calories per tablespoon.
- It has no fat.
- It has no sodium.
- It's potassium-rich, which can help fight water retention.

For now, the final word on apple cider vinegar is that it can put you on the track to good health and long-term weight loss. If you really want to shed excess pounds—and enjoy long-lasting results—start eating a good, well-balanced diet, include apple cider vinegar whenever you can, and have your doctor recommend an exercise regimen suited to your goals. (Go to Chapter 16 for more pound-paring vinegar power quickie diets.)

Apple Cider Vinegar Helps Keep Blood Pressure in Check

As a health writer always on deadline and prone to stress-induced high blood pressure, I've taken an alternative route to staying heart-healthy. Each day I make sure I get plenty of fruits and vegetables—and now, vinegar is also part of my prescription to good health.

As people age, they become more susceptible to several life-threatening diseases. According to the American Heart Association, about one out of four adults has high blood pressure. Untreated high blood pressure can bring on a deadly stroke or heart attack.

Rather than opt for medication, apple cider vinegar can aid in the prevention of high blood pressure, and today, doctors know that potassium—which we already know ACV is rich in—is needed to counteract the damaging effects of sodium—including high blood pressure.

Health Fact!

If your blood pressure is under 120/80, there is little need for you to be overly concerned about a moderate salt intake.

The American Medical Association found that potassium lowers blood pressure. The results of 33 studies showed that potassium lowers blood pressure in patients with hypertension, and it can also help prevent hypertension by lowering blood pressure levels. While all the research was based on potassium supplements, the lead author, Dr. Paul Whelton, a professor and dean of the Tulane University School of Public Health in New Orleans, believes that this is not the only way to obtain the desired level. Many fruits and vegetables are potassium-rich, and eating five or six a day can fill the recommended intake of potassium.

Good Potassium-Rich Fruits for Keeping Your Blood Pressure Lower

Vinegars can be made from the various fruits below. (See Part 4, "Other Natural Vinegars.")

1 apple = 159 mg	1 orange = 237 mg
3 apricots = 313 mg	1 peach = 171 mg
1 cup blueberries = 129 mg	1 pear = 208 mg
1 cup cranberries = 67 mg	1 plum = 113 mg
1 lemon = 80 mg	1 pomegranate = 399 mg
1 mango = 322 mg	1 cup raspberries = 187 mg
	1 cup strawberries = 247 mg

Avoid These High Blood Pressure Culprits

Bacon	Marinated foods*	Smoked food	High-sodium canned foods
Catsup	Diet soda	Fast food	Ham
Hot dogs	Pickled foods*	Salted potato chips	Salted pretzels
Salted nuts	Fried food	Sausage	Shellfish
Fatty meats	Seasoned salts	Duck, goose	Butter

*If your blood pressure is normal, go ahead and enjoy seasoned salts, and eat marinated and/or pickled foods in moderation.

THE VINEGAR AND FIBER–CHOLESTEROL CONNECTION

Heart problems continue to be a major problem to both men and women. Apple cider vinegar can be heart-healthy too, because it contains pectin, a soluble fiber, which aids in lowering cholesterol.

Fiber-rich apple cider vinegar can contain a healthy dose of pectin when it's made from fresh, natural apples. "Soluble fiber helps reduce cholesterol by binding it with the fiber, which your body then eliminates," says Connie Diekman, R.D. This, in turn, reduces the risk of heart ailments, such as heart attacks and strokes.

The Cholesterol Puzzle

Dazed and confused about cholesterol? Here's the lowdown. The more high-density lipoproteins or HDL (good cholesterol) you have, the better. This kind we want to be high—it lowers the risk of heart disease. Oxidized (free radical–damaged), LDL (bad cholesterol) puts you at higher risk for heart disease. But you can guard against it with antioxidant vitamins that are found in apple cider vinegar.

SLASH ARTERY PLAQUE WITH APPLE CIDER VINEGAR

If you have high cholesterol, you're hardly alone. Simply put, plaque buildup in the arteries can cause heart attacks and strokes by blocking blood flow to the heart and brain. But diet, exercise, and lifestyle changes help people every day to lower their cholesterol levels.

Recent research proves that one way to lower LDL (bad) cholesterol may not be with drugs, but with apple cider vinegar. The Japanese Corporate News Network (JCNN) reported on a study that found the regular intake of vinegar (15 milliliters, or 3 teaspoons, or more per day) can significantly reduce the level of cholesterol in the blood. According to the JCNN article, "acetic acid has induced the effect." The results were presented at the 59th Annual Meeting for the Japanese Society of Nutrition and Food Science.[3]

ANTICANCER APPLE CIDER VINEGAR

Cancer: It is a frightening disease for men, women, children, and pets. And today it is a growing epidemic that may lead to heart disease in the future. So what exactly is cancer? It is a group of diseases characterized by abnormal cells that go awry. If the spread is not controlled, you can die.

Cancer is caused by external (chemicals, radiation, and viruses) and internal (hormones, immune conditions, and inherited mutations) factors, according to the American Cancer Society. But you can reduce the risk of getting cancer.

Scientists now know that dietary changes hold the key to preventing a number of cancers, and research shows that certain antioxidant-rich fruits and vegetables—especially teamed with apple cider vinegar, which contains beta-carotene, a carotenoid—can help guard against cancers.

"Moreover, carotenoids serve as the body's raw material for the production of vitamin A, another potent antioxidant, the scarcity of which has been linked, in particular, to cancers of the respiratory system, colon and bladder. Carotenoids and vitamin A work in concert to protect the body from cancers associated with chemical toxins," explains Dr. Earl Mindell.[4]

Numerous studies have found that eating fruits and vegetables cuts the risk of cancer. Medical experts know that eating foods high in the antioxdants C, E, and beta-carotene may trap free radical molecules that cause normal cells to become cancerous.

What's more, according to The Vinegar Institute, vinegar was given kudos as "Food of the Week" in May 2005. Cancer Research UK, a charity in the United Kingdom with a new "Fiver Day" campaign as part of its Reduce the Risk Program, awarded vinegar this honor for being "healing and cleansing" and because "it also contains anti-cancer elements." On the downside, another article points out that people in the United Kingdom, much like Americans, may be not getting enough fruits and vegetables.[5]

The National Cancer Institute recommends you get between 20 and 30 grams of fiber a day by eating a diet high in fruits, vegetables, and whole grains. Pectin, a soluble fiber in vinegar, helps dilute cancer-causing compounds in your body and speed cancer-causing dietary fats through the colon before they can be absorbed, according to research. In fact, studies show that a high fiber diet can kill colon cells, report British medical researchers in London.[6]

But no single food or supplement can prevent cancer. Apple cider vinegar, which contains both beta-carotene and fiber, is not a magic bullet—it's still very important to eat a variety of antioxidant-rich fruits and vegetables to reduce all cancers.

Amazingly, however, vinegar is considered a "weapon" against cancer, according to scientists at the A.P. John Institute for Cancer Research. In the early twenty-first century, a press release announced the discovery that acetic acid has a deadly effect on cancer cells because it stalls the energy-producing process in cells. The release notes "logic dictates that if you shut down glycolysis with acetic acid, cancer cells will die from starvation." Plus, it was noted, "Citric acid is converted into acetic acid in the body and when combined, prove to be valuable weapons in fighting cancer."[7]

Breast cancer and prostate cancer are among the deadliest cancers. And they both are very sensitive medical matters.

But the good news is both hormonally driven cancers are preventable—and almost always curable when caught early.

• **Breast Cancer:** Risk of breast cancer, reported the American Cancer Society (ACS), is linked to various factors that affect circulating hormone levels throughout life: age of menstruation, number of pregnancies, breastfeeding, obesity, and physical activity. Here's the best dietary approach to risk reduction:

A low-fat diet (one with 30 percent or less of total calories coming from fat) may keep "bad" estrogen (a female hormone) levels down, limiting exposure to the type of estrogen that leads tumor growth.

Instead of unhealthy high-fat toppings and unhealthy high-fat food (there are good fats, including olive oil), pile your plate with fruits and vegetables and use vinegar when it's palatable. Remember the label on ACV? It shows that this product can help you to lower your caloric intake and maintain a low-fat diet.

As an alternative to high-fat meat, try soy foods. Genistein, a compound in soybeans, may be able to inhibit the spreading of cancerous tumors. It is believed that it inhibits the growth of new blood vessels which nourish cancer cells. So start snacking on more soy nuts, soy milk, soy burgers, and miso soup.

Eating more vegetables. For added protection, follow the NCI guidelines to eat five or more servings of fruits and vegetables—especially vegetables from the cabbage family, such as broccoli, cauliflower, and Brussels sprouts. In fact, studies show that cruciferous veggies have a chemical called indole-3-carbinol which helps to decrease the levels of the "bad" estrogen like a low-fat diet does. And note, teaming fruits and vegetables with beta-carotene-rich apple cider vinegar may prevent cancer, too.

• **Prostate Cancer:** Scientists know that prostate cancer is connected to male hormones, but they are unclear as to the exact mechanism that causes the cancer. Here's the best dietary approach to risk reduction.

The best preventive measure, according to the American Cancer Society, is to limit intake of foods from animal sources, especially saturated fats and red meats. Lean poultry such as turkey and chicken with whole grains such as brown rice and pasta are good substitutes. And note, our meal plans boast slim and healthy eating with flavorful apple cider vinegar.

Switching to low-fat fare based on fresh vegetables and fruit that are chock-full of the antioxidant vitamins C, E, and beta-carotene (again, which is present in apple cider vinegar) will help protect against prostate cancer by trapping cancer-causing free radical molecules.

• **Cervical Cancer:** The rates of cervical cancer have plummeted over the past decades, according to the American Cancer Society. The lower rates are due to the Papanicolaou (Pap) test, which was introduced in the 1950s.

Recently researchers at Johns Hopkins University in Baltimore and the University of Zimbabwe found vinegar could screen for cervical cancer where Pap tests aren't available. The low-cost technique could improve the chances of detecting cancer in developing countries such as Asia, Latin America, and Africa.

Nurse-midwives used the vinegar technique to screen 10,934 women at primary-care clinics in Zimbabwe. Precancerous cells turn white when swabbed with an applicator soaked in a solution of acetic acid, the main ingredient in vinegar. Pap smears were also performed on the women and the vinegar test was more likely to pick up precancerous or cancercous cells than the Pap smear.[8]

While cervical cancer in the United States has decreased, about 4,800 women are expected to die of it each year. The study's coauthor Paul Blumenthal often sees patients with an abnormal Pap smear. He may repeat the Pap smear, but he will also splash vinegar on the cervix as a backup test. To me this is good news. As a DES daughter (DES, a synthetic estrogen given to about 4.8 million women in the United States between 1938 and 1971, has been linked to a rare form of cancer in their daughters), I know what abnormal Pap smears are all about. Who would have thought vinegar could be used as a "second opinion"?

In conclusion, according to the American Institute for Cancer Research, scientists have not yet pinpointed how dietary fat promotes cancer development. However, it seems that fat is involved in both the early abnormal cell changes that may lead to cancer and in helping existing tumors to grow. For now, research shows that dietary changes are one of your best safeguards against cancer.

ACV Cancer-Prevention Nutrients

While apple cider vinegar contains beta-carotene, vitamin C, and calcium, it can also be paired with these cancer-fighting nutrients found in foods in our recipes:

Nutrient	Found in	What It Does	Protection
Beta-carotene	Carrots, salad greens	Beta-carotene in the body can change into retinoic acid, a substance used to treat cancer of the blood and bladder	Stomach, larynx, lung, esophagus, breast
Vitamin C	Broccoli, strawberries, red and green peppers	Boosts protective white cell activity	Breast, stomach
Calcium	Tofu	Calcium, in association with vitamin D, binds to fats in the intestine, reducing ability to promote cancer	Colon

Scientists' Anticancer Marinade

So you probably know that meats cooked at high temperatures on a grill form cancer-causing compounds, right? Well, I bet you don't know that a recipe from researchers at Lawrence Livermore National Laboratory in California offers a solution. While studying the effects of chemicals in our diet, they found a new way to lower "bad" compounds called heterocyclic amines.

"When we barbecued market-fresh meat, we found startlingly high levels of heterocyclic amines," says Jim Felton, Ph.D., division leader in molecular and structural biology. But when Felton and his colleagues coated chicken with a special marinade before grilling it, the results changed. They still don't know exactly how it decreases the heterocylcic amines—but it works.

Here's the scientists anticancer marinade: ½ cup packed brown sugar, 3 cloves crushed garlic, 1½ teaspoons salt, 3 tablespoons mustard, ¼ cup cider vinegar, 3 tablespoons lemon juice, and 6 tablespoons olive oil.

YES! VINEGAR HELPS YOU BEAT TYPE 2 DIABETES

This may come as a surprise: Apple cider vinegar may be just the remedy to help you stave off type 2 diabetes, which usually develops after age 40. This all-too-common disease is characterized by elevated levels of blood sugar, or glucose, which result from the body's inability to make enough insulin, a hormone needed to convert sugar, starches, and other food components into energy.

The symptoms of diabetes include hunger, unusual thirst, blurred vision, frequent urination, weight loss, and fatigue. According to the American Diabetes Association, millions of Americans have diabetes (mostly type 2).

The upside, however, is that most of the people who have type 2 diabetes, much like people with high cholesterol, can control the disease through diet and lifestyle changes. And that's where ACV comes into play again.

Researchers at Arizona State University found that including apple cider vinegar in the diet may help to slow the rise of blood sugar after a high-carbohydrate meal. ABC News reported the story on its website on January 26, 2005.

In the study, type 2 diabetics, prediabetics, and healthy people consumed either 2 tablespoons of apple cider vinegar in a glass of water sweetened with saccharine or a placebo prior to eating a breakfast containing a whopping 87 grams of carbs. Dr. Carol Johnston, a researcher at Arizona State, discovered that vinegar slowed the spike of blood sugar in all three groups up to 34 percent.[9]

It may be beneficial to improve your diet, too. Here are some more ways diet teamed with ACV (in the form of either taking 2 tablespoons in water or including it in your meals) and lifestyle changes can help lower your risk.

- *Eat more fiber-rich foods:* Dietary fiber has been associated with reduced insulin requirement in many studies over the past several
decades. It is linked with blood sugar control.

- *Lower dietary fat:* A high-fat diet seems to increase the risk of diabetes. Eating five or six mini low-fat, high-fiber meals will help you
maintain satiety throughout the day to avoid hunger pangs.

- *Get a move on:* Regular exercise can help you keep your weight in
check, and help make your insulin work more efficiently, like maintaining a computer so it will last.[10]

APPLE CIDER VINEGAR BEATS BONE LOSS

The facts are frightening. Countless women and men over age 50
may have an osteoporosis-related fracture in their lifetime. But as scary
as this seems, we are not powerless. The right nutrient-dense diet—
teamed with apple cider vinegar, which contains bone builders such as
boron and calcium—can help lower our risk.

Evidence shows that boron, a bone-buddy mineral, plays a role in
utilizing calcium and magnesium—other bone builders. Still, most
Americans are probably not getting enough boron, which is found in
apple cider vinegar.

Boron also helps the metabolism of calcium and magnesium—and
boosts blood levels of the bone-building hormones estrogen and
testosterone, according to research. Your best bets: Eat soy, prunes,
and apples.

In addition, most women don't get the recommended daily al-
lowance of bone-building calcium in their diet.

But apple cider vinegar comes to the rescue again. If taking a tablespoon of vinegar in water doesn't appeal to you, try more calcium-rich
recipes that include broccoli and dairy, including yogurt and milk paired
with apple cider vinegar.

BOOSTING YOUR MEMORY WITH APPLE CIDER VINEGAR

Iron, a mineral found in apple cider vinegar, may strengthen brain
power. Since iron is involved in distributing oxygen to brain cells (and

every other cell in the body), when you lack this mineral you find it hard to concentrate.

In the early 1990s, Harold Sandstead, M.D., professor emeritus of preventive medicine at the University of Texas, discovered that women whose diets lack zinc and iron experienced more difficulties on standard exams than women with an adequate dietary supply. In his study of women aged 18 to 40, Sandstead found that giving these women more zinc and iron raised their scores on memory tests an average of 20 percent.

Boron plays a crucial part in memory function, too. Scientists at the USDA's Human Nutrition Research Center have linked boron deficiencies to chronic lethargy and fatigue. In brain studies, they found that the electrical activity of the gray matter in the boron-deficient indicated increased drowsiness and mental sluggishness.

Food for thought? Your best food sources for these two nutrients to help strengthen your mental powers: Boron: apples, broccoli, cabbage, cauliflower. Iron: ground beef, turkey, spinach, and peas. To get you started, try our apple cider vinegar recipes, including these iron-rich foods.

VINEGAR—A VIRUS FIGHTER?

I am intrigued by the fact that vinegar has been used in China to prevent the spread of a virus such as SARS (severe acute respiratory syndrome) and other deadly respiratory illnesses. Remember seeing people on TV in China wearing masks in fear of contracting SARS?

An anonymous source noted that on February 13, 2003, an outbreak of pneumonia in several cities in southern China's Guangdong province had been controlled. According to press conferences held by various government officials, emergency strategies were required to control the prices of vinegar and other antiviral medicines, which had skyrocketed due to their effectiveness in curing this disease.

Viruses, like SARS, come and go. As a kid, I recall tuberculosis (TB) was the health scare. The infectious disease is still around. Researchers in Venezuela, France, and the United States discovered the active ingredient in vinegar, acetic acid, can kill mycobacteria—even drug-resistant mycobacterium tuberculosis. One of the researchers accidentally found vinegar's ability to kill the bacteria is due to the acetic acid. Commercial white vinegar was used whenever possible (its strength at about 6 percent).[11]

Another highly infectious virus is Ebola. As we open our hospital doors to infected people working in Africa to stop Ebola, the United States is sending thousands of military personnel to West Africa. Nobody knows for sure how *exactly* it's contracted—much like in the beginning of the AIDS epidemic. But during that health crisis the government didn't listen to the infected victims. AIDS and Ebola patients often are ostracized, especially when all the facts are not clear. Some authorities believe the world is not winning the war against Ebola despite its military and humanitarian efforts to help people in West African countries.

As we continue to lend a hand our own people are coming home sick with the deadly virus. During the media hype people traveling turned to antiseptic wipes. Also, like during the Middle Ages, when vinegar was used to disinfect sick rooms, people were discussing the therapeutic remedy as a means of protection.

PROOF OF LIFE: APPLE CIDER VINEGAR

As a folk remedy, apple cider vinegar has been praised as a cure-all for treating allergies to sunburn. As you've seen so far, I do include past studies about apple cider vinegar and more recent research backing up the evidence. But finding new, improved, hard-hitting studies on humans (not lab rats or test tubes) with groundbreaking results showing that it can lower the risk of developing heart disease, cancer, diabetes 2, and obesity is a big challenge; they're not often available. But this lack of real research does not mean apple cider vinegar is all hype.

Some research has been done (you can search online and discover small published studies conducted in the past few decades), but if the work is conducted with a baker's dozen of people instead of a thousand or more people, the results are not earthshaking or groundbreaking in the health world; and red-flag words "further research is needed" often follow findings.

But note, apple cider vinegar shows promise in obscure studies (using lab rats instead of ten humanoids) that do make the news. The end result: Acetic acid—the primary compound in cider vinegar—is powerful and may indeed lower the risk of developing cancer, heart disease, and diabetes 2, as well as obesity. Still, larger controlled studies using thousands of humans, peer group–reviewed, and followed up for long-term results are ways to back up claims; or finding and using a likable heroic creature and human (as in the classic novel *Flowers for Algernon*) may suffice if and only if there are long-lasting results.

I'd love to report to you that apple cider vinegar, a potent elixir, is the ultimate answer to end global warming and provide world peace as well as stop deadly viruses and natural disasters. In reality, scientific proof linked to groundbreaking studies using humans does not exist. The good news is, vinegars—not just apple cider vinegar—contain extraordinary healing compounds that provide proof vinegar isn't just a condiment to consume like using a lucky rabbit's foot. (Refer to Part 4, "Other Natural Vinegars.") Meanwhile, take a look at some surprising apple cider vinegar remedies that may work for you with or without sign of scientific approval.

TWELVE UNEXPECTED HOME CURES: APPLE CIDER VINEGAR TRIOS

Apple cider vinegar (ACV) can and does help fight diseases as I've discussed—but mix it up with other healing superfoods, such as honey and olive oil, and what have you got? Welcome to secrets to healing pesky ailments by using double-duty unexpected apple cider vinegar combinations!

Vinegar, an ancient remedy, is touted for its amazing powers used solo. However, through trial and error I've discovered that sometimes pairing this vinegar with other healing superfoods is more realistic for staying healthy. A combo effect, in fact, can be even more useful and work faster and better. Here, take a look at some common health woes and the combo apple cider vinegar remedies that may be the trick for you.

1 ACCELERATED AGING Age is just a number if you take care of your health. Everyone has an expiration date, but that fact doesn't mean you cannot enjoy robust physical and mental energy throughout the passages in life. Apple cider proponents who use vinegar each day and maintain a healthy lifestyle are living examples of how this revital-

izing potion can help keep you ageless. If you team it with another superfood? Think a double punch of age-defying rewards.

What ACV Mix to Use: Try 1 teaspoon apple cider vinegar in an 8-ounce glass of water with a splash of fresh lemon juice and 1 teaspoon of anti-aging honey. Do this ritual each morning upon rising before breakfast.

How It Works: Vinegar, lemon, water, and honey are essential items in your kitchen and are instant health aids for keeping regular throughout the day. Potassium-rich vinegar and honey with their anti-aging antioxidants boost physical energy, and keep your immune system strong. Lemon is a natural detoxifier with plenty of vitamin C, and water will keep you hydrated and on even keel.

Testing, 1, 2, 3: By combining honey and lemon, I tried this homemade vinegar drink. A cup of hot of iced antioxidant-rich white or black tea is even better, though, and more my cup of tea. (See Part 5, "The Elixir of Youth.")

2 ALLERGIES Due to erratic climate change around the nation and world, seasonal spring and fall allergies, complete with sneezing, a runny nose, congestion, and watery eyes may follow you around longer than two seasons. Living in the Sierra Nevada we are visited by a late spring and short summer, but in recent years, thanks to the West's drought, pollen and smoky skies from wildfires linger in the air.

What ACV Mix to Use: Try combining 1 tablespoon of locally produced honey—within a fifty-mile radius—and 1 tablespoon of vinegar in a cup of antioxidant-rich black or green tea or fresh orange juice.

How It Works: Apple cider vinegar has detoxifying agents that help rid the air and your body of pollutants. Honey, tea, and oranges are nature's immunity boosters, protecting you from environmental toxins that can make you more vulnerable to allergies.

Testing, 1, 2, 3: I'm sensitive to pollutants in the environment. I use this ACV trio and, more times than not, it works. I'm not 100 percent allergy symptom–free, but better than years ago during my antihistamine days, which included a paramedic visit and appointments to the doctor, whom I would ask, "Isn't there a seasonal allergy cure without side effects?" The saline spray bottles and antihistamine boxes sit unopened in my medicine cabinet. Honey, tea, and oranges with a bit of vinegar are used up by me—a down-to-earth woman—and replaced with more of these must-have natural staples. The end result? I have fewer allergy woes.

3 ASTHMA Welcome to another respiratory problem linked to the immune system that makes it harder to breathe easy. It's often made worse by Mother Nature's wrath, whether it is life in the big city with its smog, or living the good country life when authorities warn you about unsafe air quality due to pollen or pollutants and to stay indoors.

What ACV Mix to Use: Opt for 1 teaspoon apple cider vinegar with 1 teaspoon honey twice daily, and white or green tea in the morning.

How It Works: Since apple cider vinegar is an anti-inflammatory, it can help shrink air passages to help you breathe easier (for mild asthma). Also, since honey is an immune booster, together these two healing superfoods may guard you from airborne allergens so you get a double-duty dose of protection.

Testing, 1, 2, 3: Asthma is foreign to me personally, but I've known people who battle the symptoms. Instead of trying the natural cure, they often turn to inhalers and complain about the scourge of how difficult breathing easy can be during bad days due to our environment, and daily stressors don't help.

4 BACK PAIN Since apple cider vinegar seems to help some people with asthma, due to its anti-inflammatory benefits, it just may come to the rescue for a backache. If your job entails sitting for long hours, if you over-exercise (especially the wrong way), lift a heavy object, or are carrying extra weight, you may experience a stiff upper or lower back. A chiropractor or masseuse may be helpful, but there is something more you can do when back pain may be on your back, so to speak.

What ACV Mix to Use: Try an ice-cold compress soaked in apple cider vinegar. Apply for 15 or 20 minutes. Follow with a heating pad as needed. For extra relief, massage your upper back with a mixture of olive oil and essentials oils. A heating pad and swimming followed by indulging in a hot tub is helpful. Repeat as needed.

How It Works: This apple cider vinegar home cure for an aching back is a spin-off from R.I.C.E. (rest, ice, compress, and elevate). The vinegar can soothe inflamed muscles, tissues, and nerves, and boost blood flow. The ice also is good for lessening inflammation. Heat can

feel super comforting and loosens up tight muscles. The multipur-
pose vinegar remedy soothes the pain. Olive oil contains a chemical,
oleocanthal, that can stop inflammation, much like painkillers.

Testing, 1, 2, 3: A nagging upper back pain pays me a visit from time
to time, especially when I am writing books. I personally can attest
that all of the ACV trio—not just apple cider vinegar—takes away the
ache so you can keep on moving and exercise, which is also helpful to
stay in shape and maintain a healthy back.

5 BRAIN FOG Ever felt mental fuzziness? Like chronic fatigue, fibromyalgia, and back pain, brain fog is now acknowledged by medical
researchers. If you didn't get adequate shut-eye, suffer from jet lag, or
perhaps are overextended you may fall victim to brain fog. To feel
more alert and get a brainpower surge, apple cider vinegar teamed
with two more super-powered superfoods may be the answer to your
problem.

What ACV Mix to Use: Try a cup of coffee, 1 tablespoon apple cider
vinegar, and 1 teaspoon raw honey.

How It Works: A cup of java can enhance brainpower because of its
caffeine. Apple cider vinegar does include potassium, which may
boost your mood and physical energy. Honey is an instantly energizing
superfood. This trio can give you the desire to get a move on; in turn,
you will likely be more clearheaded.

Testing, 1, 2, 3: Due to having two dogs, one senior and one pup,
I'm awakened at five to six A.M. most days of the week. I have tried
this natural concoction and yes, it does get rid of the fog so I can think
without feeling tired.

6 CAFFEINE WITHDRAWAL Like a skin cut, abruptly cutting
caffeine from your daily diet comes with a sobering tsunami of side effects. A headache, irritability, lack of concentration, muscle aches, and
anxiety are just a few of the symptoms that'll haunt you and leave you
wondering, "Is it worth it?" If you want to be rid of caffeine for good,
the best way to do it is to taper off, but if for some reason your supply
comes to a halt, vinegar and honey are super healing foods that may
help you.

What ACV Mix to Use: Take 1 tablespoon vinegar with 1 8-ounce
glass of water. Drink 6–8 glasses of water daily. Add 1 teaspoon honey

as needed. (Note: Tapering off slowly from caffeine is best. If you have to stop caffeine for a short time, once back to your regular regimen, the side effects will stop.)

How It Works: It is important to stay hydrated during the withdrawal period, which can last a few days to weeks, depending on your caffeine intake. Remember, apple cider vinegar has detoxifying components so combining water with it will help you flush out the toxins as well as help lessen high anxiety. Honey taken with or without vinegar will calm you and provide instant energy, a blessing if you're feeling lethargic or have flulike symptoms.

Testing, 1, 2, 3: One time I cut out my one cup of joe in the morning unwittingly and abruptly experienced the side effects of stopping my intake of caffeine. I was rudely awakened with insomnia (I don't have problems falling asleep), a migraine (I've never had one of these headaches), and high anxiety, which prompted me to visit my general practitioner. Once back on my one cup of coffee in the morning, and the ACV mix—I felt normal again.

7 CATARACTS Cataracts are caused by a clouding of the proteins in the lens of the eye. The result: gradual blurred vision—usually more so at a distance than close up—for reading. This eye problem can be linked to age, sunlight, smoking, and poor nutrition.

What ACV Mix to Use: Take 1 to 2 teaspoons apple cider vinegar daily. Drizzle the combination superfoods on raw vegetables or salad greens.

How It Works: Enjoying a healthful lifestyle with a nutrient-rich diet, not smoking, and using this vinegar combo (by putting it on antioxidant-rich foods) may help you lower the risk of developing cataracts. To say vinegar solo is a cure-all for cataracts is like saying vinegar will make you twenty again.

Testing, 1, 2, 3: No cataracts at this time (I have endured dry eye and an abraded cornea from walking into a ficus tree), but including vinegar, olive oil, and vegetables in my daily diet may offer me protection, so I see it as inexpensive insurance for keeping my eyesight, allowing me to continue enjoying the gift of sight.

8 CUTS Eye problems are all too common and miserable until you seek and get relief; cuts on your hands, legs, feet, or anywhere on your body (but ones that do not require stitches) can be another challenge, but apple cider vinegar—and all vinegars—can come to the rescue. Have you ever cut your finger with a knife or stepped on a nail? If so, you get it. A cut burns and throbs and isn't to be ignored.

What ACV Mix to Use: Apply apple cider vinegar diluted with cleansing water to the wound. It has both antibacterial and anti-inflammatory properties. Also, you can put a small amount of manuka honey (another excellent healer) on the wound to help get rid of the swelling and ache.

How It Works: For centuries, vinegar has been touted and used for its antibacterial powers (refer to Chapter 2). Manuka honey (ideal for skin) contains hydrogen peroxide, which has both antibacterial and antifungal properties, but it also contains a phytochemical whose healing benefits make it even more amazing. It has been used by doctors in hospitals around the world, including the United States, to treat skin infections that are antibiotic-resistant.

Testing, 1, 2, 3: I've experienced bites, stings, punctures, and cuts while living in the mountains. Once when I was barefoot walking on the deck, I stepped on a rusty nail. I didn't know about the potent vinegar, water, and honey concoction, so I headed to the doctor. One tetanus shot later I had to cope with the throbbing for a few days. If I had known about the ACV trio, the pain would have been less rather than more. I would have used it for these and other unexpected mountain mishaps from cutting my index finger in the kitchen while dicing apples like competing chefs do on the television show *Chopped* to being bit on my cheek by a spider gone AWOL from the woodpile outdoors.

9 HIGH ANXIETY Feeling on edge can be something you experience but others can't see unless they know you and may be able to sense you're uncomfortable. You don't die from feeling anxious and it's usually temporary. Life's stressors, lack of sleep, and even foods, such as those containing caffeine and sugar, can act as triggers and put you in high anxiety mode.

What ACV Mix to Use: Try an 8-ounce glass of water with 1 teaspoon of apple cider vinegar and 1 teaspoon lavender honey.

How It Works: The ingredients in honey can be calming (some medical doctors believe nature's nectar can beat insomnia) paired with soothing lavender, a known relaxer, as well as water, which can also relax you (ever notice how people in movies drink a glass of water when they are under pressure?). But it's the honey, too. The superfood may help to calm you due to its anti-stress antioxidants, minerals, and vitamins.

Testing, 1, 2, 3: One night before a national radio interview, I was anxious. As the news segment guest, my topic of overdue West Coast earthquakes was stressful especially since I was getting ready for an out-of-country trip located north to Washington and British Columbia in the shaky Cascadia Subduction Zone. So, since it was scheduled live at ten P.M., I couldn't go swim to relax. Instead, I made a quick homemade vinegar drink with ACV, lavender honey, and water. I felt at peace within minutes and nobody knew I was jittery before.

10 LIVER POLLUTION Apple cider vinegar can help rid you of toxins in the blood, metabolize fats, and keep the liver free of pollutants. Its detoxifying powers help you take charge, sort of like using a filter in a coffeemaker.

What ACV Mix to Use: Combine 1 cup water (bottled or sparkling), 1 teaspoon apple cider vinegar, ½ teaspoon fresh lemon juice, and raw honey to taste. Drink daily especially after a bout of overindulging in junk food, alcohol, a polluted environment, or taking prescription medications.

How It Works: Being proactive will help give you peace of mind. The detoxifying vinegar and its purifying added ingredients in the ACV combo will help your liver (an essential organ used to excrete toxins in the body) to get back to its healthy state.

Testing, 1, 2, 3: After a holiday event, dealing with a natural disaster such as a wildfire, or even using the fireplace too much during the cold winter months, this detoxification combo is a keeper for me; it's like changing the filter in my fish aquarium.

11 SEASONAL AFFECTIVE DISORDER This condition doesn't seem as dark as liver problems, but that's not to say it is a cakewalk in the wintertime if you live in the Northern Hemisphere. It's a condition that causes low moods and energy, especially in the winter months. Also, the farther you are from the equator, the more common SAD—or its milder form, the "winter blues"—is and it can wreak havoc on your everyday life.

What ACV Mix to Use: Mix 1 or 2 teaspoons each of apple cider vinegar and honey in a cup of coffee in the morning and afternoon.

How It Works: Apple cider vinegar can help boost the level of serotonin in the brain. Feel-good caffeine in tea, along with energizing honey, can give you a physical and mental boost. So once the vinegar, honey, and tea combo cure is taken and kicks in, it's best to use that energy drink to exercise—and that will give you that feel-good natural endorphin high throughout the day.

Testing, 1, 2, 3: I brewed a cup of joe spiked with honey and ACV. After I drank the concoction (it was a cold rainy weekday before noon), I was ready to go swim at a local resort pool. Not only did I get my water fix, along with the hot tub after, I felt lucky and played the dollar slot machines—and won. So is a java vinegar honey drink a high five for beating seasonal blues? It can be.

12 NOT BALANCED Ever notice, not unlike SAD, feeling out of sync with your body and mind can leave you feeling on overload—stressed out and not grounded? This ailment happens to both men and women (at all ages) and is an uncomfortable place to be. You need to regroup for your sanity's sake. Then you will be able to find your comfort zone—or Zen—and return to inner peace

What ACV Mix to Use: Try mixing 1 tablespoon apple cider vinegar with a calming tea, such as chamomile, lavender, or white tea with vanilla, and add 1 piece of dark chocolate.

How It Works: The vinegar will boost your potassium levels putting your sodium-potassium ratio back on track so you will feel energized and not drained. Soothing teas will calm your busy mind and racing thoughts, due to the anti-anxiety herbs, and chocolate with its mood-enhancing serotonin, a brain chemical that can make you feel happier and improve brain power and memory.

Testing, 1, 2, 3: Sometimes, you, perhaps like me, may have a problem of saying no and play the role of the Cat in the Hat—but when taking the ACV combination remedy, it helps to get centered and prioritize things to do while staying in the moment and knowing that being hit by a wave of challenges is temporary.

Cobb Salad

❖ ❖ ❖

¼ head iceberg lettuce
½ bunch watercress
½ head romaine lettuce
2 cups baby spinach, chicory, or
   endive
1 or 2 avocado, sliced
6 slices Canadian bacon
¾ cup Roquefort cheese, crumbled

2 cups cooked turkey or chicken,
   cubed
2 hard-cooked eggs, sliced
1 cup red or yellow grape tomatoes
2 scallions, chopped
1½ cups bocconcini (small
   mozzarella balls)

Line large serving platter with greens. Top with 1 row each avocado, bacon, cheese, turkey, eggs, tomatoes, scallions, and bocconcini.

Dressing

2 tablespoons chives
¼ teaspoon tarragon
2 garlic cloves, minced
½ cup Marsala olive oil
¼ cup apple cider vinegar

1 tablespoon Dijon mustard
4 strawberries
¼ cup pineapple or orange juice
salt and pepper to taste

Place all ingredients (herbs, oil, vinegar, mustard, fruit and fruit juice, spices) in jar of blender. Blend until well mixed. Hollywood's Brown Derby restaurant made this salad famous.

(Courtesy: *Cooking with California Olive Oil: Recipes from the Heart for the Heart* by Gemma Sanita Sciabica.)

VINEGARY HEALING HINTS TO PRESERVE

ACV KEEPS THE DOCTOR AWAY

Disease	How ACV Works
✓ Overweight	Fiber in ACV provides bulk/curbs appetite; keeps sodium-potassium ratio in balance so you're less hungry and decreases bloating and water retention.
✓ High blood pressure	Potassium in ACV helps reduce high blood pressure.
✓ High cholesterol	Insoluble fiber in ACV reduces cholesterol by binding with fiber, which is eliminated by body.
✓ Cancer	Beta-carotene in ACV helps fight cancer-causing free radicals in the body and boosts the immune system; acetic acid in vinegar helps detect cervical cancer.
✓ Osteoporosis	Boron in ACV helps metabolize bone-builders calcium and magnesium; calcium helps keep bones strong.
✓ Impaired memory	Iron and boron in ACV are needed to keep mental functioning at its best.

In the next chapter, I'll show you how apple cider vinegar is hardly alone. You may think ACV is the one and only vinegar to have and to hold until death do you part—but it's time to widen your circle of vinegars because others boast health perks, too.

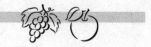

PART 3

RED WINE VINEGAR

The Red Wine Vinegar Chronicle

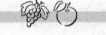

*Beware of vinegar of sweete wine, and the anger of
a peaceable man.*
—John Florio, First Fruits[1]

There's no denying that I was an audacious child who grew up to be a
daring teenager in the kitchen by following fad diets. On a chilly, overcast Sunday afternoon the rebellion arose. Sitting in my room I read
Seventeen and was inspired by skinny Twiggy-type models. I sensed
they lived on salads drizzled with vinegar.

That night when dinner was served, it was a feast. Our parish priest
was a guest. As he talked to my parents, I didn't touch the food on my
plate. Instead, I created my own diet of vegetables with a real vinaigrette of red wine vinegar and olive oil, like Julia Child would make.
My mother, a natural-born cook, didn't understand my resistance to
eating pork chops with gravy, scalloped potatoes with cheddar cheese,
asparagus with hollandaise sauce, and Boston cream pie.

She asked me, "Why aren't you eating?" I munched on the green
spears, pushing the sauce to the side, and drizzled red wine vinegar on
the stalks. My craving for exercise soared as I chatted about riding a
ten-speed through California and hiking the Pacific Crest Trail. And
that evening was the beginning of my diet phase, which included fat-
burning vinegar—a dieter's best friend.

While apple cider vinegar may hold forefront in U.S. history, wine vinegar, its ignored counterpart, was commonly used as well in the past centuries. Wine vinegar, naturally, is made from wine—red, white, or rosé—and is medicinal from head to your ten toes as well.

In 5000 B.C., the Babylonians used grapes to make vinegar. Hippocrates used wine vinegar as an antibiotic to treat his patients in 400 B.C. The Four Thieves used vinegar during the plague in Marseilles. Throughout time, wine vinegar, like apple cider vinegar, was a cure-all folk remedy.

Generations of families, rich and poor, have used wine vinegar to help remedy a wide range of ailments—both inside and outside the body. Red wine vinegar, a sacred and mysterious cure-all for thousands of years, has been a medicine, a preservative, and a primary cooking ingredient to the folks of the Mediterranean.

At the opposite corner of Castile (due south of the Basque country) in Rioja is the region of Spain's best red wine vineyards. This is one of the original places where red wine vinegar is made. Yet while folk medicine has been busy touting apple cider vinegar throughout American history, it has ignored the vast virtues of its forerunner—red wine vinegar, an ancient medicinal miracle, too.

A NEW LOOK AT AN OLD VINEGAR

Red wine vinegar was used centuries ago for its antiseptic and anti-bacterial healing qualities. In the past, I eagerly spoke to vinegar aficionado Lawrence Diggs, author of *Vinegar*, who chatted up some new ideas on old wine vinegars.

Which doctors, besides Hippocrates, turned to red wine vinegar for its healing power? "Who knows," he says. "If you have a fine red wine vinegar, you're probably not going to be using it to clean out your stomach." However, he adds, doctors might resort to wine vinegar for treatment if that's all they had on hand. "But they would probably use vinegar from a cheaper thing. Because all you need is an acetic acid. That's what's working in terms of antiseptic."

According to Diggs, Hippocrates did not use apple cider vinegar. "It was wine vinegar." The odds are good that the good doctor used wine vinegar as an antibiotic to treat his patients, he says. "One would guess it was wine vinegar because the Greeks and Romans were into wine."

For example, it has been reported that vinegar was part of the reason that the Roman army succeeded. It is believed that Spartianus, a Latin historian, documented that vinegar mixed with water was the drink that helped the soldiers survive battle as well as the various climates they endured in Europe, Asia, and Africa. Undiluted vinegar was easier to transport than wine, and also more sobering.

Red wine vinegar also should be given credit for the Middle Ages. Remember the four robbers who were able to rob from the dead and dying without getting sick by dousing themselves with Four Thieves Vinegar? Well, apple cider vinegar may not have been the key life-saving ingredient, after all.

"I think it was wine vinegar because that was the common vinegar in that time and place—in most of Europe. The place people talk about The Plague is France and Italy, and those places have a lot of wine," says Diggs. "We know that the vinegar that was most common at that time was wine vinegar. Now whether it was *red wine vinegar*, we don't know."

Vinegar for Self-Preservation

In 1803 Ivan Gyodorovich Kruzenshlern, a Russian navigator and explorer, set out on an exploration of the globe. To prevent scurvy, he had a large amount of vitamin C–rich cabbage pickled in barrels and brought them onboard his ship before he left for sea.

In 1806 he and most of his crewmen were in good health. The secret? Vegetable oil and cabbage soaked in vinegar. There was no record of what kind of vinegar he used to make pickled cabbage. It was believed, however, that he used natural wine vinegar since there was no synthetic vinegar made of petroleum alcohol at that time.[2]

RED WINE VINEGAR: THEN AND NOW

I remember as a young girl growing up in the fifties that red wine vinegar and oil were mainstays on our kitchen table. My mom was a wonderful cook who made meals from scratch. She saw to it that our family ate a salad with oil and red wine vinegar every day. And there's more.

When I was nine years old, my mother went to Europe for three weeks. She went to France, Italy, and Rome. When she returned, the gourmet cook inside her came out of the closet. Our family was served a vast variety of dishes from the Mediterranean world. From snails to fettuccini, wine vinegars became a permanent fixture on our table.

And today, the foods that sustain the Mediterranean table—bread, olive oil, red wine—and of course, red wine vinegar—have become mainstays of American restaurant tables and are even making it into the homes of American families—not just mine.

I can personally attest to this. Not only have I noticed small Italian restaurants boasting all-white or red-and-white-checkered tablecloths, but on each table, big or small, sure enough, there's a glass container of olive oil and red wine vinegar. And now, at home on a glass kitchen table I have the same. It adds a worldly European flair, and naturally, it's for health's sake.

While we know that apple cider vinegar is a beloved vinegar for eating, red wine vinegar is a popular specialty vinegar, vinegar company workers tell me. And doctors in America are using red wine vinegar, too, for extra flavor—*and* for health's sake.

Allan Magaziner, M.D., for one, is aware of the possibility that red wine vinegar may contain resveratrol—like wine. And since he doesn't drink, he gets the potential health perks of red wine vinegar without the ill effects of alcohol. He believes that red wine vinegar, like apple cider vinegar, contains healthful ingredients—and perhaps even more that scientists will discover in the future.

Peasant Salad with Red Wine Vinegar

❖ ❖ ❖

If you're looking for a down-to-earth, year-round fresh salad, this recipe comes to the rescue. Its main stars include greens, tomatoes, cheese, seeds, olive oil and vinegar. This concoction has been tagged "country salad" and "peasant salad." As a hardworking mountain woman with a city heart, I would say this recipe has my name on it. After all, I am a vegetarian with aspirations of becoming a vegan. Some folks believe salads are mere side dishes or rabbit food. I disagree. A salad with superfoods can be a satisfying and delicious meal in itself.

1 cup tomatoes, diced
2 cups baby spinach, chopped
1 cup cheddar cheese or Monterey
   Jack cheese
½ cup Fuji apples, chopped, or
   dried cranberries
½ cup sunflower seeds or pecans,
   chopped

1 tablespoon Heinz Red Wine
   Vinegar
3 tablespoons olive oil
¼ teaspoon sea salt
½ teaspoon freshly ground black
   pepper

In a bowl, combine tomatoes, spinach, cheese, apples or cranberries, and seeds or nuts. Drizzle vinegar and oil over the salad mixture. Sprinkle with salt and pepper. Serves 3–4.

VINEGARY HEALING HINTS TO PRESERVE

✔ Wine vinegar was used as an antibiotic as early as 5000 B.C.
✔ Wine vinegar was used in the Middle Ages in Europe to fight the plague.
✔ Red wine vinegar was derived from Spain's best red wine vineyards.
✔ Wine vinegar preserved food and lives back in the early 19th century.
✔ Today doctors use red wine vinegar regularly for its healthful antioxidant compounds.

These days, doctors, nutritionists, and chefs know all too well that red wine vinegar not only contains healthful compounds, but its varied uses—not just for vinaigrette—make it well worth having it in your pantry, just like its counterpart, apple cider vinegar.

The Old and New Healthful Ingredients

*You drink vinegar when you have wine at
your elbow.*

—Thomas Fuller[1]

Once I hit age seventeen, I started my trek on the road and it led me into Vinegar World—a place I tagged that means going out of a comfort zone and discovering vinegar diversity. There was more to my life than apple cider, red, and white vinegar. I rode my ten-speed bicycle from San Jose to Los Gatos, a progressive region south of San Francisco. One afternoon I stopped at a health food store on the main street. Mesmerized by all the superfoods, I was like a kid at a new, improved candy shop. My days of eating twentieth-century American fare, including TV dinners and fast food, were done.

In the morning, I embraced the Grapefruit Diet. Hollywood dieters swore by the slimming power of this pounds-off plan. My diet for the next day's menu include half a grapefruit and black coffee for breakfast; half a grapefruit, one hard-boiled egg, one cucumber (sliced and drizzled with red wine vinegar), and black Lipton tea for lunch; and one whole grapefruit, two hard-boiled eggs, half a head of lettuce (drizzled with red wine vinegar), one tomato, and tea for dinner.

My dad understood what I was doing. He would fast during the week and indulge in my mom's meat and potatoes, plus cakes and pies on the weekends. But my mother, who received pleasure from cooking, baking, and plating meals for our family, was confused by my need for the food imbalance. I could have had my cake and eat it, too, according to her. I didn't listen and delved into a new relationship with food—including red wine vinegar, which turned out to be a superfood.

The finest red wine vinegars are believed to be made by the slow, or Orleans, process. Some vinegar companies make chemical- and additive-free red wine vinegars. They come from wines that are grown with all-natural fertilizers and without chemical pesticides, and contain no sulfites, a common food additive.

The best part is that these red wine vinegars may retain healthful nutrients. While the best red wine vinegars contain no unhealthy ingredients, they have many recognized ingredients and even "hidden" ones you should know about.

RED WINE VINEGAR NUTRITION FACTS

If you take a look at a nutritional label of natural, organic red wine vinegar, you will be pleasantly surprised. It will tell you that it comes from fine Italian red wines to provide a full-bodied vinegar with exceptional flavor. It reads that it's slowly aged without added sulfites. Also, it does not contain added sugar or artificial colorings. Plus, it is organically grown and processed in accordance with the California Organic Foods Act of 1990.

Per serving size—1 tablespoon—a common brand of red wine vinegar label will tell you that it contains no calories, no fat, 0 milligrams of sodium, no carbohydrates, and no protein. It is not a significant source of cholesterol, dietary fiber, vitamin A, vitamin C, calcium, or iron.

Keep in mind, however, if you analyze 3½ ounces, almost one-half cup of red wine vinegar, there will be other ingredients, based on a product data sheet by a national vinegar company:[2]

- Water: 89 grams
- Calcium: 8 grams
- Phosphorus: 10 milligrams
- Sodium: 6 milligrams
- Potassium: 80 milligrams

A NEW CLASS OF NUTRIENTS

So are you now wondering where's the good grape–red wine stuff in red wine vinegar? No one knows for sure. "It's possible that there could be some antioxidants in red wine vinegar," says UC Davis wine chemist Andrew Waterhouse, Ph.D.

"What we're looking at is a new class of antioxidants which don't have, according to governmental nutritionists, any nutritional value. And what we're trying to do, is establish whether or not they have some nutritional or health benefit," says Dr. Waterhouse.

"There's also some dispute among the people studying this whether these things could ever be called nutrients because of the definition of nutrient," adds Dr. Waterhouse. And up to now, no one has ever included these nutrients in Western medicine.

In addition, some of these new disease-fighting nutrients on the block may or may not go astray during the vinegar-making process. Because vinegar is made with a lot of oxygen and air exposure, a lot of the antioxidants found in wine are broken down, explains Dr. Waterhouse. "But I don't know how much."

He does theorize, however, that red wine vinegar, like red wine, does contain some good stuff. "The phenols that are in the grapes are probably the best for you." And past research shows exactly that.

The Grape Stuff

Wine vinegar has grapes as its raw material. Keep in mind that red wine vinegar comes from red grapes. And grapes, whether fresh, juiced, or fermented, are an excellent source of flavonoids—phenolic compounds that act as powerful antioxidants.

Flavonoids: powerful disease fighters, may help to fight viruses, allergies, carcinogens, and inflammation. In addition, these super antioxidants may also help to reduce your cholesterol level and prevent the oxidation of LDL cholesterol.

Proanthocyanidin: a flavonoid abundant in grapes.

Quercetin: a flavonoid that appears in red wine grapes, for instance, may be one of the most powerful anticancer agents ever found. It may reverse tumor growth by blocking the conversion of normal body cells to cancer cells; improves pancreas function, and levels the release of insulin; it may help prevent some problems linked with diabetes (cataracts, blindness, nerve damage, and kidney damage).

Resveratrol: another natural compound in grapes that may play a role in producing healthy cholesterol levels, reduces unhealthy fats in the blood, and prevents blood clotting in arteries narrowed by years of eating a high-fat diet.

In two European studies on the phenolic composition of high-quality wine vinegars (including "El Condado" wine vinegars and sherry vinegar) produced in the south of Spain, researchers found a variety of phenolic compounds—and a few compounds not identified in other traditional wine vinegars. However, much more research must be done.[3]

Meanwhile, "People are trying to associate red wine vinegar with red wine. They figure that the stuff is in the red wine so the logical extension is that it must be in red wine vinegar. And they're right," says Lawrence Diggs.

"The question is," he adds, "does it change when it reacts with acetic acid. Does it have the same benefits? If you put acetic acid on a sore, it will kill a lot of bacteria. However, if you drink it, the body neutralizes the acetic acid as it's on its way down. So is it as good as red wine? Who knows? We don't have the studies."

Fact: Red Wine Polyphenols Are Good for You

We know red wine is chock-full of polyphenols—those powerful antioxidants that guard against heart disease. How? Polyphenols block the oxidation of LDL or the "bad" cholesterol. Studies show that red wine polyphenols can slow down blood clotting. That means it can help lower the odds of blood clots forming which are the culprits of heart attack and stroke.

Research at the University of California at Davis also shows that red wine polyphenols slowed the formation of tumors in mice bred to develop the types of cancers that strike humans.

> Also, scientists at U.C. Berkeley have shown that red wine is rich in the new class of polyphenols, powerful antioxidants that help neutralize free radicals which damage DNA, alter body chemistry, and destroy cells.

RESVERATROL

Resveratrol (pronounced *res-VER-a-trawl*), is found in both red grapes and red wine. It's another flavonoid that covers the skins of grapes and fights disease. It's also a natural fungicide that helps protect grapes from bacteria.

Grapes are one of the richest sources. "Grapes and anything made from grapes that include the grape skin or some effective extraction of the grape skin contains resveratrol. The usual example is that the resveratrol is low in white wine, not because all white grapes are low, but because the skins are discarded when white wine is made. The amount in grapes, juice and wine is different in years, locations and varieties," explains Dr. Leroy Creasy, Ph.D., emeritus professor of fruit and vegetable science at Cornell University College of Agriculture in New York.

New research indicates that resveratrol may be the ingredient in red wine which helps lower cholesterol. Resveratrol also seems to prevent blood platelet aggregation, and reduced blood clotting in arteries narrowed by years of eating a high-fat diet.

Resveratrol may also be a powerful cancer inhibitor. It may cause precancerous cells to return to normal, according to a 1997 University of Illinois study. John Pezzuto at the University of Illinois at Chicago screened about 1,000 plants for anticancer activity. He discovered one active ingredient—resveratrol. In lab tests, resveratrol zapped both cancer-inducing free radicals and inflammation.[4]

When I first spoke with Dr. Creasy, he believed that there was a good chance that red wine vinegar would indeed contain resveratrol. "Red wine vinegar made strictly from wine would probably have as much as the wine. Unless it's broken down by the bacteria and we don't know that yet." And so I waited . . .

THE TEST RESULTS

"I analyzed a cheap red wine vinegar," reports Dr. Creasy. "There was no resveratrol. The red wine vinegar profile looked like diluted red wine. Apparently diluted 10 times. It is quite likely that red wine vinegar from different producers will be distinct in phenolic composition."

The good news is, Dr. Creasy said that analyzing one red wine vinegar sample doesn't mean that much. "Because if you had pure red wine vinegar it could be there. That's based on my experience with the wine people. There isn't anything that could be absolutely certified as being 100 percent vinegar."

He added, "It is still possible that the Acetobacter organism can break down resveratrol. Resveratrol does inhibit some bacteria and possibly some have developed the biochemistry to destroy it. So it may have been there at the start but might be gone. No one knows." Currently, whether or not red wine vinegar contains resveratrol remains a very controversial topic and has not yet been scientifically proven.

OTHER ANTIOXIDANTS AND RED WINE VINEGAR

Dr. Waterhouse does not know for certain if red wine vinegar does contain resveratrol. But he does know that there are a lot of polyphenols in red wine vinegar, as in red wine. "Some of the polyphenols have a good research history, other ones are called antioxidants—but they don't have any medical effect whatsoever. Antioxidants are important for health, but which specific ones are still under investigation," he says.

U.C. Davis research involves the wine compounds—tannins, quercetin, and resveratrol—found in red wines. Their studies showed that tannin-rich wine was able to reduce platelet aggregation and increase HDL cholesterol levels, suggesting that tannins may help protect against heart disease.

Can red wine vinegar do what red wine does—and more? "Certainly. In test-tube studies," answers Dr. Creasy. "Quercetin, tannins in red wine occur in all plants, including grapes, wine and probably vinegar."

In fact, for people like Dr. Creasy who don't drink alcohol, he believes including red wine vinegar in the diet would be good. "It adds up," he says. "You're supposed to eat five fruits or vegetables a day and I heard that 95 percent of Americans don't get that per day. Most people can't eat a lot of vinegar, but if you put it on veggies and your five a day you're on the healthy track."

Red wine vinegar is also the vinegar of choice for Connie Diekman, R.D. "I do use that as a seasoning on chicken, fish, salads, and marinades." Does she use it for health reasons? "I do it more as a flavoring. Because that is what we *know* it can do. And that gives pleasure to eating," she says. "But it does come from the grape and I am picking up some of the potential antioxidants."

Mediterranean Vegetable Soup

❖ ❖ ❖

Soup's on! A cool day or night is a perfect time for hearty vegetable soup. Think plenty of fresh, seasonal vegetables and wholesome stock for a chunky semi-homemade dish. Garlic and onions, carrots and celery—fresh tomatoes—with whole grain rotini make a pot of soup on the stove top a crowd-pleaser as a comfort food in your bowl for lunch or dinner.

This recipe is inspired by my mother's homemade vegetable soup. My version is like her batch, but it's meatless and filled with fresh ingredients (not canned or frozen staples popular in the twentieth century)—except for the vegetable broth. Fast-forward to the twenty-first century. When I came home from a trip to Canada, I was visited by a cold-flu bug. It was rest, juice, herbal tea, and vegetable soup that helped soothe the aches and cure the sniffling. I turned to premium canned soup varieties, but vowed to make my own soup from scratch when I was back with the living. I hit the kitchen one afternoon. Using an all-natural, organic, store-bought broth was amazing, especially with flavorful vinegar. Not only was it easy, the aroma in my cabin was sublime.

½ tablespoon extra virgin olive oil
   or European-style butter
¼ cup yellow onion

2 cloves garlic, finely chopped
1 carton (32 ounces) organic
   vegetable broth

2 cups mixed fresh vegetables,
  chopped (broccoli, cabbage,
  carrots, celery, green bell
  pepper, jicama, radish)
1½ tablespoons Heinz Red Wine
  Vinegar
1 teaspoon Nakano Natural Rice
  Vinegar
1½ cups uncooked whole grain
  rotini

5 Roma tomatoes, peeled, chopped
½ cup fresh spinach, chopped
sea salt and freshly ground black
  pepper, to taste
½ cup finely shredded Parmesan
  cheese
garnish

In a skillet, heat olive oil or butter over medium heat; add onion and garlic. Sauté for a few minutes. Pour into a large pot. Add broth and bring to a boil. Add vegetables and vinegar. Bring to a bowl again, then reduce heat to low. In another pot, boil pasta for seven minutes until cooked. Add pasta and tomatoes to vegetable mixture. Stir in spinach. Sprinkle with salt and pepper. Simmer for about 10 minutes. Serve hot with sprinkled Parmesan cheese. A bowl of this soup pairs well with slices of a fresh, warm baguette. Serves six.

I love this soup. A splash of vinegar gives it a nice tangy flavor. Not only is it easy to put together, it's easy on the eyes and palate. It's also time to blast soup myths: You can use fresh tomatoes; forget canned goods. Some folks say broccoli and spinach in your soup can create a bitter taste. I disagree. Follow the broth box directions and do not dilute. Add any of your favorite fresh herbs for extra flavor. It's not your mom's soup—it's fresh and whipped up quickly to maintain the good-for-you antioxidant-rich ingredients.

VINEGARY HEALING HINTS TO PRESERVE

✓ The best red wine vinegars are made by the slow Orleans process.
✓ Red wine vinegar is no-cal, fat-free, and low in sodium.
✓ Red wine vinegar may contain disease-fighting antioxidants and maybe resveratrol.
✓ By teaming red wine vinegar with vegetables, you will get more antioxidants in your total diet.

RED WINE VINEGAR'S POTENTIAL
DISEASE-FIGHTING INGREDIENTS

Ingredient	What It Does	May Help Prevent
Catechin	Blocks LDL (bad) cholesterol from entering the artery walls, inhibits blood clots, relaxes blood vessels, inhibits tumors.	High cholesterol, stroke, cancer
Polyphenols	Slow down blood clotting by its antioxidant action; inhibit formation of cancer-causing carcinogens.	Heart attack, stroke
Proanthocyanidins (PCOs)	Block the formation of cholesterol deposits on artery walls.	Heart disease
Quercetin	Reverses tumor growth by blocking the conversion of normal body cells and cancer cells; improves pancreas function, and levels the release of insulin; free radical scavenger.	Cancer; diabetes complications (e.g. cataracts and kidney damage)
Resveratrol	Prevents blood platelet aggregation and reduces blood clotting in arteries; lowers cholesterol.	Heart attack; stroke
Tannins	Reduce platelet aggregation and increase HDL cholesterol levels.	Heart disease

In the next chapter I'll show you exactly how red wine vinegar complements the intriguing French paradox and its good-for-you fat. Like red wine, it also has other benefits that you should know about and be ready to incorporate it into your diet.

Tapping Into the French Paradox

*The French are not sloppy about their eating
habits. They have discipline in their diet, and
include plenty of fresh fruits and vegetables.*
—Elisabeth Helsing, Ph.D.,
World Health Organization in Europe[1]

At nineteen, I conformed and attended college in San Jose. It was a
time I bonded with my father. As an insurance salesman, he traveled
to clients in San Francisco. One weekday I was invited to come along.
As a gift, he offered to let me clothes shop at the factory outlets, followed by lunch after. We met at a restaurant on San Francisco's famous Fisherman's Wharf. Views of the Golden Gate Bridge, Russian
Hill, and the fishing fleet and harbor were impressive—foreshadowing
for me later attending San Francisco State University. I ordered a Bay
Shrimp Louie with a house lemon-and-red-wine vinaigrette *and* slices
of warm, fresh French bread and pats of real butter.

At the time, I felt guilty indulging in the dressing and bread paired
with real butter. But I told myself, "It's a special occasion." Later when
I discovered the French paradox, it made sense. If you indulge in a little bit of high-fat fare—like the French do—it can help fill you up and
not out. And you beat unhealthy Cookie Monster cravings (the vinegar seemed to stave off the need to overindulge) that can lead to
health woes later in life.

Did you know that heart attacks, strokes, and cancer are the three deadly diseases that account for the majority of diseases in the United States? That is why it is important for you to understand the term "French paradox"—especially when it may be one of the red wine vinegar wonders.

Medical researchers thought that reducing the fat intake and boosting the carbohydrate intake in your diet would lower your risk of heart attack and strokes. Yet the number of fat-loving diseases soars. Scientists concluded that people just consumed too much of the typical American high-fat fare. However, in France, even though the typical French citizen eats a diet richer in fat—much of it artery-clogging saturated animal fat—there is a significantly lower rate of heart disease in that country than in America where it is the Number 1 killer. This apparent inconsistency was called "The French Paradox" back in 1991 by Serge Renaude, M.D., Director of the French National Institute of Health and Medical Research.[2]

It's no secret that the French enjoy their rich sauces and fat-laden cheese. Renaude believed that part of this so-called French paradox was linked to their consumption of red wine.

Keep in mind, however, the French diet also includes a lot of antioxidant-rich garlic, fruits, and vegetables. Mealtime in France is a time for relaxing—and the French do not overeat the way men, women, and children do in America. Food portions are smaller, and the French don't eat as many Big Macs and fried chicken as Americans do.

There's More to the French Diet

According to medical experts, the French paradox is more likely due to a variety of reasons. The French eat plenty of fresh fruits and vegetables (see Chapter 14, "Combining Vinegars and Garlic, Onions, and Olive Oil"); eat in a relaxed, family-style environment; and exercise.

Researchers have now discovered that the red wine savored by the French people contains healthful chemicals such as tannins, quercetin, oligo, proanthocyanidin, catechins, and epicatechins. However, it's resveratrol that may be able to prevent the inflammation of the blood vessels and blood platelets from clumping.

But the question remains, does red wine vinegar have the same potential health effects as red wine? "Because it is derived from red wine it probably is still going to have some of the benefits as red wine, perhaps not as strong," says Dr. Allan Magaziner, one of the leading authorities in nutritional and preventative medicine. "I know red wine is studied more at this time. In the years to come, perhaps we'll find much more beneficial effects of red wine vinegar."

RED WINE VERSUS RED WINE VINEGAR

Okay, so red wine has some good health benefits. Let's look at the benefits of drinking red wine: According to the late Robert Crayhon, M.S., certified nutritionist, copper-containing substances are sprayed on French vineyards. Copper is a heart-healthy nutrient which helps keep cholesterol levels in normal ranges. Red wine contains powerful antioxidants. It can help relax you. It is often drunk in a social environment of friends and family, which is healthful.[3]

Wine Labels Tout Health Benefits, Sort Of

These days, the government is allowing winemakers to advertise that wine may be good for you. But the wording is very evasive. The label reads, "The proud people who made this wine encourage you to consult your family doctor about the health effects of wine consumption." This is a hint that, for some folks, wine may be healthful.

But alcohol is not perfect. I remember what it was like when I was a teenager with parents who were alcoholics . . .

This was a far cry from the harmonious home of my early childhood. I saw firsthand how alcoholism could change people. My father, once so kind and caring, now only critized me. Meanwhile, my mom, who had always wanted only the best for us, was now often too drunk to take care of herself, much less our family. Violent arguments usually took place at the dinner table. My mother would end up crying and retreat to bed with a book in one hand, a drink in the other, while my angry father left the house for hours.

That was decades ago, and today I still find myself with painful memories of that time.

I am hardly alone. There are millions of adult children of alcoholics.

Sons of Alcoholics

It is no surprise that adult male children of alcoholics are more likely to become alcoholics than men raised in nonalcoholic families. Worse yet, alcoholism is not the only problem with which adult sons may contend.

According to experts, sons of alcoholics may fall victim to lack of self-esteem, relationship problems, and fears of inadequacy.

Building up self-confidence is a must for adult sons who want to find the road to recovery. Here are five tips for adult children of alcoholics: Break the silence; form healthy male relationships; find a mentor; seek spiritual guidance; and stop drinking if you have a problem.

According to the National Institute on Alcohol Abuse and Alcoholism, millions of people abuse alcohol or are alcoholic. Of that number, more men than women are alcohol-dependent or have alcohol-related problems.

While red wine can be good for your health, it can also be harmful. Alcohol depletes nutrients zinc and magnesium in the body; it can up the number of free radicals in the body; it can cause liver damage; alcohol drunk by pregnant women can lead to low-birth babies with lower IQs; social drinking can progress into alcoholism; alcohol damages the brain; it impairs the function of the digestive tract; and it may up your risk of breast cancer.[4]

What's more, wine can pack on the fat, which is not heart-healthy. One 4-ounce glass packs 100 calories. That can add up. Also, if you're migraine-prone, it's best to stay clear of red wine, which is one culprit. And the American Cancer Society reports that alcohol can cause serious liver damage.

Sadly enough, I know this can be true. At 74, my father became ill. I can tell you from my heart that it was the most painful ordeal he and I have ever experienced. My dad was in great physical pain for weeks. He died on February 28, 1998. On his certificate of death it reads: *Immediate cause: liver failure; Due to: liver abscess; Due to: liver cancer.* And to this day, since alcoholism runs in my family, I have never drunk alcohol—not a sip.

THE ALTERNATIVES TO RED WINE FOR HEALTH

If you are drinking red wine for health benefits, think twice. "There are less toxic ways to get the benefits of the antioxidants, polyphenols, and other substances found in red wine," says Crayhon. "Fruits, veg-

---

Grape Juice Works Like Wine

One study at the University of Wisconsin Medical school, led by John D. Folts, reveals that three glasses of purple grape juice equal the blood-clotting stopping power of a glass of wine. He believes that it's the flavonoids, not the alcohol, that help ward off heart attacks among people who drink red wine.

---

etables, garlic, spices, herbs, and supplements can give you just as much antioxidant benefit if not more." And so can red wine vinegar.[5]

And now red wine vinegar, like grape juice, is being considered as a tradeoff for red wine. "Actually, red wine vinegar is just red wine that has soured," says Dr. Mindell. And does he believe it has any resveratrol in it? "Yes! It's a healthy thing to use."

Healthy indeed. As a nondrinker, I'm hardly alone. In fact, Dr. Magaziner admits that he is not a big drinker. He said to me, "I'm like you—I just don't enjoy alcohol. But I do eat a lot of red grapes." And I consume red grapes, grape juice, and red wine vinegar for the nonalcoholic protection.

UC Davis Enologist Turns Wine to Vinegar

Imagine this: You're the department winemaker and cellar master at the University of California–Davis department of viticulture and enology. The wine they produce is for research—not to drink or sell. So, when a study is done, rather than toss the good stuff out, it's put in a vinegar barrel. Ernie Farinias does just that.

Farinias, like other small-time vinegar makers (retired Chef Sal Campagna creates his vinegar, too), insists that it's easy to do—and he's been making homemade red wine vinegar for more than a quarter of a century.

If you have leftover red or dry white wine, get a vinegar

barrel (a 1-gallon glass jar will do) and wash it well. Then, round up mother of vinegar (available in some wine specialty shops) and distilled water. Mix the mother with the wine in your clean container. Add one part water to three parts wine. It will dilute the wine and "cut the alcohol"— according to Farinias. Cover the container with cheesecloth and secure with a rubber band. Let it sit at room temperature for about two to three weeks. Then, siphon the vinegar out of its container and pour into a clean bottle with a metallic lid.

Want more vinegar? Put this new batch in a clean 5-gallon oak barrel. Each time you have leftover wine, dilute it just like you did before. But use caution, nutritionists say homemade vinegar is unpredictable and should never be used for canning or preserving—for safety's sake.[6]

Spaghetti with Red Wine Vinegar Sauce

✦ ✦ ✦

Spaghetti is classic Italian cuisine often served with a chunky tomato sauce, including herbs, olive oil, vegetables—and red wine vinegar. I can get this sauce at a restaurant, or go to the grocery store and grab a box in the frozen foods aisle. Also, I have used a store-bought marinara sauce. But going back to basics and doing it yourself for the flavor of it all is worth the effort and will take your taste buds on a European getaway. . . .

Instead of letting it simmer for hours as my mother did back in the twentieth century, it was my goal to make this recipe fast to maintain the integrity of nutrients in the tomatoes and other ingredients. Vivid images of the character in *Eat, Pray, Love* come to mind. When the traveler was in Italy and ordered a simple plate of spaghetti, it was an unforgettable feast for one.

2 tablespoons extra virgin olive oil
¼ cup yellow onion, chopped
1 clove garlic, minced

sea salt, ground pepper, nutmeg to taste

5 Roma tomatoes, peeled, chopped
1 zucchini, chopped
1 package uncooked whole grain
  spaghetti
1 tablespoon oregano vinegar

1 tablespoon Heinz Red Wine
  Vinegar
¼ cup fresh basil, chopped
grated cheese, for topping

In a skillet, drizzle olive oil to sauté onion and garlic. Add spices and tomatoes. Cook for about 10 minutes. Add zucchini. While the sauce is simmering, boil water in a large pot and cook pasta for several minutes. Drain pasta. Drizzle vinegars on cooked pasta. Dish up and top with sauce and cheese. Garnish with basil. Serves 4. Pair with a rustic baguette and olive oil or butter.

VINEGARY HEALING HINTS TO PRESERVE

✓ Red wine vinegar contains polyphenols—and maybe resveratrol.
✓ Red wine vinegar is fat-free.
✓ You can add red wine vinegar to fruits and vegetables and get additional antioxidants.
✓ Red wine vinegar does not cause liver damage.

I chewed the fat about fatty foods and red wine and its potential health perks with doctors around the nation. They were not surprised by its workhorse powers and were eager to discuss the merits of the alternative—vinegar that comes from grapes—not apples. Red wine vinegar teamed with good high-fat cuisine paired with red wine (in moderation) can be good for you, but can it battle diseases and boost your lifespan? Turn the pages to discover what it can do.

Is Red Wine Vinegar Good for You?

*The bitterer the salad of endives, the stronger must
be the vinegar.*

—Palestinian Proverb[1]

Restless as a young college student in the suburbs I craved more of a life experiences type of education. I majored in physical education, but feeling trapped, I dropped out to face challenges in different places like trying different vinegars from different places. So, I turned to hitching and hiking with a dog across the country. On the road, eating healthy was a challenge. I had a fully stocked backpack stuffed with granola, peanut butter, and nuts. But when my stash was depleted I was at the mercy of people who offered me rides and eats. At truck stops, roadside cafés, and homes, main-dish salads with vinegar were a staple for me.

On the West Coast red wine and olive oil were readily available. But in the Deep South and Midwest, it was a different story. I admit, even though it was an era of bean sprouts and yogurt, some big-city folks were not on the health bandwagon. One young musician in New York, for instance, offered me his apartment for the night. He left to stay with his fiancée. I was tired and famished.

When I opened the fridge it was bare except for the box of fried chicken that greeted me. No fish. No fresh salad with a red wine and olive oil dressing like I ate with my dad back in the days of San Francisco by the Pacific Ocean. "Should I eat it?" or "Should I not eat it?" went through my mind. Instead of dying of starvation I caved and devoured a leftover chicken thigh and wing without the flavor that vinegar—any kind—can provide. On the couch with a scratchy blanket, instead of counting sheep while worrying about where my next meal was going to come from while traveling to Quebec, Canada, I envisioned salads with fruit, vegetables, nuts, and a vinegar dressing like I could get in the Golden State. Homesick for whole, clean, real foods I fell asleep.

Not only are red wine vinegar's specific nutrients good for preventing health ailments but it can help treat disease, too. Many health practitioners emphasize its antioxidant vitamins, which can help you stave off age-related diseases and keep you living a longer, healthier life, too.

But there is *sooo* much more to know about the hidden ingredients in red wine. Here are expert reports and anecdotes about red wine vinegar (and a few of my own experiences) to show you how this condiment, like apple cider vinegar, is a gold mine.

RED WINE VINEGAR AND HEART DISEASE

The frightening fact is, heart disease, not cancer, is the number one killer of both men—and women—in the United States.

Some risk factors for heart disease include high blood pressure, high cholesterol and a high-fat diet, and obesity. But don't despair. Red wine vinegar comes to the rescue.

For one, flavonoid-rich like wine, vinegar may help lower your total cholesterol level and prevent the oxidation of LDL cholesterol, the "bad" cholesterol, says Allan Magaziner, D.O. Translation: less risk of heart attacks and strokes.

Danish researchers found that weekly consumption of wine may cut stroke. In a 16-year study of 13,329 people, those who said they drank wine on a weekly basis—about one to six glasses per week—had a 34 percent lower risk of stroke than those who never or hardly ever drank wine. Those who said they had wine daily had a 32 percent reduction in risk. Those who drank beer or spirits did not have a significant reduction in stroke risk.[2]

One reason for wine's protective effects, the researchers say, may be its flavonoids and tannins—nutrients that may help inhibit the plaque obstructions that cause heart attacks and strokes.[3]

But note, the American Heart Association does not recommend that you start drinking to reduce your risk of heart disease and stroke. Research shows there is a higher risk of heart disease linked with drinking too much alcohol.[4] (My mother was taking blood pressure medication in between drinking bourbon and water.) Also, if red wine vinegar does, in fact, contain resveratrol like red wine—and doctors and researchers believe that it may—it can fight heart disease, too. How exactly does red wine work?

Rescarch at the University of Illinois shows intriguing data about resveratrol. "First, it inhibits the formation of blood clots, which can trigger both heart attack and stroke. Second, it plays a role in cholesterol metabolism, which may prevent the formation of artery-clogging plaque," reports Dr. Earl Mindell.[5]

Keep in mind, red wine vinegar is used in heart-healthy dishes such as salads, pasta plates, vegetables, and beans. In fact, beans are full of heart-healthy soluble fiber—the kind that helps control blood fat levels. James Anderson, M.D., a researcher based in Lexington, Kentucky, has found that eating just one cup of cooked dried beans a day can reduce artery-clogging LDL, the "bad" cholesterol, by 20 percent.

And our recipes at the end of this book include nutritious beans teamed with health-boosting red wine vinegar. This, in turn, can give you good nutrition such as you'll find at the Pritikin Longevity Center in Santa Monica, California (now in Miami, Florida).

Pritikin's former director of nutrition services, Susan Massaron, says they do indeed include low-sodium vinegar (red wine, balsamic, and rice) in their meal plans. Why? "We use it as a seasoning," she says.

"Since our participants are on a low-sodium eating program, we try to keep our sodium very, very low. We find that the acidity from the vinegar gives an underlying sharpness to the food. It gives an edge to the food that substitutes very nicely for salt. It gives the illusion of salt without actually adding the sodium," adds Massaron. And note, Pritikin does not use seasoned vinegars because of the sodium content.

Why is it so important to have a low-sodium diet? "Primarily what we're keeping the sodium low for is to ward off hypertension or to correct hypertension or high blood pressure," says Massaron. Plus, for many people, she adds, by reducing their sodium intake, they will significantly reduce their blood pressure.

I remember when I was in college, my diet lacked nutrient-rich foods. In fact, while I had classes scheduled back to back, I didn't allow myself a chance to eat a proper diet. I was living on diet soda and salted sunflower seeds. Then, one day I took my blood pressure at one of those self-service tests at drugstores. It was 150/90! I was shocked. I immediately stopped my high-sodium diet. And in no time my blood pressure was back to a healthy 120/80.

RED WINE VINEGAR AND CANCER

Another benefit of red wine vinegar is its flavonoids, which can help guard against cancer. "Most of the studies performed on flavonoids have demonstrated their effectiveness in the prevention and treatment of various cancers. Some of the compounds that display anti-tumor effects are quercetin, hesperidin, genistein, rutin, naringin, catechin, and Pycnogenol," reports Dr. Magaziner. And red wine vinegar may contain many if not all of these disease-fighting compounds.[6]

Research suggests that resveratrol inhibits the development of cancer in animals as well as prevents the progression of cancer. However, the jury is still out on how effective resveratrol is as an anticancer compound since human research is still needed in this area.

Another big benefit of flavonoid-rich red wine vinegar: paired with vegetables and fruits high in antioxidant vitamins C, E, and beta-carotene, you can prevent a number of cancers. These vitamins trap the free-radical molecules that cause normal cells to become cancerous. According to the American Cancer Society, studies show that a diet high in vegetables can lower cancer risk.

In addition, munching on more veggies and fruits and eating less meat may help stave off breast cancer, according to a past study. Researchers examined a link between intake of meats, vegetables, and fruits with levels of oxidative DNA damage in 21 healthy women (who had a high risk because they had a close relative with breast cancer) while consuming their usual diet or a diet low in fat.

Follow the ACS's guidelines to eat five or more servings of fruits and vegetables a day—especially vegetables from the cabbage family, such as broccoli, cauliflower, and Brussels sprouts. Studies show that phytochemicals (found only in plant foods) known as indole-3-carbinols found in cruciferous vegetables help to lower estrogen-causing cancer.

Plus, beans are superhealthy for you too. Beans also contain many compounds, such as phytoestrogens, phytates, and isoflavones, that are believed to have cancer-fighting properties. In fact, studies have shown that a diet rich in beans can reduce the risk of breast, lung, and pancreatic cancer. Try bean recipes teamed with red wine vinegar to help you get back on the healthy, five-a-day track.

CANCER-FIGHTING VEGETABLES

A diet high in a variety of nutrient-rich vegetables teamed with red wine vinegar may help prevent certain cancers. Here is a look at popular vegetables and the protection they may offer:

Superfood	Cancer-Fighting Substances	Protection For
Artichokes	Vitamin C, an antioxidant that stimulates tumor-attacking cells	Stomach, esophagus, larynx
Asparagus	Vitamin C and carotene, shown to fight cancer tumors by boosting white blood cell activity; selenium, a nutrient that activates infection fighting cells	Stomach, larynx, esophagus, lungs
Bell peppers	Vitamin C	Stomach, larynx, esophagus
Broccoli	Quercetin, an antioxidant that stimulates tumor-fighting cells; indole-3-carbinol, a chemical that helps prevent "bad" estrogen that causes cancerous mutation in cells; and vitamin C	Lungs, colon, breasts

Corn	Protease inhibitors, which, according to research, may be potent cancer fighters	Breasts, colon
Green beans	Fiber, which may help decrease levels of cancer-promoting "bad" estrogen by escorting estrogen-contributing dietary fats out of the system	Breasts, colon
Salad greens	Beta-carotene, which may boost white blood cells; vitamin C	Stomach, larynx, esophagus
Tomato	Lycopene, an anticancer agent that helps destroy free radicals	Stomach, colon, mouth, throat

RED WINE VINEGAR AND BODY FAT

Dr. McBarron knows firsthand about fat-fighting red wine vinegar. She usually eats low-fat fare. Is red wine vinegar a typical condiment on her dinner table? Yes, she says. From salads to main dishes, she can count on red wine vinegar to help maintain her weight and keep her body fat in check.

"Any time we cook chicken or fish, we usually use red wine vinegar. I sauté the vegetables in it." She will also add a couple of tablespoons of red wine vinegar when a recipe calls for a liquid.

"I'm married to an Italian. He grew up having pasta seven days a week. We always have pasta on the table. I'll have it four to five times a week. My husband is extremely healthy. He was raised on a healthy diet. When I met him I always did the salad dressing on the side because I was trying to watch my weight. And he always had oil and vinegar. I thought, 'Oh, that sounds terrible.' I don't even have salad dressing in my house anymore—it's always oil and vinegar for the taste and nutrients in it."

Dr. McBarron's One-Day
Sample Vinegar Meal Plan

With the aid of Terri Brownlee, R.D., we designed a typical daily meal plan based on what works for Jan McBarron:

Breakfast

Fiber-Rich Fruit Salad: Mix ¼ cup each sliced strawberries, cantaloupe balls, grapes, and blueberries. Sprinkle with 1 tbsp organic mango vinegar.
1 cinnamon-raisin bagel
½ cup skim milk

Lunch

Slimming Stuffed Tomato: Stuff 1 medium tomato, hollowed, with ¼ cup each diced cucumber, green pepper, red onion, and cooked rice, and 1 tsp each olive oil and red wine vinegar. Broil 5–8 minutes.
½ wheat pita, toasted
1 cup honeydew or cantaloupe, cubed

Dinner

Tangy Chicken Bake: Bake 3 oz. skinless chicken breast topped with 1 tbsp each orange marmalade and raspberry or apple cider vinegar at 350° for 25 minutes.
½ cup wild rice
8 asparagus spears, steamed
½ cup mandarin oranges
Snacks: plenty of fresh fruit: blueberries, grapes, pears, and strawberries

LOSING YOUR BODY FAT

While some body fat (the yellow stuff that insulates our bodies) is "good," too much of it is "bad." Says the late Tony Perrone, Ph.D., who is well known throughout Hollywood for creating lean bodies, "Body fat makes you pudgy and hides the definition of your muscles. It tends to sag in areas that are unsightly."

Worse, too much fat can cause a host of health problems. Excess body fat puts you at higher risk for diabetes, high blood pressure, heart disease, and stroke.

Again, red wine vinegar is one solution to taking and keeping fat off. "Vinegar is an allowable free food," says Dr. Perrone, "because it doesn't contribute any significant caloric intake. It doesn't harm a person's efforts to lose body fat."

So go ahead—switch to noncaloric, fat-free red wine vinegar salad dressing. When you toss a salad of mixed greens, substitute 2 tablespoons fat-free red wine vinegar for the 2 tablespoons of regular dressing you normally use three times a week. Calories saved per week: 420. Fat grams saved: 60. Your weight loss in one year: 6¼ lbs.

Fat-Fighting Red Wine Vinegar		
Fat Dressing (1 Tbs)	Lean Dressing	Calories Saved
French dressing, low-cal	Red wine vinegar	15
French dressing, regular	Red wine vinegar	65
Mayonnaise	Red wine vinegar	100
1000-Island Dressing, regular	Red wine vinegar	80

I have witnessed people at a salad bar load up their plate with healthy, fresh vegetables and fruits. Then, they top it off with ladles of high-fat salad dressing (also high in preservatives, chemicals, and sodium). By doing this, you turn a good salad into a salad gone wrong.

LONGEVITY

So how does fat-fighting red wine vinegar help add years to your life anyhow? "Because of its antioxidant effects," answers Dr. Magaziner. "Any foods that have antioxidants in them are foods that we should incorporate into our diet because they help enhance our immune system. In turn, it helps us to feel healthier and hopefully reduce some of the diseases that we face as we get older."

When you eat a variety of foods that contain disease-fighting antioxidants, you can stall or prevent ailments associated with aging, adds antioxidant guru Jeffrey Blumberg, Ph.D., at Tufts University.

"You still get older," says Dr. Blumberg, "but you'll increase your lifespan." Medical doctors agree: the healthier you are, the younger your body stays. So go ahead—it's never too late to put these eight healthy, low-fat, antiaging foods teamed with age-fighting red wine vinegar on your menu! Just turn to our recipes in the back of this book.

Seven Antiaging Foods + RWV to Fight Father Time

1. **Carrots:** Beta-carotene-rich carrots keep your vision clear and sharp, according to studies at the USDA Human Nutrition Center on Aging in Boston.
2. **Red pepper:** Peppers, especially the red ones, are a great source of vitamin C and can enhance the body's immune function to help keep you healthy.
3. **Broccoli:** According to the American Cancer Society, studies show vegetables in the cabbage family (or crucifers) appear to protect against stomach and colon cancers. Eat more broccoli and cauliflower.
4. **Spinach:** Leafy green vegetables, which are rich in vitamin A and iron, can help keep your nails strong and healthy.
5. **Asparagus:** Low-cal asparagus is a good source of vitamin C, which works as an anti-inflammatory agent and can help fight arthritis aches and pains.
6. **Tofu:** According to the American Cancer Society, tofu can inhibit the type of estrogen that causes breast, uterine, and ovarian cancers.
7. **Fish:** Because it contains vital omega-3 fatty acids, fish can retard the aging process.

Not only is red wine vinegar plentiful with antiaging antioxidants, it's cholesterol free, sodium free, and fat free. And that without a doubt can help stave off age-related ailments such as heart disease and cancer, too.

Angelo, the health-wise man in Chapter 1, will tell you how vinegar can turn back the clock. He believes that the vinegar in his diet is one reason he has no major health problems. As a regular customer at the former Salvatore's Continental Restaurant in San Carlos, California, he always ordered red wine vinegar on the side to put on his pasta salad. "He told me vinegar is good for your health," says the retired chef, Sal Campagna, a vinegar connoisseur who made his own flavorful vinegar.

For Theresa Garrido, a woman with strong Basque roots, red wine vinegar is a handed-down folk remedy well worth holding on to. A busy young woman, she is a dental office manager in San Francisco, California, a wife, and a mom. When her fun-loving toddler, Eric, bumped his head on a door frame at her parents' house, vinegar came to the rescue. "My mom took a quarter and pushed it against the welt," she recalls. "Right after, we used red wine vinegar and salt. It takes away the inflammation and makes it heal faster, so they say." And it did.

Many health practitioners emphasize red wine vinegar's amazing anti-inflammatory components and antioxidants, which can help you deal with common ailments at any age, generation to generation; stave off age-related diseases; and keep you living a longer, healthier life, too.

Greek Salad

❖ ❖ ❖

This is my own recipe, inspired by my love for salads with California's veggies paired with a Greek flair. It can be dished up year-round, especially with our state's Mediterranean-like climate.

1 cup Roma tomatoes, halved	1 cup feta cheese, crumbled, with
¼ cups red onion, sliced in half	Mediterranean herbs
rounds (optional)	½ cup pitted ripe colossal olives
2 cups baby spinach	

1 tablespoon Heinz Red Wine
  Vinegar
3 tablespoons extra virgin olive oil
  to taste

¼ teaspoon sea salt
½ teaspoon freshly ground black
  pepper

In a bowl, combine tomatoes, onion, and spinach. Chill for an hour. Add cheese and olives. Drizzle vinegar and oil over the salad mixture. Season with salt and pepper. Serves 3–4.

VINEGARY HEALING HINTS TO PRESERVE

✓ Red wine vinegar contains flavonoids (and perhaps heart-healthy resveratrol), which can help prevent high blood pressure, stroke, and heart attack.

✓ Red wine vinegar is rich in cancer-fighting antioxidants that can help lower cancer risk.

✓ Teamed with antioxidant-rich vegetables, red wine vinegar can help fight cancer.

✓ Red wine vinegar, which is low-cal, sodium-free, and fat-free, can help you keep your body fat ratio lower.

✓ Red wine vinegar, which is free of cholesterol, sodium, and fat, can help add years to your life.

✓ Red wine vinegar can help you live longer whether you use its healing powers internally or externally.

✓ Plus, if you pair red wine vinegar with disease-fighting, antiaging foods, you can boost longevity.

Red wine and apple cider vinegars are good for you, but variety is the spice of a healthful diet. Enter rice vinegar—one that is popular in Asian countries—an up-and-coming flavorful favorite that can be paired with other vinegars for more flavor and provide some other health benefits, too.

PART 4

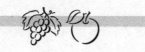

OTHER NATURAL VINEGARS

CHAPTER 10

Healthy Rice Vinegar

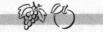

Pure rice vinegar is the best among vinegar.[1]
—Togo Kuroiwa

After traveling across America with my dog, I did end up back on the West Coast, a place touted for its fresh apples and wines—two sources of vinegars—but cities with an Asian influence, from Los Angeles to San Francisco, fed my knowledge of nature's remarkable remedy. I brought my Southern California friends up north to San Jose. During one of our road adventures on a rainy night we visited a popular Asian restaurant in Chinatown, San Francisco.

One money-minded individual of our group ordered tea. A large white teapot with six teacups and steaming hot tea was a welcome treat. The waiter took our thrifty friend's order for one (we decided earlier to share the generous portions of a single serving of each dish since we were broke). The order for one included stir-fried vegetables, rice, wonton soup, fried shrimp, and egg rolls. When we enthusiastically asked for six dishes the no-nonsense server folded his arms and took a dramatic pregnant pause. He sighed. He mumbled some Chinese words as he rounded up our menus, one by one. Alas, the food gods understood our financial plight: We were soon served a fabulous feast that was only supposed to serve one person but fed the whole group because the condiments—including rice vinegar, filled us all up.

These days, countless people like me, and perhaps you, may crave a Chinese foodfest and/or are crunching numbers to make ends meet. Flavorful rice vinegar dishes can help during a budgeting challenge. Do-it-yourself rice, stir-fry vegetables sautéed with seasoned rice vinegar (which I've discovered in the world of vinegars), tea, and Chinese cookies (purchased online or in specialty Asian stores or some grocery stores) come to the rescue. And rice vinegar isn't new—it goes back thousands of years.

For more than 3,000 years, the Chinese have been making rice vinegar. Rice vinegars come in red, white, brown, or black. They are most often used in Asian recipes that require vinegar.

The Japanese have been making vinegar since yesteryear, using rice as its basic material and utilizing the production method brought from ancient China. Yet new kinds of vinegar emerged in the 1910s in Japan. They were made of alcohol and petroleum and upstaged the traditional natural vinegar.

RICE VINEGAR IS DIET-FRIENDLY

Personally, I wasn't aware of rice vinegar and its versatility until a surprise happening. My girlfriend, a good cook, is from Taiwan. One day when I was visiting her, she was making dinner. I was surprised that she used brown rice vinegar in the soup, salad, and fish. "It is no big deal," she said. It is a staple of her Asian diet.

Rice-wine vinegar is less acidic than other types, so you can use more of it in a vinaigrette with oil. That reduces both the grams of fat and the calories per serving. They are good for flavoring with herbs. And rice vinegar contains healthful ingredients. After all, it's made from rice.

Good Grains

In the 1940s the nutritional value of rice became popular thanks to Duke University's William Kempner, M.D., who created the Rice Diet to reduce high blood pressure. He believed that the low-sodium content of the rice and fruit had a good effect on blood pressure. Brown rice is also healthful because it provides fiber, plus 5 grams of protein per cup. It also has some vitamin E, and is high in selenium.

While rice vinegar, unlike apple cider and red wine vinegars, is not high in potassium, it is higher in phosphorus and calcium—two minerals your body needs. Although it has only trace elements of vitamins A, C, riboflavin, and niacin, rice vinegar does contain other ingredients, according to a national vinegar manufacturer.[2] Per 3½ ounces:

- Carbohydrates: 3 grams
- Calcium: 1 gram
- Sodium: 5 milligrams
- Potassium: 8 milligrams
- Phosphorus: 1 milligram

But it's not just the labeled ingredients in rice vinegar that make it healthful. It's the amino acids in vinegar that are the secret of pure rice vinegar's good-for-you healing power.

AMINO ACIDS: THE REAL ESSENCE OF RICE VINEGAR

When genuine natural rice vinegar is manufactured according to the method of production available from ancient times, it will contain more amino acids than any other vinegar.

Because of the amino acids in it, natural rice vinegar is an effective healer as well as a seasoning, according to *Rice Vinegar*'s author Togo Kuroiwa.[3]

According to the Japan Food Research Laboratories, pure rice vinegar contains many of the essential amino acids, which include lysine, histidine, alginine, valine, isoleucine, leucine, and phenylalanine.[4]

Remember how acidity and strong alkali are what originate a disease and the affected region always indicates strong alkali? If pure rice vinegar is rich in amino acids, which Kuroiwa believes it is, then it can neutralize alkali in the ailing body part.[5]

"Amino acid," he adds, "therefore, is the thing itself for curing disease and injury and showing great effect on the human body. As a result, we understand very well the various effects of vinegar which have been proven in the experiences gained by so many people over so many years since ancient times."[6]

While nutritionists agree that vinegar boasts amino acids—we don't know which ones are in rice vinegar. "Rice does have protein in it. So it would have amino acids in it. But the key is, how much rice is in the vinegar," says Connie Diekman, R.D. And nobody knows the quantity.

Rice vinegar is going to add to your daily required intake of amino acids. "The big question mark is," adds Diekman, "protein is digested in acid. So are we losing the amino acids because of the acidity of the vinegar?"

Herbal vinegar writer Maggie Oster adds, "Because the grain remains present throughout the fermentation and vinegar-producing process, this rice vinegar has a significant amino acid content. The medical claims made for Japanese rice vinegar include the ability to neutralize lactic acid in the body, alkalinize the blood, and generally promote good health."[7]

A GARDEN VARIETY OF RICE VINEGARS

Type of Vinegar	Description	Tried-and-True Uses
Brown rice	Golden colored, like apple cider vinegar. Mellow. Made from brown rice and water.	Mainstay in salad dressings, pickling mixtures, and marinades, it also perks up vegetable dishes, sauces, dips, spreads, and entrées.
Black rice	Popular in China. Dark colored. Rich flavor. Made from rice, wheat, millet, or sorghum.	Braised dishes, dipping sauces; substitute for balsamic vinegar.
Red rice	Dark colored, but lighter than black rice vinegar. Tart and sweet.	Noodle soup, and seafood dishes; substitute for black rice vinegar.
White rice	Colorless. Mild flavor.	Stir-fry and sweet-and-sour dishes.

BOOSTING YOUR RICE VINEGAR SMARTS

So, do you know where in the world rice vinegar has been making a big splash? Do you get the difference between original rice vinegar and seasoned rice vinegar? Are you watching your cholesterol? Read on, and find out the answers straight from Mizkan Americas, Inc., to these questions about rice vinegar.

Q. *What is the history of rice vinegar?*
A. Rice vinegar is a by-product of sake (Japanese rice wine) and is used heavily with sushi in Japan. About 20 years ago, rice vinegar was introduced to the U.S. market.

Q. *What is seasoned rice vinegar?*
A. Seasoned rice vinegar is rice vinegar blended with sweeteners and salts. Rice vinegars are popular because they are sweeter, milder, and less acidic than traditional white vinegar.

Q. *What is the difference between original seasoned rice vinegar and flavored seasoned rice vinegar?*
A. Both are lightly flavored with sugar and salt for a smooth, mellow taste. The flavored seasoned rice vinegars have been infused with a special blend of seasonings that may include Italian herbs, red pepper, roasted garlic, basil, or oregano. All are great for splashing on your favorite food as a flavor enhancer or as a versatile recipe ingredient.

Q. *Can you use natural or seasoned rice vinegars for pickling?*
A. This is not recommended, since these vinegars are very low in acidity and may not be able to inhibit microoganisms that cause spoilage, which would ruin your cucumbers or make them unsafe. If you'd like, you can pour some seasoned rice vinegar on the cucumbers and store them in the refrigerator, but for no longer than 24 hours.

Q. *Are rice vinegars fat-free and cholesterol-free?*
A. Yes.

Q. *How do I use seasoned rice vinegar?*
A. Seasoned rice vinegar is so versatile that you can use it in almost any of your favorite recipes. Use it straight on salad, mix it with oil to

make a salad dressing, use it as a marinade, or splash it on any grilled meats or vegetables, just to name a few things you can do.

RICE VINEGAR SUCCESS STORIES

In his book, Kuroiwa provides various real people who reveal exactly how rice vinegar worked wonders.[8]

Jyosuke's Story: "Good for a Broken Bone"

"It seems to me that rice vinegar is good for dislocation of bones and sprains. This is a case of a broken bone.

"My brother-in-law called on our home after getting a diagnosis from his doctor that he had a crack in his shoulder blade. He complained of not being able to lift his shoulder and claimed he had a high temperature.

"I had then heard of how good rice vinegar was for such a case. I decided to give him a rice vinegar wet dressing. I used about 0.3 pints of wheat flour to knead it with a wine cupful of vinegar and water and applied it all to the affected region.

"He said he felt very well and had no shoulder ache that night. He had a good night's sleep because of the wet dressing. He found the packing sheet completely dry the following morning. He changed it two or three times since then and found himself in good condition in his shoulder."

Kazuko's Story: "Good for Constipation"

After a stomach operation this woman suffered from lack of bowel movements. While someone told her that fasting was a solution, she decided to try rice vinegar enemas instead.

"I gave rice vinegar injections into the bowels three times a day—morning, midday and evening. I did that everytime I had a bath. On the third day after I started giving myself rice vinegar injections, I had a bowel movement . . . Three times a day, I had rice vinegar, each time sipping one wine cup full of it. I poured four or five tea cups full of rice vinegar into the bathtub and took a bath three times a day. After I had easy bowel movements."

Shizue's Story: "Good for Rhinitis"

"I heard that rice vinegar was good for rhinitis (inflammation of the nasal mucous membranes), and I thought I should try it. First, I had a tablespoon of vinegar in a cleaning device and cleaned my nose. I did this twice or I used 10cc of rice vinegar.

"I repeated this for three months. The mucous in my nose began to disappear. At the same time, I felt very good after cleansing the nose. Previously, if I didn't clean my nose for a week, I would have had a hard time with my nose closed up. Now, the nose stays the same even if I didn't wash my nose.

"It has been about a year since I started using vinegar. I cleanse my nose at least once a week. I feel wonderful and feel as if I have finally cured my nose. For your information, I think the amount of rice vinegar I use for cleaning my nose is just about right for me."

Seasoned Rice Vinegar Bell Peppers

❖ ❖ ❖

In the twentieth century, stuffed peppers included white rice, hamburger, bread crumbs, and tomato sauce on top. As a kid, I did enjoy these as well as porcupine meatballs (covered with rice). My mother used to create these little guys using meat, canned sauce, and dried herbs. My choice of foods as a West Coast native has morphed throughout the years—and meat is a memory.

During the early part of the twenty-first century while new to Lake Tahoe, I went through an anti-cooking phase. Frozen food entrees were my best friends. One afternoon during a snowy day, at the grocery store in the frozen food aisle I stared through the glass cases at ready-made stuffed green bell peppers with meat. I did get nostalgic and almost caved to savor the meaty treats like the ones my mom used to make. But I got the idea to put a meatless pepper on the table that's wholesome, filling, and full of deliciousness.

These stuffed peppers can be a side dish or an entrée. For me, it was a light dinner. The aroma lingered in the kitchen. What's more, I felt better that I cooked a meatless dish. I still get flashbacks of hamburger, but going vegetarian always wins. Novelty can be unsettling, but once you take the plunge it can be a blessing in disguise.

1½ cups brown or wild rice,
  cooked
2 tablespoons European-style
  butter or olive oil
¼ cup yellow onion, chopped
¼ cup fresh baby spinach,
  chopped

2 teaspoons herbs, your choice
2 bell peppers, red, yellow, or green
½ cup Roma tomatoes, sliced
4 tablespoons Parmesan cheese
2 tablespoons rice vinegar or
  Nakano Seasoned Rice Vinegar

In a pan, cook rice according to instructions. Meanwhile, in a skillet, melt butter, sauté onion. Pour into cooked rice. Add spinach, and herbs. Set aside. In a microwave dish with 1/2 inch of water put two sliced, seeded peppers. Microwave about 5 minutes. Remove and stuff rice mixture. Top with tomatoes. Bake at 350 degrees for about 25 minutes. Top with cheese. Drizzle with vinegar. Serves 2.

VINEGARY HEALING HINTS TO PRESERVE

✓ Amino acid–rich rice vinegar helps to balance the pH in the body.
✓ Rice vinegar can help fight aches, congestion, and constipation.
✓ Rice vinegar is a good flavoring with herbs in nutrient-dense foods.
✓ Rice vinegar users believe it really works.

The rice vinegar demand is here to stay. But that's not all. Take a look in the upcoming chapter on the "balsamic boom" and you may see why I see a boom with this special vinegar that's growing in popularity, whether it is on TV cooking shows, in restaurants, or in your own kitchen.

The Balsamic Vinegar Boom

This vinegar tastes like it's got oil in it![1]
—Richard Simmons

My lack of knowledge was replaced by hunger for learning about exotic vinegars and paved the way for vinegar adventures in the eighties. As an undergrad back in the San Francisco Bay Area, I was living on a shoestring budget. The foodie roommate in my life with Italian roots was in tune to Mediterranean fare, including red wine, olive oil, and fine vinegars I hadn't tried. On Christmas one year his parents invited us to a classy restaurant with Continental cuisine. I ordered lobster. A tossed green salad with balsamic vinaigrette (I didn't know what it was then, but sensed it took a sophisticated palate) was served with a basket of French bread and butter. The salad dressing was new to me since apple cider, red wine, and white were the vinegar staples in my life. Each bite was different, but special. Dinners like this one were treasured since, as a student, living at the Student Union Potato Bar and Bagel Sandwich Shop was all I could afford.

Generous gifts like this meal with an olive oil and balsamic dressing were a luxury. (I was clueless that years later balsamic vinegars, including black cherry, cranberry, and white varieties, would be sitting in my pantry waiting to be paired with citrus olive oils, such as blood orange olive oil and lime olive oil.)

Back home in our modest garden apartment, I put a doggie bag of salad and pricey shellfish into the old fridge. That night, we stayed up like two kids, playing with our new toys and munching on the balsamic vinaigrette salad. The dressing was put in a small container; it was decadent. I felt like an adopted daughter who'd entered food heaven and was obliged like Cinderella to face fine dining like it was commonplace at the ball before the clock struck midnight. Centuries ago, other people from regions around the world appreciated balsamic vinegar too.

For 1,000 years, balsamic vinegar coined "Aceto Balsamico" has been considered for its medicinal properties.

In the seventeenth century, people used it as a gargle, tonic, and air purifier against the plague. The word "Balsamico" in Italian means balm, which connotes a healing, soothing medicine. And it was.

In the twenty-first century, the belief that balsamic vinegar is nature's miracle worker still remains. Today, it is very popular both in Europe and the United States. However, many people are clueless as to why it is so good. They just know it is.

AN ITALIAN THING

Balsamic vinegar is traditionally made in Modena, Italy, and historically made from Trebbiano grapes grown around the hills of Modena. The grapes are allowed to ripen until they are supersweet before harvest time. The juice is then filtered and poured into a progression of casks made from a variety of woods—such as oak, chestnut, ash, cherry, and mulberry, from which it reaps a deep reddish-brown color.

Vinegar that gets the grade "traditional vecchio" is aged at least 12 years, while the variety called "tradizionale extra vecchio" is aged at least 25 years—and can cost more than $100 per bottle.

"In Modena, balsamic vinegar is not just vinegar, it is a symbol of sophistication, a good investment, and a way of life. The prices range from a few dollars per bottle to more than $300 for a 7½ ounce bottle from a batteria dated 1730. This makes vinegar a very extravagant and pricey condiment," reports the Vinegar Man, Lawrence Diggs.

"In Italy, it is so highly prized that sometimes it is not sold at all. It is saved by the family for special gifts for dowries. The very best balsamics may be reserved for close associates and family," adds Diggs.

Balsamic vinegar as a treasured gift? Absolutely, says chef Sal Campagna, who is of Italian descent. His parents were born in Sicily. And for their seventy-fifth wedding anniversary, Sal turned to balsamic vinegar. It's true. A bottle from Modena (priced at $120 for 8 ounces) was part of the anniversary dinner package. At his restaurant, Salvatore's, which specializes in Continental cuisine, he provided an extravagant celebration dinner. For dessert, the creative chef drizzled the rich vinegar over vanilla ice cream for forty people.

What's more, when he told me this story, I just had to indulge. After my dinner at Salvatore's (salad with red wine vinegar and olive oil dressing, salmon, and a baked potato), I indulged in the balsamic vinegar decadent delight. And to my surprise, the Italian dessert was *magnifico!*

The two kinds of balsamic vinegar are the real stuff (*Aceto Balsamico naturale*), like the vinegar I had at Salvatore's, and the industrial or imitation. The industrial version is boiled-down Trebbiano grapes that have been mixed with regular vinegar, then flavored and colored with carmelized sugar, herbs, and other ingredients. It is aged about a year.

Bob Rubinelli, founder of Rubinelli, Inc., in Cicero, Illinois, explained it to me, which has a more Italian flavor to it: "I traveled to Modena, Italy, to find out firsthand about balsamic vinegar. My hosts were two local producers, Mr. Aggazzotti and Mr. Galletti, who graciously took me through the entire production process at their acetificio and explained to me the two basic types of vinegar.

"First there is 'Traditional Balsamic Vinegar of Modena.'" He wasn't disappointed to see the legend of this product, dating back nearly 1,000 years. He passionately raves about the Trebbiano grapes, transferring the unfermented juice to wooden barrels, and the forever-long aging process.

"The second balsamic vinegar product is the commercial/industrial version. This is the version we so commonly see on the grocery store shelves. It is an imitation produced by adding sugar and flavoring to a small amount of strong wine vinegar," he explains. "It is an affordable, versatile, delicious vinegar that imparts some of the same characteristics of the traditional and is the basis for a fine salad dressing, marinade, or cooking ingredient. This commercial balsamic vinegar sells for under four dollars per seventeen-ounce bottle."

Diggs agrees that the inexpensive balsamic vinegar has its place.

"I like vinegar cookies but I prefer the extra tartness and the flavor stability of the industrial balsamics in these cookies," he says. "And in any recipe which calls for a lot of vinegar, e.g., a cup, you may not want to use vinegar that costs over $100 per bottle. Tradizionale is something for special occasions. Industrial balsamics are for everyday use."[2]

Adds Rubinelli: "There is a third type of balsamic vinegar that will vary according to the producer—this is a blend of traditional and commercial. Aggazzotti, for example, produces a product that is five percent traditional and costs under $10."[3]

The fact remains, balsamic vinegar—real and imitation—has soared in its popularity due to the American discovery in the 1970s and 1980s. But just how nutritious is it anyhow?

GOOD STUFF

Not everybody is going to buy the expensive balsamic vinegar. A lot of folks will, however, purchase balsamic vinegar at food specialty shops, grocery stores, and health food stores. And that's where you can get a bottle of organic balsamic vinegar. On the front label it may read: "Product of Modena, Italy. Produced in wooden casks. No added sulfites." Sounds good to me.

Then, turn that balsamic vinegar bottle around and you'll be greeted by this: "Following centuries of Italian tradition our Organic Balsamic Vinegar is carefully blended from grape must and wine from Trebbiano and Lambrisco grapes. Produced in wood, the result is a richly flavored vinegar with intense aromas and delicately balanced sweet and sour taste."

So what happens if you check out a bigger quantity of balsamic vinegar. One national vinegar production company did just that.[4] Here's what you get for 3½ ounces, or almost a half cup:

- Calcium: 12 grams
- Carbohydrates: 30 grams
- Fat: 0
- Sodium: 20 milligrams
- Potassium: 70 milligrams

- Sugars: 30 grams
- Phosphorus: 20 milligrams

It also has trace elements of ash, vitamin A, thiamine, riboflavin, niacin, iron, and vitamin C. But there's more to it.

SECRET INGREDIENTS

As with red wine vinegar, the labeled contents aren't the entire story. Balsamic vinegar, like its grape-filled counterpart, contains powerful antioxidants that protect against heart disease by blocking the oxidation LDL—the "bad" cholesterol—and may even fight cancer.

Upon my request and interest, Dr. Leroy Creasy analyzed a bottle of his personal balsamic vinegar. Indeed, like other wine vinegars, it was high in polyphenol activity, he reported. More scientific research is required before we know just how potent balsamic vinegar is in fighting disease.

THE BALSAMIC BANDWAGON

Meanwhile, Italian restaurants use it. Celebrities use it. Doctors use it. And even health spas and Food Network chefs use this dark vinegar with a mellow, slightly syrupy taste.

Richard Simmons, a well-known fitness expert, says balsamic vinegar is one of his Top 10 favorite foods. "I love salads, but most fat free dressings aren't palate-pleasing. This vinegar tastes like it's got oil on it! I use it on salads or to marinate. I've even used it in casseroles."[5]

BALSAMIC VINEGAR AND OLIVE OIL

Is balsamic vinegar and olive oil a good and healthy mix? "Olive oil provides your monounsaturated fatty acids. So if you're looking for a salad dressing option—it's wonderful," says Connie Diekman, R.D. "The major thing that I hear from people is that the flavor combination is so full it almost feels decadent." And that's not all.

Chef Campagna told me that he used to plan menus for San Francisco's World Champion 49ers and their former coach, Bill Walsh.

Often, the salad dressing of choice would include balsamic vinegar. Balsamic vinaigrette was their favorite dressing, and Sal would use different ratios of olive oil.

If you marry balsamic vinegar and olive oil, does it make a pleasant and healthy mix? Absolutely, say chefs, nutritionists, and doctors. Not only will you get the cancer-fighting, antioxidant-rich polyphenols in vinegar, but heart-healthy monounsaturated olive oil that forms its base in a vinaigrette can help to lower your cholesterol levels, too. (See Chapter 14, "Combining Vinegars and Garlic, Onions and Olive Oil.")

THE BALSAMIC VINEGAR PARADE

When I wrote the first and second editions of *The Healing Powers of Vinegar*, balsamic vinegar was a "mysterious elixir" to me. This time around, in the third edition, I noticed flavored balsamic vinegar is well liked by chefs on the Food Network, specialty olive oil and vinegar sellers offer a wide selection online and in their retail stores, and the vinegars are making a big splash with consumers like me, too.

My pantry not only includes the basic vinegars—apple cider, red wine, and white—but it also a wide variety of balsamic vinegars that are fun to use in cooking and baking. I'm talking flavors, including dark chocolate, lavender, honey ginger white, champagne, sweet potato—the list of flavors (much like honeys and coffees that I love) is infinite. You'll find I include some of these flavored balsamic vinegars in my recipes.

You, like me, may be eager to enjoy making a balsamic vinegar reduction—just like the Food Network chefs do. Simply put, a balsamic vinegar reduction is a process of boiling down balsamic vinegar, resulting in syrup that can be used in sweet and savory dishes. You can mix the balsamic vinegar with honey (be careful so it's not too sweet) on high heat to a boil, then turn down to a low simmer until the vinegar has reduced several minutes.

A vinegar reduction makes a nice sauce or glaze for entrees to desserts. Balsamic reduction can be drizzled over fresh fruit, cooked vegetables, poultry, or fish. It's often used on green salads, tomatoes, and may liven up sauces. It's rich, decadent, and is an awesome way to give life by a quick drizzle of deliciousness.

So, the question is, do these flavored balsamic vinegars have health perks? When paired with the Mediterranean diet foods, including vegetables, fruits, poultry, and fish, flavored balsamic vinegars make nutrient-dense dishes tastier. And that's not all. When adding raw honey and fresh herbs and spices, you've got nature's finest ingredients to enhance healing foods. It's a sublime superfood that can do no wrong for your dishes year-round as you put your imagination to work.

And, like red wine vinegar rich in polyphenols (those compounds that act as disease-fighting antioxidants), balsamic vinegar drizzled on nutritious foods just makes it more nutritious and bursting with flavor so you'll get the healthful antioxidant effect. (See Part 4, "Other Natural Vinegars," to discover more healing powers of balsamic vinegar.)

MORE VINEGARS, PLEASE

- *Beer vinegar:* Made in Germany, Austria, and the Netherlands. It is said to have a "malty taste." The vinegar from Bavaria is a light golden color, with a sharp flavor.
- *Coconut vinegar:* Derived from the sap of the coconut palm, coconut vinegar, another specialty vinegar, is popular in the cuisine of Southwest Asia (especially the Philippines) and in some dishes of India. It's cloudy white in color and boasts a sharp taste.
- *Distilled vinegar:* White vinegar is praised for its many household uses, from washing windows to cleaning coffeemakers. Unlike apple cider vinegar, which boasts 240 milligrams of potassium per cup, distilled white vinegar has a mere 36 milligrams per cup of this mineral.
- *Malt vinegar:* From Europe's beer breweries comes malt vinegar, which is made from fermented malted barley. It's especially "in" in England, the place where it's "in" to sprinkle it on fish and chips. In fact, these days you can even buy potato chips that contain malt vinegar.
- *Sherry vinegar:* Derived from the southwest region of Spain, sherry vinegars are made like balsamics. They're aged for several years before bottling, and they cost more, too.
- *Ume plum vinegar:* Ume plum vinegar comes from what else? Ume boshi plums. Since it is made with salt, you can add less salt to your foods. (See Chapter 13, "Fruit-Flavored Vinegar Craze.")

Balsamic Vinaigrette

◆ ◆ ◆

¼ cup balasmic vinegar
6 tablespoons water
1 tablespoon Dijon mustard
1 tablespoon freshly ground
   black pepper

½ teaspoon minced dried
   basil
2 tablespoons olive oil (or
   canola oil)

In a small mixing bowl, whisk together balsamic vinegar, water, Dijon mustard, black pepper, and dried basil. Vigorously whisk in a thin stream of olive oil. Store vinaigrette in refrigerator until ready to use. Will keep up to 2 weeks in the refrigerator. Serves 12. Health perks: 23 calories per tablespoon; 2 g total fat; 0 cholesterol; 6 IU vitamin A; 32 mg sodium.

(*Source*: Chef Michel Stroot of the Golden Door Spa.)

VINEGARY HEALING HINTS TO PRESERVE

✓ Balsamic vinegar is high in antioxidant polyphenols.
✓ Balsamic vinegar is fat-free.
✓ Balsamic vinegar is high in potassium.
✓ Balsamic vinegar is tasty.
✓ Balsamic vinegar and olive oil are the dressing of the new millennium.
✓ Balsamic vinegar is popular, but try other vinegars, too.

The balsamic boom is here to stay. In the past decade its popularity has grown on cooking shows, in magazine recipes and specialty vinegar shops, and in my own kitchen, and perhaps yours, too. Sure, apple cider and red wine vinegars are popular, but balsamic is exotic. These days it's not uncommon to find it used in appetizers, entrees, and desserts. Herbal vinegars, like balsamic, are finding their way into the kitchen around the globe. In the next chapter, come along and I'll show you that there's more to vinegar than just a salad dressing.

12

Healing Herbal Vinegars

From sublime sage and majoram to zesty jalapeño garlic, flavored vinegars are a treat for both the palate and the eye.
—Heinz U.S.A.

After surviving a feast-or-famine lifestyle with vinegary exotic restaurant meals, no-cooking salad and baked potato bars (sprinkled with vinegar) at college, I recall one Mother's Day. I was a magazine journalist living and working in San Carlos. On deadline for completing articles for a woman's magazine, I felt lonely and disconnected from the world. I tried to forget that it was a celebration for women with kids, despite my being a mindful mom to four fur children.

In between inputting words, in my study I wolfed down nuked bland manicotti-in-a-box (the kind found in the grocery store frozen-food aisle). The sound of an incoming fax grabbed my attention. The paper greeted me with a colorful drawing of my three cats, one dog and me smiling amid trees and a bungalow with three words: "Happy Mother's Day." A knock on the back door hours later was another surprise. My landlord "fairy godmother" said, "You have to eat." I left my work to escape into another world: an Italian restaurant that served pasta with authentic flavorful sauce to live for.

These days, when time is short, I cook whole grain pasta, use my own fresh tomato marinara sauce, spices, and a splash of herbal vinegar (available at online specialty food stores, or I borrow Alton Brown's flawless Tarragon Chive Vinegar recipe or use one of the herbal recipes in this chapter) to mimic the sauce like that night at the special bistro, an oasis.

Combine herbs, berries, flowers, and vinegar and what do you get? Healthful herbal or infused vinegars that can be an extra boon to your health, too.

Dioscorides, who reportedly traveled through Egypt with Nero's army, found that Egyptian medicines included vinegar combined with honey, brine, thyme, or squill, and this mixture was used for many health ailments.[1]

Like healing vinegar, herbs—such as parsley, sage, rosemary, and thyme—have been shown to contribute not only to good lyrics, thanks to Simon and Garfunkel, but to good health. You can make your own herbal vinegars and reap a host of therapeutic effects from these herbs mixed with wine, rice, or apple cider vinegar. Think about using some of these herbs steeped in vinegar for the therapeutic benefits you can obtain both outside and inside your body:

CHAMOMILE *(Anthemis nobilis)*: Chamomile, a common folk medicinal herb, has been used to treat a variety of health ailments. The dried flowers brewed in a tea help combat anxiety (a brew without licorice root is best), gastrointestinal symptoms, minor infections, and skin disorders.

Recent research shows that chamomile contains apigenin, a flavonoid which has antioxidant properties and may inhibit skin tumor formation. Thus it could be beneficial in sunscreens.[2]

COMFREY *(Symphytum officinale)*: The herb comfrey may aid in healing cuts and help soothe minor burns and swelling faster.

ECHINACEA *(Echinacea angustifolia)*: This infection-fighting herb can help kill bacteria, fungi, viruses, and other germs. Echinacea contains a natural antibiotic called echinacoside and a germ-fighting compound called echinacein. It is also used externally for cuts, burns, and cold sores.

EUCALYPTUS *(Eucalyptus globulus)*: This herb relieves runny noses and helps clear the sinuses and respiratory system. It's used in many saunas to help people breathe easy. I personally use fresh eucalyptus in my shower for the wonderful aroma. It also has antiseptic, antiviral, and decongestant benefits.

FENNEL *(Foeniculum vulgare)*: Some mainstream doctors find that the use of herbs can treat everyday ailments. Fennel used in a tea has been known to relieve symptoms of abdominal discomfort, such as gas, bloating, and belching.

HORSETAIL *(Equisetum arvense)*: Both the American Indians and the Chinese use silicon-containing horsetail to stop bleeding and to help wounds and broken bones heal faster. It's the solubility of silica in fluids of wounds or in the poultice materials, and its absorption directly into blood and cells at the site of the wound, that makes horsetail work, according to herb expert Daniel B. Mowrey, Ph.D.[3]

European research reveals that horsetail stops bleeding and helps build up the blood. It has good antibiotic action, too. "Silica acid, or horsetail tea," adds Dr. Mowrey, "causes a slight rise in white blood cell count, and thereby enhances nonspecific resistance to diseases of many types."[4]

JUNIPER *(Juniperus communis)*: The dried fruit and leafy branches have been used as an antiseptic, and act as a diuretic. Also, juniper has been used as a detox and body cleanser, as well as for reducing muscle pain.

LAVENDER *(Lavandula angustifolia)*: This fragrance is used in aromatherapy for relaxation. Also, you can drink lavender tea, which acts as a mild sedative. It is also used to help heal scars, minimize stretch marks, and soothe insect bites.

MINT *(Mentha spp.)*: Mint is beneficial for normal skin, refreshes, and cools. Peppermint not only can soothe tense muscles, but can be used to cure an upset stomach.

NETTLE *(Urtica spp.)*: To stave off allergies, congestion, watery eyes, and other hay fever symptoms, nettle may do the trick.

OREGANO *(Oregano vulgare)*: Oregano oil is both antiseptic and anti-inflammatory. Not only does it kill bacteria, viruses, fungi, and other germs, it also fights infection, from colds to the flu. Also, oregano contains carvacrol, a type of phenol that is potent as an antiseptic.[5]

As an anti-inflammatory, oregano can be rubbed on aching muscles to relieve strains, and used externally to help heal burns and wounds, reports Dr. Mindell.[6]

PARSLEY *(Petroselinum crispum):* This cleansing herb is packed with disease-fighting antioxidant vitamins A, C, and E. Also, it boasts plenty of iron. Parsley gets its good reputation, however, for its diuretic action. Plus, it's believed to ease PMS symptoms, including cramps, hormonal mood swings, and bloating.

"Parsley does not allow salt to be reabsorbed into body tissues and literally forces debris out to the kidneys, liver and bladder. It is this ability which has saved lives—especially in cases where urine was backing up and poisoning the kidneys and liver," reports Laurel Dewey, an herbalist in Glenwood Springs, Colorado.[7]

RED CLOVER *(Trifolium pratense):* This herb is phytoestrogen-rich, which is believed to be soothing and healing.

ROSEMARY *(Rosmarinus officinalis):* This ancient therapeutic herb contains calcium, magnesium, sodium, and potassium, all of which help balance fluids surrounding nerves and heart tissues.

In fact, rosemary may help to lower blood pressure. The rosemary leaf may have other positive cardiovascular effects owing to its rosemaricine content, and the flavonoid pigment diosmin.

Rosemary may also be known as the cancer-fighting herb. A research project at Penn State proves this to be true and shows that rosemary could reduce the risk of cancer in rats given a powerful carcinogen.[8]

SAGE *(Salvia officinalis):* Herbalists claim sage is a natural astringent and antiseptic. It's recommended for gingivitis and to soothe a sore throat. But caution: pregnant women should not take it.

THYME *(Thymus vulgaris):* Thyme is a delicate herb which is a natural source of iron, magnesium, silicon, sodium, and thiamine. Its power is as an antiseptic and a general healing tonic. It is believed to be helpful in cases of anemia. It can also subdue coughing and relieve intestinal ailments.

Make Your Own Therapeutic Vinegar

Just start with dry whole herb sprigs—from thyme to rosemary. Place a couple of sprigs in a sterile pint jar. Heat two cups of vinegar to a simmer in a small stainless steel or ceramic saucepan. Pour the steeped vinegar into the jar (use a funnel) and allow to cool. Let stand for seven days before using. It's recommended to store it at room temperature.

CREATE YOUR OWN FLAVORED VINEGARS

You can make your own flavored vinegars by blending your favorite herbs, fruits, and spices. The following recipes are courtesy of Heinz.

- **Basil Garlic Vinegar:** Place ½ cup coarsely chopped basil leaves and 2 cloves peeled, split garlic in a sterilized pint jar. Heat Heinz Wine or Distilled White Vinegar to just below boiling point. Fill jar with vinegar and cap tightly. Allow to stand 3 to 4 weeks. Strain vinegar, discarding basil and garlic. Pour vinegar into a clean sterilized jar, adding fresh basil for garnish if desired. Seal tightly. Use in dressings for rice, pasta, antipasto salads, or in flavored mayonnaise.
- **Herb Vinegar:** Make a bouquet of 3 to 4 sprigs each parsley, sage, marjoram, and thyme, and place in a sterilized pint jar with ½ teaspoon whole black peppercorns. Heat Heinz Distilled White or Wine Vinegar to just below the boiling point. Fill jar with vinegar and cap tightly. Allow to stand 3 to 4 weeks. Strain vinegar, discarding herbs. Pour vinegar into a clean sterilized jar, adding sprigs of fresh herbs for garnish if desired. Seal tightly. Use in marinades for mushrooms or artichokes, or in dressing for tossed green or pasta salads.
- **Lemon Thyme Vinegar:** Remove peel (colored portion only) from 1 lemon in a thin spiral and place in a sterilized pint jar with 4 to 5 sprigs of thyme or lemon thyme. Heat Heinz Distilled White Vinegar to just below the boiling point. Fill jar with vinegar and cap tightly. Allow to stand 3 to 4 weeks. Strain vinegar, discarding peel and thyme. Pour vinegar into a clean sterilized jar, adding fresh thyme sprig and peel for garnish. Seal tightly. Use in dressings for tossed green salads or marinades for vegetables.

- **Jalapeño Garlic Vinegar:** Cut a few small slits in 2 small jalapeño peppers and place in a decorative bottle with 2 cloves peeled garlic. Heat Heinz Wine or Apple Cider Vinegar to just below the boiling point. Fill bottle with vinegar and cap tightly. Allow to stand 3 to 4 weeks. Use in dressing for taco, tomato and onion, or avocado salads, or when making salsa.

Health Fact!

Food Safety Alert: It is difficult to determine the exact shelf life of homemade flavored vinegars which include oils. American Dietetic Association (ADA) nutritionists question the safety issue since we do not know if we can prevent food-borne illnesses.

According to the ADA, millions of Americans yearly contract food-borne illnesses. The home is a common place for food-borne illness to occur. But the ADA is constantly at work learning how consumers can protect themselves and their families from the threat of food-borne illness.

Mac and Cheese with an Herbal Vinegar Twist

❖ ❖ ❖

These days, traditional macaroni and cheese gets a bad rap for its cheese, margarine, and white pasta, a "bad" carb. It's time to shed some light on these ingredients, which can be enjoyed in moderation, and tweak the dish. Welcome to my new age macaroni and cheese—a "mainstream America" dish that can please the kid in you.

Back in the day when I was younger and living in the burbs, my mother dished up two varieties of macaroni and cheese. On busy work and school weeknights we'd get the Kraft dinner in a box ruined with hot dog chunks that was cooked and served in several minutes. During some chilly winter weekends, we got macaroni and cheese with TLC that was made from scratch with whole milk, cheddar cheese, and bread crumb topping. The difference in taste and texture of the two meals was like comparing the temperature of night and day in the Sierra.

I have tried Lean Cuisine as well as Amy's all-natural frozen mac and cheese for instant meal gratification that would take me back in time to the homemade stuff. I got the idea to healthy up a feel-good, old-fashioned comfort food. Here it is with a new Italian twist.

3 tablespoons European-style
    butter (set aside 1–2 teaspoons
    to grease baking dish)
1⅓–1½ cups mixed cheese
    (cheddar and Gruyere), grated
½ cup organic half-and-half
½ cup organic 2 percent reduced-
    fat milk
1 teaspoon fresh basil
2 teaspoons seasoned herbal
    vinegar (I used Etruria Thyme
    Vinegar)

2½–3 cups whole grain rotini,
    cooked and drained
½ cup each broccoli and
    cauliflower, chopped, cooked
Parmesan cheese, fresh and grated
    for topping
2 large Roma tomatoes, sliced

Preheat oven to 375 degrees. Grease with butter an 8-inch square casserole dish (or use ramekin dishes for cute single servings). Set aside. In a sauté pan melt butter. Add cheese, half-and-half, milk, herbs, and vinegar. Stir till blended well. Meanwhile, boil rotini and nuke or steam broccoli and cauliflower. Fold in cooked pasta. Pour half of the mixture into casserole; top with crucifers. Sprinkle with Parmesan cheese. Top with rest of pasta. Place tomatoes on top.

I lighten this up and delete the customary flour-and-buttered-crumb topping. Bake for about 30 minutes. Serve warm. Makes 8 servings.

The different flavors of cheese, the vegetable layer with gooey cheese, the fresh tomatoes and wholesome pasta paired with herbs, and the tang of vinegar make this a winning homemade entrée for lunch or dinner.

Vinegary Healing Hints to Preserve

✓ Chamomile   For stomach ailments, minor infections, and skin disorders

✓ Comfrey   Heals cuts, burns, and swelling

✓ Echinacea   Antiseptic, heals

✓ Eucalyptus   Antiseptic, deodorant, stimulates, soothes, heals

✓ Fennel   Soothes abdominal woes

✓ Horsetail   Heals minor wounds, antibiotic

✓ Juniper   Relieves muscle soreness, cleansing

✓ Lavender   Sedative, soothes insect bites

✓ Mint   Treats normal skin, soothes tense muscles and tummy

✓ Nettle   Treats allergies, congestion

✓ Oregano   Antiseptic and anti-inflammatory, relieves muscle soreness, heals wounds

✓ Parsley   Cleansing

✓ Red clover   Soothes, heals

✓ Rosemary   Heart-healthy, cancer-fighting

✓ Sage   Astringent, antiseptic, soothes a sore throat

✓ Thyme   Antiseptic, helps anemia, coughs, intestinal upsets

Now that I've infused some herbal vinegars into your brain, pantry, and palate, in the next chapter you'll find out how pairing popular fruit vinegars—an Asian favorite—results in one more vinegar type that may captivate you with its healing powers and amazing flavors.

Fruit-Flavored Vinegar Craze

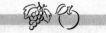

*A spoonful of honey will catch more flies than a
gallon of vinegar.*

—Benjamin Franklin[1]

I wasn't introduced to the wide variety of herbal vinegars until writing
this third edition of *The Healing Powers of Vinegar*, but fruit-flavored
vinegars is another story. I was assigned a story about wayward cats in
Kauai, Hawaii—an island with Asian cuisine, home remedies, and
vinegar powers.

I eagerly booked a flight across the Pacific Ocean to meet the cat
people. With its breathtaking beaches, green valleys, cool waterfalls,
and magnificent mountain peaks, the island of Kauai seems like a
utopia. On the second day, my fair skin was sunburned. A local cat
lady introduced me to using cactus plant for the redness and inflammation, and she concocted a cold fruit-flavored vinegary drink with
the promise of amazing properties. "Drink it. It will heal your skin
fast," she said. "It's an Asian delight with coconut, pineapple, and
guava. You'll like it." I was pain-free by the morning.

While herbs and vinegar pack a powerful punch, fruit-flavored
vinegars are something to write home about. Not only do they sing
out "taste me," these specialty vinegars are truly special. I talked to a

variety of experts to help you learn why fruit-flavored vinegars are becoming so popular.

Fruity vinegars boast health benefits, too, while adding a splash of flavor to meals. The fresh flavor of fruit vinegars—such as raspberry, blueberry, strawberry, and orange—can perk up a healthful salad or make a tasty marinade for poultry. Plus, antioxidant vitamin C in oranges, raspberries and blueberries enhance your immune system and keep disease at bay.

Blueberry Youth-Boosting Bliss

A study reported by the National Institute on Aging, U.S. Department of Agriculture, shows that animals fed a blueberry extract diet, rich in naturally derived antioxidants, had fewer age-related motor changes and performed better than their counterparts on memory tests. In result, blueberries may guard the body against damage from oxidative stress—one of the biological processes linked to aging.[2]

- *Raspberry vinegar* is a very popular wine vinegar that's been infused with fresh raspberry. It has a stunning red color and tastes like the berry. Raspberry vinegar is an acid syrup made with fruit juice, sugar, and white wine vinegar and, when added to water, forms an excellent cooling drink in summer, suitable also in feverish cases, where the acid is not an objection. It makes a useful gargle for sore throats.[3]

  "When you need the full-bodied rich flavor of raspberry in a salad or sauce, reach for this one. It will win you big points in the kitchen when you use it on salad dressings, marinades, sauces, and glazes. You can also enjoy it by just drizzling it on fresh fruit," says the Vinegar Man, Lawrence Diggs.
- *Strawberry vinegar* provides health benefits, too. Strawberry-infused vinegar, which uses balsamic vinegar, is a source of vitamins A and C, and is low in calories and free of fat, cholesterol, and sodium. Berry vinegars are good, as are citrus delights.
- *Orange vinegar* is another fruity vinegar that shouldn't be forgotten. "When you want your guest to say, 'Wow, how did you make this salad?' think blood orange vinegar. This vinegar has a deliciously deep orange taste of blood oranges. Whatever you put it

on will radiate oranges. It has a slightly sweet edge to it that works well with its orange base. This is a vinegar that inspires experimentation," Diggs told me.

• *Mango honey vinegar* is sherry wine vinegar with mangoes added. This infused vinegar contains 6 mg of vitamin C, has a whopping 266 IU of vitamin A, and is fat and cholesterol free and has 23 calories and 1 mg of sodium per serving.

Try these fruit vinegars, and for your health's sake, enjoy.

JAPANESE FAD, DRINKING VINEGAR

A trend in Japan that has hit America is to consume vinegar drinks, in particular those made from fruit. As the Vinegar Institute reports, vinegar drinks seem to be popular among health-conscious people who have knowledge of vinegar's healing powers. According to Takashi Tajiri, a professor of food administration in Kinki University's agriculture department, "I think people believe that drinking vinegar is more efficient than taking it by eating dishes in which it is used as a seasoning," he said. "When foods are heated, some of the [nutritional benefits] of vinegar are lost."[4]

According to the *Japan Times*, vinegar brewer Uchibori Vinegar, Inc., has seen the average monthly sales at each of its six shops rise tenfold from two years ago. The shops offer more than three dozen types of vinegar. These are made from mangoes, pears, raspberries, strawberries, and other fruits. The managing director, Mitsuyasu Uchibori, recommends that the vinegars be teamed with water or milk.[5]

Also, Mizkan Americas, Inc., offers a black vinegar beverage, a mixed-vinegar beverage touted as "an energy drink." No telling if it will be a mainstay in the vinegar parade.[6]

DIVING INTO VINEGAR DRINKS

Fruit-flavored vinegar drinks continue to be "in" and here to stay. After all, they do go back in history, but in the twenty-first century they've made their mark too. Shrubs are popular in New York, Seattle, and Los Angeles. But that doesn't mean people in other regions of America don't enjoy these "energy" drinks served at restaurants and bars (some drinks can contain alcohol). You can even order them on-line in grocery and food categories as well as in vinegar and gourmet food specialty shops.

These vinegar drinks are healthier than sugary sodas, but they do contain a lot of sugar, too. However, they contain no fat or cholesterol, are low in sodium, and have a good amount of potassium. Vinegar-based syrups are supposed to be diluted and added to chilled bottled or sparkling water to create a soda. I tried a turmeric vinegary drink and a ginger vinegar drink, produced by Som (old Thai word for "sour") Pok Pok (made in Portland, Oregon) and available online. It's an acquired tart taste, but if created with your favorite spices and fresh fruit, I'm sure it can be savored year-round like dark chocolate (well, almost).

KOREAN DELIGHT, PERSIMMON VINEGAR

Yes, persimmon vinegar is made from persimmons, a fruit that is an excellent source of vitamins A and C, as well as fiber. Also, because persimmon doesn't have a long shelf life, it makes sense to turn this healthful fruit into a fruity vinegar, which can be stored in your kitchen pantry for a long time.

The consensus is, persimmon vinegar isn't cheap—but it's worth the money for a variety of reasons. Grace, a 25-year-old San Francisco–based woman from Korea, swears by this stuff. She says, "The taste is sour yet sweet. It's an absolutely delicious vinegar. Two tablespoons can be mixed with water and ice to be enjoyed as a drink. Although it is vinegar, it has a natural sweetness from the persimmon."

Also, Grace points out that this very popular vinegar in Korea may help to boost the metabolism and prevent the common cold due to its high vitamin C content. "It also contains tannin, which is known to be really effective for treating diarrhea as well as constipation, stom-achache, and good for the respiratory system, too.

"In Korea, though, it is mainly popular because it has the ability to break down fats and helps you digest food better. This drink first be-came popular at Korean saunas and spas because people would drink this and go into saunas to sweat. They are only sold by the bottle itself—and you have to mix it with water and ice—so even at the sauna they make it for you. It doesn't come in a bottle already made. You want to put just a few tablespoons in a glass of water because it is very sweet and sour. However, the acidity level is much lower than in regular vinegars, so it is not difficult drinking it at all," she explains.

Adds Grace, "I have been drinking this for two years now, and I feel it is effective. I always drink it before going into a sauna or exercising, and I believe that it aids in breaking down fat. You also sweat a lot more, which is good."

Persimmon vinegar is made from Korean persimmons. The fruit is aged for a few years and exported to Japan, European countries, and America. Also, while it isn't easily found in the United States, it may be found at larger Korean supermarkets.

Other fruit-flavored vinegars include blackberry, black cherry, black fig, cherry, ginger, key lime, mint, mint and celery, peach, pineapple, pomegranate, and sun-dried apricot.

OTHER SUPER-SPECIAL VINEGARS

- *Shanxi vinegar:* Shanxi province of China is touted for its vinegar making. In fact, the natives make a variety of Shanxi vinegars, which are believed to lower blood pressure, increase energy, and add years to your life. So naturally, this ancient vinegar is valued by its people in China. "They've been making vinegar since about 700 B.C. in that little region in China. They make it out of barley and peas. As far as healthy vinegars are concerned, if you're looking for nutrients, that's going to be one of the vinegars with a higher nutrient value than the others just from what it's made from," says the Vinegar Man, who uses it in foods such as salads. "It has a very smooth front end; it's not so harsh. You take it like cough syrup," he adds. Many people in China, in fact, will take a tablespoon before meals. They also marinate their fish in this healthful vinegar, and dip their vegetables in it, too.
- *Spicy pecan vinegar:* "You can use the rich nuttiness of this vinegar to add an unexpected depth to almost any dish. You can use it as a dressing for a salad of bitter greens and fresh herbs, or mixed into pasta, wild rice, or barley for a surprising twist. You will certainly want to try it in vinegar cookies and vinegar pie," Diggs says

with enthusiasm. (See his tasty cookie recipe in Chapter 16, "Fat-Burning Vinegar.")

- *Cane vinegar*: A specialty vinegar and Philippine delight, mellow cane vinegar is made from sugar cane juice. It is also made in France and America. It varies from dark yellow to golden brown in color, and is similar to rice vinegar.

Steen's cane vinegar is one of America's best vinegars, according to Diggs. "Steen's is actually in the business of producing superior sugar cane syrups, but several years ago, they tried their hand at making sugar cane vinegar." The Vinegar Man makes it a goal to include it in any vinegar tasting.

Plus, he touts it as great for cooking and recommends it as a "house" vinegar for homes and restaurants "because it is a taste that you won't get tired of quickly. And, of course, it goes with any Cajun cooking that calls for vinegar."

Mango Honey Vinegar

❖ ❖ ❖

1½ cups sherry wine vinegar
1½ cups fresh orange juice
½ cup honey
10 ounces ripe mangoes (1½ to
2 cups), peeled, small dice

2 teaspoons chili sauce, with
garlic
2–3 tablespoons fructose

In a medium-sized saucepan, bring sherry wine vinegar and orange juice to a boil. Stir in honey, mangoes, and chili sauce. Let cool. Push through fine sieve. Add fructose, if needed. Transfer to sterilized glass container. Keep refrigerated.

(*Source:* Chef Michel Stroot of the Golden Door Spa.)

THE VINEGAR CURE

Thanks to vinegar's stores of multiple compounds and its potent bioactive effects, scientists report a wide variety are believed to have healing powers. Studies show the therapeutic properties of vinegar, which include antibacterial activity, lowers the risk of heart disease and diabetes. But it's the potent antioxidant activity in different vinegar varieties that affect human health.

To date, most of the studies on vinegar and health have been small-scale, as noted in Chapter 5. Folklore and anecdotal evidence shows vinegar can cure a wide range of health ailments and may help stall diseases and aging. But a collection of studies, many in the early twenty-first century, and published in the *Journal of Food Science*, shows how different vinegars hold healing virtues, giving credit to the antioxidants.

A group of vinegars, including apple cider, grape, plum, persimmon, rice, sherry, and traditional balsamic, share many of the same disease-fighting phenol compounds. In the circle; of antioxidant studies, caffeic acid, catechin, epicatechin, gallic acid, and cholorgenic acid are also noted among many other compounds with scientific names. While the research in this journal is impressive, further studies linked to health effects of consuming vinegar by humans are necessary. But for now, the idea of vinegar touted as ancient folk medicine turned modern miracle continues to gain popularity around the world, as everyday people have faith and personal proof that it's a powerful healer.[7]

VINEGARY HEALING HINTS TO PRESERVE

✓ Fruit-flavored vinegars have a wide variety of health benefits, just like apple cider vinegar and red wine vinegar.
✓ Fruit vinegar drinks are popular in Japan.
✓ Persimmon vinegar, rich in vitamins A and C, is "hot" in Korea and good for the total body.
✓ Shanxi vinegar, made from barley and peas, is a nutritional bonanza and appreciated in China.

In the next chapter, in Part 5, you'll discover that vinegars teamed with fresh garlic, onion, and olive oil—in both cooking and baking—provide even more health perks for you, as well as feed the senses, including aroma and taste.

PART 5

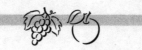

THE ELIXIR OF YOUTH

14

Combining Vinegars and Garlic, Onions, and Olive Oil

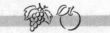

Our Garrick's a salad; for him we see
Oil, vinegar, sugar and saltiness agree.
—Oliver Goldsmith[1]

After the trip to the islands, I was more open-minded to healing superfoods. Being a California journalist for national women's magazines kept me on the inside track of nutrition, but I was the go-to West Coast writer (who was believed to be a nature girl living on the beach munching on trail mix). I noticed red wine vinegar was used in some dishes, including fresh salads and hearty soups (created by Midwest and Deep South nutritionists I was teamed with), but fruit-flavored vinegars (as well as wine, balsamic, and herbal kinds) were ignored.

One early spring, I traveled from the San Francisco Bay Area to British Columbia, Canada. I fell in love with Pacific Northwest city cuisine and wanted to explore it; my traveling friend did not. The best part of the trip was dinner. The Pacific Northwest fish was tangy and savory. Back home we went to the store and picked out salmon fillet to bring our traveling food experience home for a repeat. When my friend cooked it (I didn't have confidence to make fish back in those days), I thought: "One day I will go back solo to B.C." I savored each bite of the cold-water fatty fish. While the relationship did not last, I did preserve his tasty recipe tricks: raspberry vinaigrette, fresh garlic, onion, lemon, and ground pepper. It brought me back to Canada and I could almost taste a future trip and the Pacific West Coast food, vinegar included.

Vinegar is one of the oldest known ingredients used in cooking (as I note in Chapter 2), going back centuries. And health-wise it can stand alone as a healthy condiment. But by teaming other superhealing foods—garlic, onions, and olive oil—with apple cider, red wine, balsamic, and rice vinegar you've added a powerful punch to any recipe.

In umpteen recipes you'll find vinegar paired with garlic, onions, and olive oil. It's common in the Mediterranean world and now in the United States, too. Not only do these extra vinegar ingredients help add flavor to food, but research continues to show that this trio can enhance your health—and boost longevity, too. All three—and vinegars—help fight heart disease, cancer, obesity, colds, aging, and much, much more.

GARLIC AND VINEGAR

Garlic (*Allium sativum*) has been touted for its extra-special health properties, today and yesterday. It's hot stuff. For at least 3,000 years, garlic, dubbed "the stinking rose," has been used medicinally.

Garlic has a long history. Louis Pasteur, bacteriologist, used it for its antibiotic effects. Albert Schweitzer treated dysentery. In World Wars I and II, the British military used it to control infection and gangrene. Pliny wrote that it cured tuberculosis. Hippocrates believed it eased the pain of stings and bites. And people in 1918 used it to fight off the flu epidemic.

Today, the therapeutic uses of garlic have been noted in more than 1,000 scientific studies. Garlic has been found to lower cholesterol and high blood pressure, as well as ward off infections and cancer.

And research shows garlic and vinegar provide super benefits to our health taken together or alone. Either way, this powerful duo enhance the immune system, prevent heart ailments, and much more.

SUPERPOWER INGREDIENTS

Garlic is chock-full of healthful nutrients. Here, take a close-up look at one average clove of garlic, which the U.S. Department of Agriculture did:

- .01 mg B_1
- .004 mg B_2
- 1.4 mg calcium
- 1.5 carbohydrate
- .07 iron
- .02 niacin
- 10 mg phosphorus
- 26 mg potassium
- .31 g protein
- .9 mg sodium
- .75 mg vitamin C

It's these very compounds that fulfill the ancient Telugu proverb— "Garlic is as good as 10 mothers."[2] And it very well may be that garlic is that good and even better. Here's why.

Garlic vs. Cancer: For many years, the National Cancer Institute has been studying how common foods can help safeguard against cancer—and garlic figures are high on their list. It may stall tumor growth, due to its therapeutic perks.

Garlic vs. Infection. Garlic contains allicin, which is a strong antibiotic. It is believed that eating garlic can help ward off colds, flu, and bronchitis. It may be the antioxidant mineral selenium in garlic that protects cells from damage and fights off disease and infection.

A study at Boston City Hospital found that allicin was effective against a wide variety of bacteria including salmonellas, streptococcus, and microbes that cause influenza and pneumonia.[3]

Garlic vs. Heart Disease. Like red wine vinegar, garlic can help lower cholesterol. Even better, garlic can raise good cholesterol (HDL, high-density lipoprotein), which fights hardening of the arteries, according to a variety of studies.

Medical experts say that the French eat plenty of heart-healthy garlic. "In fact, the beneficial side of their alcohol consumption may be its ability to help the body absorb more of the beneficial substances in garlic," reports nutritionist Robert Crayhon.[4]

ONIONS AND VINEGAR

For centuries, doctors, philosophers, and common folk have praised the onion (*Allium cepa*) with curative powers. Hippocrates prescribed onions as diuretics, wound healers, and pneumonia fighters. In the Far East onions were used to treat infections. General Ulysses Grant believed onions were good for dysentery. And today, in the U.S. we believe onions are a healing food.

Onions Are Historically Healthy

There are more than 500 varieties of onions produced commercially around the globe. Most likely, the onion originally came from central Asia. And they have made their mark in history more than you'd ever imagine.

Ancient Greeks and Romans ate onions. Antony and Cleopatra (who had vinegar smarts) worshipped onions. They believed onions were a symbol of eternity. Why? Because of the circles that make up their structure.

Grecian athletes praised onions, too. Herodotus advised the first Olympic athletes to eat onions to "lighten the balance of the blood." To firm up their muscles, Gladiators were rubbed with onion juice.

In the Middle Ages, doctors prescribed onions as a remedy for headaches, snakebites, and hair loss.
(*Source:* National Onion Association.)

Like garlic, onions—"the rose among roots," according to Robert Louis Stevenson—are part of the healthful allium family of vegetables. Research shows that medical benefits from eating onions regularly include reduced risk of cancer, heart disease, diabetes, and even asthma. And you can give credit to its nutrients.

According to the National Onion Association (NOA), there are few other vegetables that provide such high flavor and low calorie content. Onions combined with garlic, olive oil, and vinegar make a food recipe complete.

And garlic and onions are Mother Nature's healing combination.

Research by Chinese scientists and the National Cancer Institute shows that eating more garlic and other bulb foods can lower the risk of getting stomach cancer. And that's not all.

Not only are onions healing with garlic, they are healthy solo, too. Good-for-you onions are low in sodium, contain several B vitamins, and like apple cider and red wine vinegar, are a good source of potassium—an important mineral for total good health.

Nutrition per Serving
of Onions

Nutrient Composition

Serving Size: 1 large (150 grams, about 5.3 ounces)
Calories: 60
Protein (g): 174
Carbohydrates (g): 12.95
Total Lipid (Fat) (g): 0.24
Cholesterol: 0.0*
Sodium (mg): 4.5
Potassium (mg): 235.5
Vitamin A (mcg): 0.0
Vitamin C (mg): 9.6
Thiamin B_1 (mg): 0.06
Riboflavin B_2 (mg): 0.03
Niacin (mg): 0.22
Vitamin B_6 (mg): 0.17
Folate (mcg): 28.5
Calcium (mg): 30.0
Iron (mg): 0.33
Phosphorus (mg): 49.5
Magnesium (mg): 15.0
Copper (mg): 0.09
Dietary Fiber (g): 2.7

*Information on cholesterol content is provided for individuals who, on the advice of a physician, are modifying their total intake of cholesterol.

(*Source:* National Onion Association; Information provided by the USDA.)

Onions vs. Cancer. According to the NOA, quercetin, a powerful antioxidant, is also present in onions. Quercetin neutralizes free radicals in the body, and protects the membranes of the body's cells from damage. Preliminary research shows that quercetin may work to prevent cancer cells and blood clots from forming, adds the NOA.

In addition, the National Cancer Institute (NCI) believes that a variety of chemicals in onions appear to inhibit the growth of cancer cells, especially of the gastrointestinal system, which means it can help prevent stomach cancer. Plus, according to reports, people in China's Shandong province, who eat large amounts of garlic and onions, cut their risk of stomach cancer as much as 40 percent.

Onions also can play a role in the five-a-day program, supported by the NCI, which is designed to help boost our intake of fruits and vegetables to at least five servings each day.

Here's how onions do their part, according to the NOA:

- Eat five servings of fruits and vegetables a day. (5½ ounces, uncooked, is considered one serving of onions.)
- Eat at least one vitamin A–rich selection each day. (Onions enhance other vegetables such as carrots, spinach, beets, or winter squash.)
- Eat at least one vitamin C–rich selection each day. (Onions are a source of vitamin C.)
- Eat at least one high-fiber selection each day. (Onions provide 2.7 grams of dietary fiber per serving.)
- Eat vegetables from the cabbage family several times a week. (Combine onions with cabbage in cooking or in salads and coleslaw.)

Onions vs. Heart Disease: Quercetin also seems to prevent blood clots from forming, which means onions can lower our risk of a stroke. Also, according to the NOA, onions have blood-thinning abilities because they contain another natural chemical, adenosine, which has been shown to lower blood levels of LDL or "bad" cholesterol in the blood. Plus, many heart patients are now advised to eat raw onions because they help increase blood circulation and reduce blood pressure and clotting.

Onions vs. Allergies: Red and yellow onions may boost your immunity to the allergic response. It's the anti-inflammatory compound quercetin—it acts a lot like the antihistamine cromolyn, that helps lessen allergies and asthma attacks.

OLIVE OIL AND VINEGAR

The olive tree was first cultivated in the Mediterranean countries 6,000 years ago. Since then, olive oil has played a therapeutic role in the diet and provides amazing healing powers, especially when combined with vinegar.

Olive oil is beneficial for the digestive system, brain power, and bone mineralization. It also protects against gallstones and stomach ulcers and helps relieve minor constipation, lower cholesterol levels, and guard against cancer, according to research by the International Olive Oil Council (IOOC).

Olive Oil and Your Health	
Protection for	**What It Does**
Liver and gall bladder	Helps to produce evacuation of the gall bladder toward the intestine.
Intestines	Helps intestinal ingestion of fatty foods; oleical acid changes the fats' makeup so that they are assimilated in the intestine.
Arteries	Antioxidant vitamin E in olive oil fights free radicals and reduces the buildup of platelets, which helps prevent arteriosclerosis.
Skeleton	Oleical acid is vital for composition and growth in human bones.
Brain	Vitamin E, linolenic acid, and alpha-linolenic acid protect the brain from aging.

Olive Oil vs. Heart Disease: Because of its biological effects, olive oil is the preferred fat by health experts for its cardiovascular benefits. Olive oil, which is 74 percent monounsaturated fat, is believed to increase the good cholesterol HDL, and lower the bad cholesterol LDL.

Olive Oil vs. Cancer: Olive oil, especially when included in the Mediterranean diet of vegetables, omega-3–rich fish, and fresh fruit, has been shown to help lower the risk of breast cancer.

While olive oil can help stave off heart disease and cancer, it seems to have antiaging effects as well. In the past, I did research for a *Woman's World* article on actress Loni Anderson's diet and how it keeps her young.

For one, the actor eats her greens. "I love a big leafy salad with olive oil," says Loni. Certain green vegetables, including Loni's favorites—broccoli, asparagus, and spinach—are full of antioxidant vitamins that may reduce wrinkles caused by repeated exposure to ultraviolet light, says Tufts University's Jeffrey Blumberg, Ph.D.

"I also throw garlic into practically everything,." Garlic is rich in the mineral selenium, an antioxidant that can help stall the aging process.

Good Fat versus Bad Fat

Saturated Fats	Monounsaturated Fats
• Fats from meats and poultry	• Peanut oil
• Palm kernel oil	• Olive oil
• Coconut oil	• Canola oil
• Fats from dairy products	

TYPES OF OLIVE OIL

- *Extra virgin:* Extracted from the highest-quality olives. It must have less than 1 percent natural acidity. Its "fruity" flavor is intense and great in salads.
- *Virgin:* Processed mechanically (pressure) and without heat, which changes the oil's acidity to 1 to 5 percent. It's recommended for use in salad dressings and marinades.
- *Pure:* A mix of refined olive oil (treated with steam and chemi-

cals) and virgin oils and is less costly. Acidity ranges from 3 to 4 percent. It's most often used in cooking.

- *Extracted and refined:* Made from whole cull olives and extracted during a second pressing with a chemical solvent; virgin oil is added for flavor.
- *Pomace:* Made by a chemical extraction of the residue leftover after crushing and second pressing of the olives. It contains 5 to 10 percent acidity; virgin oil is added for flavor.

I prefer to use extra virgin olive oil because it is the "crème" of the crop, so to speak. It makes my tossed green salads extra-special.

MEDITERRANEAN DIET

Garlic, onions, and olive oil—Mediterranean cuisine staples—are part of traditional and contemporary menus. We know Mediterraneans' diet includes these healthful ingredients which are key to helping reduce the risk of heart disease and cancer. And combined with red wine vinegar, their dishes are even healthier.

"Pastas, risottos, focaccias (Italian flat pizza bread), hefty salads— all those favorites at the local Italian restaurant—are just what the doctor ordered for good health and longevity. When travelers return from the Mediterranean crazy about the local food, they have fallen in love with Mother's Nature's own medicine," reports Nancy G. Freeman in her article on the Mediterranean diet.[5]

Ah, the Mediterranean diet. I can relate. For the past decades I have practiced the traditional healthy Mediterranean diet without knowing it. I eat plenty of breads, pasta, fruits, vegetables, olive oil, yogurt, fish, and poultry. And I eat very little sweets and red meat. I am a healthy woman. It's got to be my diet and lifestyle (and luck).

Just chew on these pro-Mediterranean facts[6]:

- Women of Greece have the lowest rate of breast cancer in the world.
- People living in countries that border the Mediterranean Sea have less cancer and heart disease than people in northern Europe and the United States.

- Mediterraneans live longer lives than northern Europeans and Americans.

Did you know that studies initiated by nutritionist Ancel Keys in the 1950s coined it the Mediterranean diet? Its typical foodstuffs include carbohydrates, fresh vegetables, fruits, salads, soups, fish, small amounts of red meat, and wine with meals.[7]

Also, Mediterraneans nix processed foods, forgo butter, and opt for olive oil, which accompanies salads, veggies, and is even used as a dip for focaccia. Keep in mind, however, it's not just what they eat—it's how they do it.[8]

Remember how it was in the fifties in America? We'd have regular, sit-down, *Leave It to Beaver* and *Ozzie and Harriet* meals. Three times a day. It was a time to eat and share with family and relatives. Well, now in 2000 we are a fast-paced society and eat on the run—kids and adults. But Mediterraneans do as we did. And it apparently has good health effects.

The Mediterranean diet—rich in vegetables, fruits, grains, beans, and fish—has once again been proven to be heart-protective. Researchers report that participants in the Lyon Diet Heart Study who had previously suffered heart attacks and who switched to the omega-3 fatty acid–rich diet had 47 to 72 percent lower risk of suffering a second heart attack or stroke.[9]

We know that fruits, vegetables, and whole grains—the crux of the Mediterranean diet—are brimming full of cancer-fighting antioxidants A, C, E, and other healthful compounds, too.

In fact, according to the American Cancer Society, vegetables and fruits are complex foods containing more than 100 beneficial vitamins, minerals, fiber, and other substances. And it's specific vitamins, minerals, fiber, and phytochemicals (again, those chemical compounds created by plants, such as carotenoids, flavonoids, termpenes, sterols, indoles, and phenols) that may help lower cancer risk.

Grains—which are part of the Mediterranean diet—contain folate, calcium, and selenium, which are linked with a lower risk of colon cancer. And beans or legumes, another food Mediterraneans eat, are rich in vitamins, minerals, protein, and fiber, which may help guard against cancer and are a healthier high-protein option to meat.

Research is still in the works. Until we know exactly how each fruit and vegetable provides protection against cancer, the ACS recommends

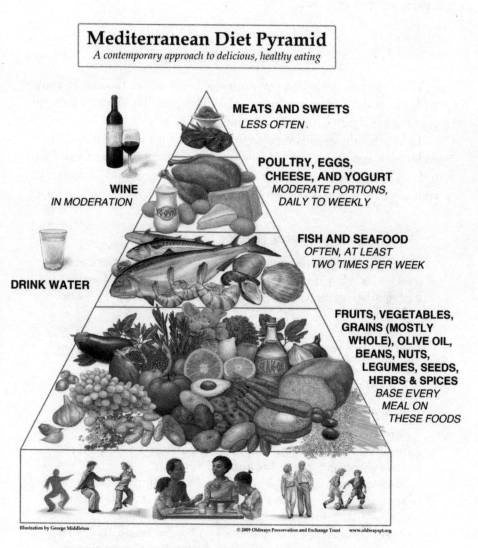

Mediterranean Diet Pyramid
A contemporary approach to delicious, healthy eating

MEATS AND SWEETS
LESS OFTEN

WINE
IN MODERATION

**POULTRY, EGGS,
CHEESE, AND YOGURT**
*MODERATE PORTIONS,
DAILY TO WEEKLY*

FISH AND SEAFOOD
*OFTEN, AT LEAST
TWO TIMES PER WEEK*

DRINK WATER

**FRUITS, VEGETABLES,
GRAINS (MOSTLY
WHOLE), OLIVE OIL,
BEANS, NUTS,
LEGUMES, SEEDS,
HERBS & SPICES**
*BASE EVERY
MEAL ON
THESE FOODS*

Illustration by George Middleton   © 2009 Oldways Preservation and Exchange Trust   www.oldwayspt.org

BE PHYSICALLY ACTIVE; ENJOY MEALS WITH OTHERS

we eat five or more servings of fruits and vegetables a day, and six to eleven servings of grains.

VINAIGRETTE, MADAM?

What do you get when you combine olive oil, wine vinegar, mustard, and a dash of ground pepper? Vinaigrette. The French will tell you that vinaigrette is the traditional salad dressing.

Today, this dressing is very popular because it's easy to make, tasty, and health-enhancing, too. While monounsaturated olive oil can help to keep your cholesterol levels in check, the vinegar adds a punch to your taste buds and will stave off a craving for salt.

Vinaigrette Tips for You and Yours

Basic Vinaigrette: Mix ½ cup olive oil, 3–4 tablespoons red wine vinegar, ½ teaspoon Dijon mustard, and a dash of freshly ground pepper. Stir before putting on salad greens.

Storing Vinaigrette: A basic vinaigrette will stay fresh for up to 2 weeks in a sealed container in the refrigerator.

Storage Tips for Garlic, Onions, and Olive Oil

Garlic: Keep garlic in a cool, dry place with good circulation—not the refrigerator. Fresh garlic may keep for months. A bonus tip: Easy peeling? Plop a whole garlic clove in boiling water for about 5 seconds.

Onions: Keep onions, whole ones, in a cool, dry place with good ventilation—not the refrigerator. Wrap scallions and cut onions tightly in plastic wrap and refrigerate.

Olive Oil: You can store extra virgin olive oil up to 1 year after opening. Store it in a cool, dark place. Do not refrigerate it, but keep it away from heat.

Balsamic Potato Salad

❖ ❖ ❖

1 medium red onion
1 medium red bell pepper
1 clove garlic (crushed)
2 ounces balsamic honey vinegar
2½ teaspoons salt
2 pounds fingerling or small
   potatoes

2 ounces olive oil
½ cup chopped Kalamata olives
½ cup chopped mint
¼ cup chopped Italian parsley
2 tablespoons oregano
1 tablespoon black pepper

Dice red onion and red bell pepper. Toss with garlic, balsamic vinegar, and salt. Place potatoes in a pot of cold water and bring to a simmer. Cook until desired tenderness. Drain and run cold water over potatoes. Toss olive oil, olives, herbs, and pepper over the potatoes. Refrigerate for at least one hour. Serves 8–10.

(*Source:* Honey Ridge Farms.)

VINEGARY HEALING HINTS TO PRESERVE

✓ Garlic's cholesterol-fighting organosulfur compounds can help keep heart disease at bay; may reduce risk of stomach cancer.
✓ Onions are heart-healthy due to the organosulfur compounds; and onions can help stave off stomach cancer because of their antioxidant quercetin. Onions may even help relieve asthma attacks.
✓ Olive oil contains squalene and has a high monounsaturated fat content—both are good for the heart.
✓ The Mediterranean diet, which combines garlic, onions, and olive oil, is a healthful, heart-smart, anticancer way to eat.

As you can see, garlic, onion, and olive oil are good disease fighters, including heart disease and cancers; and by including these with vegetables you're getting more protection and lowering your risk of developing health woes. I continue to explain to vinegar fans that any vinegar is not a magic bullet. But how can you go wrong by pairing this mighty trio with vinegar? On the next several pages, you will find out more why vinegar can be the potion to heart health.

CHAPTER

15

The Liquid to Heart Health

*As he taketh away a garment in cold weather, and
as vinegar upon nitre, so is he that singeth
songs to an heavy heart.*[1]
—The sacred scriptures of Judaism and Christianity

Surviving an unexciting trip to Canada with a dictatorial traveling partner (despite his exciting choice of a salmon vinaigrette entrée) was a challenge, but nothing like a decade of unpredictable Lake Tahoe winters I endured in the future. I am hip to a variety of fair-weather friends who pass on visiting me during this season—but sometimes they attempt the journey like a character out of *Star Trek*. There's one expedition of a health magazine editor, a New York brainiac.

In February, our cruelest season, this long-time contributing editor of a health magazine arrived at San Francisco Airport en route to Lake Tahoe to meet me. In the midst of a snowstorm, I put together a heart-healthy whole grain pasta (with red wine vinegar) and chicken, a salad masterpiece with superb vinaigrette, French bread, and a home-baked custard pie. I built a big, crackling fire in the rock fireplace and bought new Boston ferns and scented vanilla candles to give my cabin a down-to-earth ambiance amid towering pine trees and a snow-covered deck.

Then, a flurry of phone calls rolled in, one by one, with snow and traffic reports:

"The snow is coming down."

"Chains are required and visibility is almost zero."

"It's bumper-to-bumper traffic."

The deal-breaker was when he said, "I'm turning back. Have you ever been to Berkeley? I'm here for three more days."

Mr. East Coast Editor was a no-show. It was just me, a winter gourmet dinner—thanks to versatile vinegar—the dog and cat, and a Sierra snowstorm.

Whenever I think of heart health, I get images of my mom complaining about heart murmurs. For years, I wondered if I had inherited her heart problems. I wasn't sure. I do know that I have abstained from alcohol and cigarettes. I eat healthy, try to stay active, and consciously de-stress. (Note to self: Must work on getting more physical and chilling out better.)2

Mom's doctors had her taking blood pressure medication. But with the help of the heart-healthy Mediterranean diet and lifestyle, I am keeping my blood pressure down naturally. And so far, my heart is healthy. (Yes, twice I have been put on a slab, studied like a frog in biology class, and given an electrocardiogram.) Still, I continue to read in the health news that baby boomers (people born 1946 through 1964), like me, are either in denial or fighting common ailments such as high blood pressure, cholesterol, type 2 diabetes, and obesity, which can shorten the lifespan.

So, how exactly can vinegar come to the rescue for aging seniors and elderly folks who face all-too-common health problems?

DESPERATELY SEEKING A HEART-HEALTHY DIET

Take my Northern California friend Kim, also a baby boomer. She struggles with her weight and is searching for a healthful diet that is practical and works. And it seems like her sister needs to find a heart-healthy diet ASAP.

"A few months ago, we got a real scare from my little sis," recalls Kim. "She's in her mid-forties and, for nearly a year, had an ongoing back pain that just wouldn't go away. The night before she was to fly down to visit our little brother in Westwood, her back pain was so bad, she couldn't catch her breath. She rushed herself to the hospital.

"The doctors discovered her heart was ninety percent blocked! They did angioplasty and removed the blockage. She's feeling better than she has in years. They put her on meds because her cholesterol is too high. They also are trying to regulate her blood sugar with medication. The doctors told her it's hereditary. She's technically my half sister. My sister's medical scare motivated me to go in for a checkup. I hope this doctor will tune into this and work with me to devise a new health plan."

After hearing Kim's story about her sister's health and her own potential health problems, and knowing that I'm prone to stress and high blood pressure thanks to my genes, I am happy that I've already been an advocate of the Mediterranean diet. (But I'm trying to also incorporate heart-healthy vinegars into my daily diet regime.) As far as Kim is concerned, she told me, "I've heard about the Mediterranean diet. Not sure what it is, though."

It's time baby boomers learn and follow the vinegar diet of the twenty-first century, which works wonders.

METABOLIC SYNDROME HITS HOME

Although I have my weight under control (and have had it that way for years with my Mediterranean-style diet), writing *The Healing Powers of Vinegar* gave me a wake-up call that it's not too late to do more to turn back my biological clock.

I am hardly alone. Stacks and stacks of research show that graying Americans like me are fighting the battle against metabolic syndrome. This syndrome affects millions of Americans—especially baby boomers. The syndrome, which is often a "silent killer," is a deadly combo of obesity, high blood cholesterol, insulin resistance, and high blood pressure.

But the battle can be won if diet and lifestyle changes are made. Research shows that the Mediterranean diet may be part of a good game plan for reducing metabolic syndrome. A study was conducted at a university hospital in Italy. People with metabolic syndrome (99 men and 81 women) followed a Mediterranean-style diet and were taught how to up their daily intake of whole grains, fruits, vegetables, nuts, and olive oil.

The results: In two years, researchers found that the Mediterranean diet group had lowered their weight, blood pressure, and levels of glucose, insulin, total cholesterol, and triglycerides, and boosted their HDL (good) cholesterol. The authors believe that the Mediterranean-style diet might indeed be useful for metabolic syndrome.[3]

A TOAST TO THE MEDITERRANEAN LIFESTYLE

Dietary data from the Mediterranean region in the recent past show the lowest recorded rates of chronic diseases and the highest adult life expectancy in the world, and reveal a pattern like the one illustrated in the list below, according to Oldways, a food issues think tank that touts the traditional Mediterranean diet pyramid.

Here are ten diet and lifestyle strategies that may help you to beat age-related diseases and add healthier, happier years to your life.

1. Opt for an abundance of food from plant sources, including fruits, and vegetables, potatoes, breads and grains, beans, nuts, and seeds. (Vinegars can enhance the flavors of these foods so you will be sure to eat them in abundance.)

2. Emphasize a variety of minimally processed and, whenever possible, seasonally fresh and locally grown foods, which often maximizes the health-promoting micronutrient and antioxidant contents of these foods. (Vinegars include healthful anti-aging compounds.)

3. Use olive oil as your principal fat, replacing other fats and oils (including butter and margarine). (Vinegars pair well with oil[s].)

4. Strive to maintain a total fat range of 25 to 35 percent of calories, with saturated fat making up no more than 7 to 8 percent of calories. (Vinegars offer flavor instead of fat.)

5. Keep your daily intake of cheese and yogurt low to moderate (and opt for low-fat and nonfat versions when you do consume them). (Vinegars enhance calcium-rich recipes.)

6. Consume low to moderate amounts of fish and poultry each week. Recent research suggests that fish should be somewhat fa-

vored over poultry. Limit yourself to a few eggs per week (including those used in cooking and baking). (Vinegars drizzled on egg salads are rich in protein.)

7. Eat fresh fruit as your typical dessert. (Vinegars with fruit are super nutritious.)

8. Enjoy red meat only a few times per month. Recent research suggests that if red meat is eaten, its consumption should be limited to a maximum of 12 to 16 ounces per month. Lean cuts are preferred. (Vinegars splashed in meat dishes provide natural goodness.)

9. Up your exercise to a level that promotes a healthy weight, fitness, and well-being. (Vinegars—apple cider—can boost the energy you need.)

10. Consume wine in moderation, normally with meals, limiting intake to one to two glasses per day for men and one glass per day for women. Wine should be considered optional. (Vinegars are a good substitute for wines in cooking.)

Now that we've put the Mediterranean diet on the table, let's talk to a guy who dishes it up for himself and his celebrity clients.

A Little Bit of Vinegar and . . .

New York–based celebrity personal trainer Joe DiAngelo vows that he has achieved great results with the Mediterranean diet.

"I am a European guy, born and raised in Mediterranean Europe. Our diet is different from the diet in the U.S.A. and northern Europe. In many European countries, there are only few people who are overweight. Europeans have access to many healthful foods. In the Mediterranean, we eat an abundance of fruits, vegetables, fresh fish, lean meats, and olive oil. Studies have shown this diet can result in a long, healthy life."

DiAngelo offers some tips on how to eat healthy—the Mediterranean way:

- Take some time for breakfast. Do not eat breakfast while you are running to get to your job. Relax and enjoy 30 minutes for breakfast. You deserve it. Eat cereal, fruit salad, and yogurt for breakfast.
- Lunch should be your biggest meal of the day. Americans make a big mistake and have a big dinner when they come home. No, my friend, your metabolism is slow at 7:00 P.M. Your dinner should be very light in calories and low in carbs. A perfect dinner would be grilled chicken salad with Italian dressing and one glass of red wine. Researchers are honing in on how a glass of red wine can offer more than just holiday cheer, but also protection against heart disease. Scientists had always wondered why the French have had a relatively low rate of heart disease, despite a diet that often includes rich foods laden with artery-clogging fat. Other studies have shown that drinking red wine may boost the blood levels of HDL cholesterol, the good cholesterol. [If you are a nondrinker, include red wine vinegar in your diet to get some of the same heart-healthy benefits.]
- Do not eat dinner after 7:00 P.M. If you get hungry, snack on fruit and nuts.
- Avoid fast food restaurants. We Europeans celebrate summer. Dear God gave us many fruits and vegetables. Take advantage of it. Go to a local farmer's market and buy fresh, organic vegetables.
- Grill your vegetables: peppers, mushrooms, eggplant, tomato, onion, zucchini, and cauliflower.
- Eat tons of salad. Avoid heavy dressings. Use virgin olive oil and apple cider vinegar as your dressing.
- Cook all foods with virgin olive oil. The health and therapeutic benefits of olive oil were first mentioned by Hippocrates, the father of medicine. Never fry food. The traditional Mediterranean diet delivers an abundance of fat, yet the associated incidence of cardiovascular diseases is significantly decreased. As a monosaturated fatty acid, olive oil does not have the same cholesterol-raising effect of saturated fats. Olive oil is also a good source of antioxidants.
- Eat fish. Mediterranean people love fish. Oh my God, there's nothing better than grilled fish with a good Italian wine. My favorite food is grilled calamari. Fish oil will assist you with weight loss and heart disease.

- Avoid stress. Stress will slow your metabolism and will make you eat more. More stress equals more stored fat on your body.
- The people of the Mediterranean incorporate physical activity into their everyday lifestyle—walking, swimming, basketball. Remember to exercise.
- Eat minimally processed foods. The Mediterranean diet, with its emphasis on fresh fruits and vegetables, crusty breads, whole grains, and a reliance on olive oil, is really a composite of the cuisines of several countries—including Spain, southern France, Italy, Greece, Crete, and parts of the Middle East. Now you know why people in this part of the world have a lower incidence of cancer, obesity, and cardiovascular disease than we see in other parts of Europe and Americas. It's not just the olive oil my friend.[4]

So now you know more about what the Mediterranean diet can do.

Cabbage Slaw

❖ ❖ ❖

1 cup white wine vinegar
¼ cup Marsala olive oil
¼ teaspoon celery seeds
2 teaspoons grainy mustard
1 teaspoon sea salt
3 cups finely shredded green
   and/or red cabbage

1 apple or pear, shredded
1 medium carrot, shredded
1 cup crushed pineapple, drained
1 cup mandarin orange sections
¼ cup cilantro, chopped

Whisk vinegar, olive oil, celery seeds, mustard, and salt in a medium bowl. Add cabbage and remaining ingredients (apple, carrot, pineapple, orange, and cilantro), stir to combine. Serve at room temperature. Keep refrigerated until ready to serve. (One serving is ½ cup.)

(*Source: Cooking with California Olive Oil: Recipes from the Heart for the Heart* by Gemma Sanita Sciabica.)

VINEGARY HEALING HINTS TO PRESERVE

✓ People of all ages, especially baby boomers and seniors, need to adopt a healthful diet plan and lifestyle to stave off obesity, diabetes, and heart disease.

✓ The Mediterranean diet, which includes fruits, vegetables, grains, fish, and olive oil (which can be teamed with vinegars), is proven to help lower your risk of developing cancer, obesity, and heart disease.

✓ Remember, the Mediterranean diet is more than just olive oil (and vinegar). It is a lifestyle.

In the next chapter I'll show you how vinegars, especially apple cider vinegar, are excellent fat fighters. That's right: You can lose unwanted body fat and pounds by turning to fat-burning vinegar.

Fat-Burning Vinegar

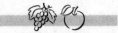

To make a good salad is to be a brilliant diploma-
tist—the problem is entirely the same in both
cases. To know exactly how much oil one must
put with one's vinegar.

—Oscar Wilde[1]

Making Mediterranean diet–type dinners, as I did for the editor who didn't come to dinner, is what I do for myself. Taking care of your ticker with whole, simple food is good for your ticker as well as keeping your weight in check. But sometimes, life's challenges can blindside you and cooking is not a top priority. The Household Renovation Diet, for instance, is not my favorite vinegar diet plan, but it will do the trick.

When the old bathroom was in need of a new shower, toilet, and floor, according to the handyman, it was estimated to be a two-to-three-day job—five days maximum. On day three of the Renovation Diet I was experiencing severe withdrawal from the comfort foods of home. I ended up moving into my sibling's mini cabin—ideal for a man, not so perfect for a fussy woman. I canceled a trip to the Pacific Northwest—as I told the airline phone guru: "There's no fresh organic produce, vinegar, honey, chocolate . . . coffee and tea are nonexistent. I can't eat." The voice told me I'd fit perfectly in my skinny jeans after the renovation was over. My canine duo was kenneled for creature comforts; it was me and the cat, Zen. But I was not Zen-like—I was hungry for fresh eats.

I survived on bottled water and Italian subs from a deli. I ordered each one with the request of drizzling olive oil and red wine vinegar on top of the spinach, lettuce, tomatoes, black olives, onions, and provolone cheese. On day thirteen, the nightmare was over. I'd lost two weeks, and was no longer a size four but a size two. I gave partial credit to vinegar for the pound-paring feat.

Folk writers tout the amazing virtues of apple cider vinegar as the cure-all for paring pounds and melting away fat. Excess body fat puts you at risk for high blood pressure, heart disease, stroke, and diabetes. These diseases are of concern to all people, but especially to baby boomers and seniors. (The fact is, these facts are worth repeating.)

It's well known that obesity is a worldwide epidemic. Blame it on an increase in high-fat foods and sugar, and a decrease in exercise.[2]

So the question remains, if an inexpensive and all-natural remedy like apple cider vinegar can help you stay lean and fit, isn't it time to put it to work?

IMPORTANT FAT-FIGHTING VINEGAR QUESTIONS FOR ANN LOUISE GITTLEMAN, PH.D., C.N.S.

Ann Louise Gittleman's books revolutionized weight loss by introducing the concept of detoxification and cleansing to mainstream America. She is on the cutting edge of health, and is known as the "First Lady of Nutrition." Her website (*www.annlouise.com*) offers a forum in which participants can get daily advice, inspiration, motivation, and fat-flushing tips free of charge. Currently living in Post Falls, Idaho, Gittleman discusses how apple cider vinegar can help you to fight fat and lose unwanted pounds.

Q. How can apple cider vinegar help you to burn fat instead of store it?

A. Apple cider vinegar is a notable fat burner because of its ability to keep sodium and potassium levels balanced. As a potassium-rich food, a couple of ounces of apple cider vinegar a day will put the lid on your appetite because you will be far less hungry and far less bloated.

Q. *Can using apple cider vinegar help you to lose inches faster than pounds?*

A. Many individuals boast that they shed inches more quickly than they pare pounds. This is again due to the high potassium levels, which help to flush out water-logged tissues, created by excessive amounts of water-retaining sodium. Bye-bye, bloat!

Q. *Does apple cider vinegar rev up the body's fat-burning power?*

A. Acetic acid, the primary ingredient in vinegar, has long been believed to boost metabolism and dissolve fats. How does this work?

Acetic acid has the ability to blunt carbohydrate metabolism and thus slow down the absorption of carbohydrates into the system, preventing them from being stored as fat. Acetic acid also can lower blood sugar by as much as 30 percent, resulting in low insulin levels, which in turn inhibit fat metabolism.

Q. *How can vinegar help you get rid of fattening toxins and safely lose pounds fast and keep them off for good?*

A. The acetic acid in vinegar acts as a blood purifier and detoxification agent, enabling toxins to be more easily transported and excreted from the body. Used on a daily basis—in salad dressings, for example—apple cider vinegar acts as a culinary fat burner.

Q. *What different types of vinegar are best for weight loss, and why?*

A. I believe that apple cider vinegar is the best vinegar for weight loss because it contains the highest amounts of purifying and health-promoting potassium, which acts as a fat-flushing agent.

Q. *Why is teaming vinegar and olive oil, like you do in your recipes, a good way to get rid of fattening toxins and to lose weight?*

A. Both vinegar and oil are blood sugar–stabilizing elements.

Q. *How do you personally use vinegar to stay fit and trim?*

A. I drink two tablespoons in filtered water at least once or twice per day.

Q. What is your favorite weight-loss vinegar tip?

A. Apple cider vinegar makes cellulite go away. Since elevated blood sugar stimulates insulin production and insulin is a fat-promoting hormone, anything that keeps blood sugar levels low will keep insulin in check and therefore inhibit fat promotion.

Speaking of melting fat with vinegar . . .

CHOOSING THE RIGHT CARBS

It's no secret that I'm an advocate of good-carbohydrate foods, which include whole grains, fiber-rich fruits, and vegetables. Also, I love potatoes, which are considered a "bad" carb because they are a high-glycemic food. So, what are high-glycemic foods?

There is a system called the glycemic index that rates how fast certain foods raise blood sugar levels and how quickly the body responds by bringing the levels back to normal. You don't want your blood sugar level raised because this will trigger the release of insulin, the fat-storing hormone. (And it's not a good idea to eat high-glycemic foods if you are diabetic or pre-diabetic.)

Vinegar may be beneficial for potato lovers who want to burn fat. In a study, 13 healthy people at Applied Nutrition and Food Chemistry, Lund University, Sweden, agreed to eat four meals: freshly boiled potatoes, boiled and cold-stored potatoes, boiled and cold-stored potatoes with vinaigrette sauce (olive oil and white vinegar, which is 6 percent acidic), and white bread. The results showed that cold potatoes teamed with vinegar had a lower glycemic index than regular potatoes. So, perhaps potato salad made with vinegar and olive oil can be included in a fat-burning diet plan.[3]

THE QUICKIE SEVEN-DAY DETOX VINEGAR DIET

No need to worry about losing those extra 5 or 10 pounds or detoxing your body after the holidays. I worked with personal trainer Chrissie Gallagher-Mundy, author of *Fat Burner Workout* and *Bikini Fit: The 4-Week Plan* (both published by Hamlyn), to develop a program to help slim down in just one week.

For an extra healthful edge to this diet plan, every day before each meal, plus in the mid-morning and mid-afternoon, drink 1 to 2 tablespoons of apple cider vinegar in an 8-ounce glass of water. Add 1 to 2 tablespoons of honey, if desired.

Make sure to check with your doctor before starting. Take a multi-vitamin-and-mineral supplement daily, drink at least eight glasses of water each day, and do the diet for only one week.

DAY ONE: Liquids Only

Combine energy-boosting fruits and vegetables to make yummy, pound-paring drinks. For all seven days, follow this basic meal plan, adding the new foods listed each day.

Breakfast: Raspberry-peach juice. In a juicer, combine ½ cup raspberries with 2 peaches. Add an apple or two if the juice is too thick. (Try different fruit combinations throughout the week.)

Lunch: Apple-carrot juice. In a juicer, combine 4 carrots and 2 green apples.

Dinner: Veggie juice. Juice your favorite veggies.

Diet Tip: "If you start off by detoxifying, you're giving your body a head start," explains Gallagher-Mundy. "It will be cleansed via the elimination of unwanted waste."

DAY TWO: Liquids and Fruits

You can eat sweet, juicy, whole fruits as often as you like today.

Diet Tip: Try apples, pineapple, mango, grapes, and watermelon, all of which help to neutralize the acidic waste that is produced when the body begins to detoxify.

Shape-up Strategy: Make the switch from walking to skipping or running. Both increase calorie burn and are fat-burning activities.

DAY THREE: Raw Veggies

Add raw vegetables to your plan. Treat yourself to a bowl of salad greens with lunch and dinner. Toss in some dandelion leaves or parsley, both of which are natural water-weight busters. (Add 1 to 2 tablespoons of red wine vinegar.)

Diet Tip: By consuming three meals and three snacks per day, you'll boost your metabolism and lose pounds faster, according to the diet pro.

Shape-up Strategy: For tummy toning, try the rope-climbing exercise. Lie on your back on the floor. Tighten your stomach muscles as you roll up to a half-sitting position. With knees bent and arms stretched out, loosely clench your fists, then raise one arm above your head, lower it, raise the other arm, and lower it. Repeat 8 times.

DAY FOUR: Cooked Veggies and Rice

Welcome cooked vegetables and brown rice into your program. To get the best nutritional value, cook the veggies quickly in a little water. (Add 1 to 2 tablespoons of seasoned rice vinegar.)

Diet Tip: Try eating an artichoke today. It will help stimulate the liver and speed up digestion.

Shape-up Strategy: To flatten your tummy, try roll-ups. Lie on your back, legs stretched out, knees slightly bent, with your arms at your sides. Flex your stomach muscles and buttocks, hold 15 seconds, and relax. Repeat 4 times.

DAY FIVE: Beans, Lentils, Nuts, and Seeds

Add beans, lentils, nuts, and seeds to your meal plan. These foods high in the healthy essential fatty acids help speed up digestion. Just make sure they're not salted or cooked.

Diet Tip: "Don't eat these with the rice at this stage. This makes complete protein and can slow digestion," recommends Gallagher-Mundy.

Shape-up Strategy: Repeat roll-ups from day four.

DAY SIX: Grains and Yogurt

Indulge in some grains and yogurt today. "Make sure the grains are whole," advises Gallagher-Mundy. "Oats are great long-term energy releasers."

Diet Tip: "Avoid wheat grains," she adds. "They are a known irritant or allergen to some people."

Shape-up Strategy: Pump up your exercise plan with muscle building to help fight body fat. Stand with legs apart, squat down, and come back up as you press a 12-pound dumbbell forward and back. Repeat 25 times.

DAY SEVEN: Fish

Get your protein fix with fish. "Fish and brown rice make for a very satisfying meal," says the diet expert. Add lemon and lime to seafood for extra oomph. (Also add rice vinegar.)

Diet Tip: The slower you eat, the better. It takes about 20 minutes for your brain to recognize that your stomach is full.

Shape-up Strategy: Get moving by bounding. Stretch your muscles and then either walk briskly or jog for 20 minutes. Push off each foot so you're spending more time in the air between each step.

HEAD-TO-TOE VINEGAR TIPS

Making some small lifestyle changes can boost your "beauty assets" from head to toe big-time.

- **Feed Your Hair.** Drink plenty of water with apple cider vinegar and eat iron-rich protein and green vegetables for a shiny, thick mane.
- **Brush Your Body.** Give yourself an all-over glow by brushing with a loofah and apple cider vinegar to help stimulate circulation and fight cellulite.
- **Stop Cellulite.** Shake the salt habit and steer clear of toxic food additives, caffeine, and alcohol. Sip a glass of water spiked with one tablespoon apple cider vinegar (each morning).

BLAST BELLY FAT + WITH VINEGAR

As a diet and nutrition columnist for *Woman's World* magazine in the mid-1990s, I penned a diet each week, such as "Lose 100 Pounds in One Week on the Cabbage Soup Diet" and "Dump Ten Dress Sizes in 21 Days on the Protein Diet." I'm exaggerating, but staying up to midnight to find studies to meet my deadline, week after week, was surreal because I ate what I wanted and stayed skinny. In hindsight, vinegar shrubs may have given me an extra kick instead of diet soda.

To survive *The Devil Wears Prada* demands, I'd go to the gym, hit the rowing machine, play racquetball, and walk home. I'd often order a vegetarian pizza (and pile fresh lettuce drizzled with red wine vinegar and olive oil on top), and drink lots of H_2O or go out to dinner with my octogenarian European-loving best friend and order a chef's salad with a vinaigrette before I'd return to my diet story for the week.

Research (despite the lack of huge hard-hitting studies using humans) continues to confirm indulging in vinegar may actually blast fat (and pounds), Japanese scientists report in the twenty-first century. Within three months, the acetic acid in apple vinegar led to both body fat and weight loss, and lower triglycerides in a study of 175 obese women and men (25–60 years old). The study-backed daily dose: one to two tablespoons of apple cider vinegar after breakfast and dinner.[4]

Nowadays, you'll find dozens of quickie books on the virtues of apple cider vinegar and how to lose pounds. If you think I'm going to hop on the bandwagon and tell you take one tablespoon of ACV and in twenty-four hours your tummy will be flat as a twenty-year-old supermodel—sorry, this is the wrong book. But I do believe vinegars paired with superfoods can indeed help you to dump stubborn pounds and whittle that tummy, sort of. The truth is, I've been told by medical doctors throughout the years as a health journalist, if you have a protruding stomach the cause may not be linked to your love for peanut butter cookies and chilling on the sofa. A pouch belly may be in your genes. Blame your mom and dad or hormones.

I was afraid that after menopause I'd get that spayed female cat look, unwanted pounds and a protruding tummy. Worse, when I started cooking and baking for my Healing Powers series, when a recipe worked I sometimes ate the whole thing. (Putting the tasty muffins or casserole in the freezer doesn't always work in the real world.) So, I went back to vinegars—not just apple cider vinegar—for extra flavor teamed with skinny fat-burning foods (fresh fruits and vegetables) that help fill you up and not out. Here are several tips I abide by to keep lean—and blast those last stubborn pounds (gained after overindulging) without trying:

1. **Vinegar Belly Blaster Rx: Go Natural.** Foods full of chemicals and high in refined sugars are calorie-dense and can pack on belly fat. Stay clear of diet sodas and high-fat meat, and stock up on fresh fruit, vegetables, and whole grains. To add flavor to a fruit salad, drizzle a bit of apple cider vinegar with honey on it. Ditto with vegetables, but use

red wine vinegar and olive oil. These superfoods offer variety and taste good. No reason to guzzle ACV.

2. Vinegar Belly Blaster Rx: Lose the Salt. Salt can cause water retention and may make you feel bloated. Also, fat-free and low-fat processed foods (such as cookies and salad dressings) can contain sodium with a capital S. Forget the saltshaker when cooking and baking. Instead, use herbal vinegars for cooking, and try balsamic vinegar when baking. You'll stay clear of salt but still get the taste.

3. Vinegar Belly Blaster: Beer and hard liquor can block your body's ability to burn fat for energy. To achieve a flatter tummy, drink alcohol in moderation. Enter apple cider vinegar, honey, and lemon. Drink a cup of hot or iced tea with this cocktail. The trio of vinegar, nature's sweetener, and citrus will energize and calm you. The end result: You will feel naturally high and avoid a "beer belly."

4. Munch on Mini-Meals: Grazing will help fight belly fat because you will lessen the amount of insulin made, which means less stored fat. Instead of three big square meals like we consumed in the twentieth century, switch up your eating style. No need to reach for that apple cider tonic when you can enjoy a variety of good-for-you foods— whole grains, fresh fruit and vegetables. Drizzling vinegars—fruit or herbal—will provide flavor and creativity like the celeb chefs use—and you'll not be hungry but satisfied.

5. Savor Whole Nutrient-Rich Foods: Get enough nutrient-dense, potassium-rich foods to help you balance your sodium intake (it's impossible to not get salt in your daily diet), and this will help you stave off bloat. You'll find a list of potassium-rich foods in Chapters 3 and 4, but bananas and apples are two favorites, budget-friendly year-round, and are filling. Plus, if you really want an extra boost for a flatter tummy, go ahead and concoct a vinegar cocktail with water, honey, and one to two tablespoons of apple cider vinegar.

72-HOUR VINEGAR SEMI-PALEO MINI-FAST

The Seven-Day Detox Vinegar Diet works, but what if you overindulge in healthful food and only need to get back to your regular diet regime—and drop a few pounds? Sometimes when I cook or bake, I end up eating the whole thing (that's how I know the recipe works). Or, there was the time while writing *The Healing Powers of Chocolate* when I was receiving pounds of gourmet truffles on my doorstep weekly. I started to include my semi-fast foods while indulging in the chocolate and then plunged into the 72-Hour Mini-Fast.

Instead of turning to a structured diet for one week, I created a fabulous go-to mini-fast plan. Welcome to the Semi-Paleo Diet, which uses only foods that are not processed—vinegar is an exception. Paleo proponents will allow vinegar in the modern twenty-first century. The Paleolithic Diet goes back to the caveman era, and includes fish and meat. But my mini-fast is vegetarian. The menu of my spin-off Semi-Paleo Diet consists of fresh fruit, vegetables, nuts, seeds, vinegars (not varieties containing sugar or gluten), tea, coffee, and water. Also, olive oil, a staple of the Mediterranean diet (an underlying theme of the Healing Powers series)—and other oils, including olive, walnut, macadamia, avocado, coconut—are given a thumbs-up by Paleo Diet proponents; these oils are good for sautéing and for salads.

Not only am I full and satisfied (thanks to the vinegar) eating this clean food diet composed of these nutrient-dense foods—fruits and vegetables are water-dense to help you burn fat—but it's a surefire way to get rid of unwanted pounds and feel more energized, too.

Mini-fasts, which might better be described as "modified" fasts because you don't cut out eating altogether, offer super health perks. By eating only superfoods you'll be giving your body a vacation from high-fat and sugary fare. After I easily survive this vinegary clean food diet for three days, I simply go back to the Mediteranean diet and lifestyle. I slowly add eggs, whole grains, dairy, legumes, and fish (the latter two are not my first choices, but I know both are good for you). No measurements are used. Portion control is honored.

Morning: Fresh fruit, including apples, figs, oranges, pears, and strawberries. Nuts, such as almonds and cashews. Tea with 1 tablespoon each honey and apple cider vinegar.

Mid-Morning: Herbal tea with honey.

Lunch: Green leafy salad drizzled with red wine or balsamic vinegar and a splash of fresh lemon.

Mid-Afternoon: Fresh fruit and mixed nuts.

Dinner: Green leafy salad with a splash of olive oil and red wine vinegar, a variety of vegetables, fresh fruit.

Snack: Herbal tea and fresh fruit.

The Rules: I drink at least six to eight 8-ounce glasses of spring water a day, plus herbal tea. I swim and walk daily. I only use this mini-fast for a few days; repeat as needed. I don't count calories, but it's likely the calorie intake for the day doesn't go over 1,200–1,300.

SKINNY SMOOTHIES

Do you really want to drink a glass of water laced with apple cider vinegar? Yes, it can and does work to suppress appetite, detox, and energize for countless people. But if you, like me, would rather try a tastier route—why not spruce up that vinegar slimming beverage (as I did in the first chapter with the ACV Super Smoothie—sweet and creamy with nature's flavors of fresh fruit)? You'll enjoy more nutritional perks and want more not less of a healthful drink.

So what exactly is a smoothie, anyhow? It's a blended beverage created with fresh fruit. The ingredients are infinite, but they can contain ice cream, milk, and other add-ins for the health nuts, including honey and wheat germ. As a native Californian, smoothies in the 1970s were big. Back in the day, these fruit shakes were all-natural, created with good-for-you health foods.

Blackberry Smoothie

❖ ❖ ❖

¾ cup fresh blackberries, sliced, frozen
⅓ cup 2 percent organic low-fat milk
1 cup all-natural vanilla ice cream
1 capful pure vanilla extract

2 tablespoons organic strawberry preserve (optional)
1 teaspoon honey
1 teaspoon Bragg Organic Raw Apple Cider Vinegar
fresh mint leaves

In a blender, mix berries, milk, and ice cream; add vanilla, strawberry preserve, and honey. Pour into a glass. Garnish with a mint leaf. Serves two.

Health Nut Smoothie

❖ ❖ ❖

¾ cup fresh peaches, sliced (leave
    skins on)
½ cup vanilla almond milk
1 cup all-natural vanilla gelato
1 capful pure vanilla extract

1 teaspoon cinnamon
2 teaspoons toasted wheat germ
1 tablespoon Bragg Organic Raw
    Apple Cider Vinegar
2 tablespoons sliced almonds

In a blender, mix peaches, milk, and ice cream; add vanilla, cinnamon, and wheat germ. Pour into a glass. Top with nuts. Serves two.

These are two smoothies, but there are hundreds to make during the summertime. Use your imagination and try seasonal fruits and vegetables, too. No-cook treats like these will make you smile and provide you more time for whatever is on your plate.

THE VINEGAR MAN'S VINEGAR DIET

While I can personally attest that the Quickie Seven-Day Detox Vinegar Diet and beauty tips work, some folks do not include the words "fat-burning diet" in their vocabulary. The Vinegar Man, Lawrence Diggs, is one of them. He believes in a more practical approach to keeping your weight in check.

"Most people are looking for those 'Oprah' diets. But this is the ultimate vinegar diet. It is rather simple, and it will really work. So if you would rather commiserate with your friend and forever talk about losing weight, this is not the diet for you."

But if you really want to lose weight, try the Vinegar Man's 10 tips:

1. Read at least one funny joke every day.
2. Do something nice for someone every day.
3. Have at least a little fun every day.
4. Say something nice about someone every day.
5. Think positive thoughts all of the time. This will put you in the proper frame of mind to stick with the diet. If you don't do those

things, you will most likely feel sorry for yourself and give up on the rest of the diet too soon for it to take effect.

6. Eat only vegetable salads liberally doused with a tasty vinegar and no oil.
7. Chew the salad at least 32 times per mouthful.
8. Eat no more than 5 hours before sleeping.
9. Get 20 minutes of vigorous (break-a-sweat) exercise every other day.
10. This will help you lose weight. If it doesn't, nothing will. In fact, it may work too well, so check with your doctor to make sure you aren't losing too much weight too fast.

And if you want to gain some of the weight back, you can use vinegar to make vinegar cookies.

Sandwiches and salads with vinegar can help you get and stay lean, but indulging in sweet stuff, like cute vinegar cookies for that sweet tooth and a cozy comfort-food kick also can help you keep the unwanted pounds off forever.

THE VINEGAR MAN'S VINEGAR COOKIES

Without a doubt, these cookies are easy to make, and you can healthy them up with healthful ingredients—including vinegar. Says the Vinegar Man, "Vinegar cookies are the nicest cookies I have tasted. They are rather easy to make and have a unique sweet and sour taste. You don't actually taste the vinegar right away. But it is there, and it adds something really special to the taste of these cookies. Try 'em!"

½ cup butter (margarine doesn't work)
½ teaspoon salt
1 egg
2 tablespoons pecan vinegar
¾ cup sugar

Put into a large bowl and blend until the butter is soft and all of the ingredients are mixed well.

Stir these ingredients well, then add

1¼ cups flour
¼ teaspoon baking powder

Mix well. Bake at 350 degrees until slightly brown (about 10 minutes in a gas oven). Add some nuts or raisins if you like. Try different kinds of vinegar. Each vinegar has something special to offer to these cookies.

(*Courtesy*: the Vinegar Man.)

While keeping lean and fit with vinegar is essential to good health, in the next chapter you will find out that there are also other vinegar-related strategies that will help you to live longer.

VINEGARY HEALING HINTS TO PRESERVE

✓ Apple cider vinegar can help you to burn fat.

✓ Choose the right carbs—whole grains, fruits, vegetables, and fat-fighting vinegar—to help you burn fat 24 hours a day.

✓ Burn fat and lose unwanted pounds with a detoxifying, healthful diet plan that includes physical activity.

✓ Take care of your outer beauty by using vinegar externally and internally.

✓ Set realistic weight-loss goals and nourish your body, mind, and spirit every day, like the Vinegar Man recommends, if you want to lose weight and keep it off for good, as well as achieve body love.

Antiaging Wonder Food

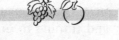

Life is like wine. The longer you take to enjoy it,
the more chance you've got of tasting vinegar.
—Anonymous[1]

Keeping slim and healthy with vinegars—not just the cider variety—is a feat I've accomplished since I wrote the first edition of *The Healing Powers of Vinegar* back in the twentieth century; I've taken the theory that the French don't get fat by embracing the Mediteranean diet and lifestyle into the twenty-first century.

When I arrived in Montreal, Canada (for the second time), I awoke at noon (thanks to jet lag). It was a chilly ten degrees and overcast. In my hotel room I grabbed the phone to ring room service while awestruck, looking out at the view of the city through the window on the twenty-eighth floor. It was too late to order blueberry waffles. We ended up making a lunch with some vinegary special requests.

Twenty minutes later, there was a knock on the door. I was greeted with food delivered by the Canadian chef. It was a grilled cheese on whole wheat (with tomatoes, spinach, lettuce, and a splash of red wine vinegar) paired with a salad I eyed in the menu ("melangees et vinaigrette mixed greens"). Once munching on the gooey cheese, warm toasted bread, and salad while anticipating a train ride to Quebec City,

I felt like a kid. The sandwich and fresh greens were comforting; I was feeling a bit seasick with waves of homesickness: dog-less and solo in a French-speaking province that I vowed to revisit when I traveled with my dog, but it spooked me decades ago.

As a child, I made grilled cheese by using a single slice of Kraft American cheese put on two white slices of Wonder bread melted with margarine. This remake of the fifties is much healthier, including whole wheat sourdough bread, fresh tomatoes, and potatoes. Traveling out of the country and turning to nutrient-dense age-defying foods—including vinegars—helps me feel younger and more energetic at any age.

I'm a California woman with a petite body (120 pounds, size 4—ideal for my 5 foot 4 inch frame). I know I look younger than old. My neighbors, and even my hypercritical brother, think I look super-young for my age. And they insist it's the vinegar in my diet. (Just kidding.) It's most likely in my genes, as well as my maintaining a healthy lifestyle—including consuming vinegar—and the Mediterranean diet.

In the twenty-first century, the average lifespan for people in America is about 77 to 81, and is on the rise. But, obesity-related diseases are believed to have reduced life expectancy by contributing to cancers, heart disease, and diabetes.[2]

I believe staying young longer is all about making choices when it comes to eating right and living a healthy lifestyle. I also know, as a health writer, that women and men in their 30s, 40s, 50s, and beyond don't have to look or feel their age. And I do give credit to Mother Nature's wonder foods—which, yes, include vinegars of all kinds.

FOUNTAIN OF YOUTH IN A BOTTLE

When I spoke with Patricia Bragg, I was impressed by her enthusiasm and youthful spirit and mind. She is one of the founders of the Longer Life, Health and Happiness Club, which exercises daily at Waikiki Beach in Honolulu. An ageless lady with boundless energy, Bragg told me that she still goes to Hawaii, a place where the longevity rate is high due to the healthful lifestyle.

According to an item on the Bragg Live Foods website (*http://www.bragg.com*), superstars Clint Eastwood, Demi Moore, Madonna, and the Beach Boys are dedicated consumers of Bragg's organic apple cider vinegar.[3]

A few days ago, I went to my local store and purchased a bottle of the Bragg raw unfiltered organic apple cider vinegar (with the mother on the label). The label says, "Go Organic!" and "Have an Apple Healthy Day!" These sayings didn't surprise me. When I've talked with Bragg on the phone, I've found her to be a down-to-earth woman. And I trusted her recommendation on the back of the bottle: "Perfect taken 3 times daily—upon arising, mid-morning and mid-afternoon. 1 to 2 tsps. Bragg Organic Vinegar in 8 oz. Glass Purified Water and (optional) 1 to 2 tsps. Organic Honey."

I admit it. I opened the bottle and smelled a strong aroma. Since I'm not a person who likes to dive into a swimming pool (I prefer to inch my way in slowly), I decided to use Bragg's vinegar step by step.

For instance, this morning, I splashed the apple cider vinegar on my face. And yes, instantly it did give me that rosy, healthy glow that women all love to have. My skin really did feel soft and supple. No kidding. And of course, I am curious to experience other ways it can make me feel younger.

I also noticed another catchy item on the ageless health guru's website. Bragg practices what she preaches. She recommends six strategies:

1. Stay clear of all refined and processed foods.
2. Eat lots of fruit and vegetables every day.
3. Begin each meal with a raw salad.
4. Try herbal substitutes for coffee and tea. (We disagree on these two superfoods.)
5. Take long walks of at least 2 miles as often as you possibly can.
6. Cleanse your body three times a day by drinking a cocktail of organic apple cider vinegar, honey, and water. Mix 1 to 2 teaspoons of cider vinegar with 1 to 2 teaspoons of honey in water.[4]

DO YOU BELIEVE IN MIRACLES?

As a journalist and health-conscious consumer, I've always been wary of "miracle" cures. And you might think that I'm pushing apple cider vinegar as one more miracle food. But when I think of miracles, I can't help but recall vinegar guru Bragg and a conversation I had with her one evening.

Bragg is a very optimistic woman, and she always seems extremely centered. One night while we spoke on the phone, Bragg sensed tension in my voice and mentioned this fact. So I told her the truth: "I'm recovering from dental surgery. I'm in pain and waiting for the stitches to dissolve."

She asked me if I'd like her to perform a spiritual prayer. There was a pregnant pause, and then I said, "Sure." I assumed she would do it when we hung up. Not so. She conducted quite a lengthy prayer, and I felt a strange chill run through my body until she was done. After a while, we said good-bye.

Minutes later, I realized I had no pain in my upper gum. I ran my tongue over the area, and the stitches were gone. They had dissolved. I vowed at that moment to believe in this woman's lifestyle, and thus I became an apple cider vinegar believer for countless uses. (But I love other vinegars, too.)

TURN BACK THE CLOCK

Stop searching for the fountain of youth. Just turn to some of your favorite foods (and vinegar) to turn back the hands of time.

When you eat a variety of healthful superfoods that contain disease-fighting antioxidants, you can forestall or prevent ailments associated with aging, explains Jeffrey Blumberg, Ph.D.

"You'll still get older," says Dr. Blumberg, the antioxidant wizard, "but you'll increase your lifespan."

Experts agree. The healthier you are, the younger your body stays. Maybe Old Man Time can't be fooled, but you can get him on your side and look forever young from head to toe. Here are ten antiaging, healthy-up, slim-down food strategies.

1 **SAVE FACE** Feeding your skin with an orange or fortified orange juice is a smart idea. This fruit contains high levels of vitamin C and heart-healthy folic acid. Vitamin C is a powerful age-defying antioxidant that can help protect the skin inside and outside your body.

Antiaging Bonus: One medium orange has just 65 calories, less than 1 gram of fat, and a good amount of fiber.

Vinegar Rx: Each morning, team that orange with 8 ounces of water and 2 tablespoons of apple cider vinegar to boost that childlike glow.

2 **CROWNING GLORY** Since your hair is 97 percent protein and 3 percent water, hair nutrition experts agree that a diet rich in protein is key to a thick, soft, and shiny mane. Protein-rich turkey builds amino acids, which strengthen hair.

Antiaging Bonus: Three ounces of white meat is a mere 133 calories, and roasted turkey breast is lower in fat than other types of meat.

Vinegar Rx: Opt for a turkey sandwich on whole wheat bread. Pile on the tomatoes, dark green lettuce, heart-healthy red wine vinegar, and olive oil (which is good for both skin and hair).

3 **SHARP BRAIN** According to research, blueberries seem to slow and even reverse many of the degenerative diseases associated with aging. Scientists at the USDA Human Nutrition Research Center on Aging at Tufts University have found that blueberries—rich in vitamins A and C and other nutrients—have a functional antioxidant and anti-inflammatory effect on brain and muscle tissue.

Antiaging Bonus: One cup of blueberries contains only 81 calories and no fat, cholesterol, or sodium. They taste great, too!

Vinegar Rx: Try a decadent and healthful dessert of calcium-rich vanilla yogurt with blueberries, and drizzle sweet balsamic vinegar or a fruit-flavored vinegar on top.

4 **CLEAR EYES** Want to preserve your sharp vision? Leutein, found in eggs, may help protect your eyes from damage caused by sunlight. Diets rich in leutein may also decrease the risk for cataracts and age-related macular degeneration.

Antiaging Bonus: One medium-boiled egg is rich in leutein and has only 69 calories. Try eating just the hard-cooked egg white—it's low in fat and calories.

Vinegar Rx: To complete your breakfast, include grapefruit, a whole grain bagel, and a hot cup of tea with a tablespoon or two of apple cider vinegar.

5 **PEARLY WHITES** It is believed by scientists and nutritionists that green tea can fight tooth decay and keep your teeth and gums healthy. Scientists believe that tea's polyphenol content destroys bacteria.

Antiaging bonus: One cup of green teas has no fat, sodium, sugar, or calories.

Vinegar Rx: Since some reports indicate vinegar might be harmful to tooth enamel, it may be wise to include green tea in your daily diet. This, in turn, may prevent potential dental problems that might be linked to acidic vinegar.

6 **HEALTHY BREASTS** Soy protein may save your breasts. Soy contains isoflavones, daidzein, and genistein, which have been linked with a lowered risk of breast cancer. The soy protein, rather than its isoflavone component, is what seems to be beneficial.

Antiaging Bonus: This popular "health food" has less than 100 calories per 3.5 ounces.

Vinegar Rx: If you stir-fry tofu with veggies, you can add rice vinegar and enjoy its flavor and healthful perks, too.

7 **YOUNG HEART** The alpha carotene in pumpkin, a fall favorite, makes this vegetable a nutritional bonanza. Pumpkin is rich in heart-healthy carotenoids, potassium, magnesium, and folate, all of which may protect you from heart disease, the number one killer of women.

Antiaging Bonus: This stay-young food has only 25 calories per half cup and no fat.

Vinegar Rx: During the cold season, a warming and healthful dessert is a slice of pumpkin pie teamed with a steaming cup of hot water spiked with a tablespoon or two of apple cider vinegar.

8 **HAPPY COLON** Tomatoes, rich in the antioxidant lycopene, may lower the risk of developing colon cancer by preventing damage caused by harmful molecules called free radicals that contribute to cancer.

Antiaging Bonus: One cup of chopped tomatoes has just 35 calories. Because of this, tomatoes are a fat-free, nutrient-rich, and versatile filler in many low-cal meals.

Vinegar Rx: Also add red wine vinegar to Italian dishes and salads with tomatoes to maintain a healthy heart.

9 **STRONG BONES** Calcium-rich yogurt can help you maintain strong bones. If your diet is deficient in calcium your body will steal it from your bones. This weakens your skeleton, and can lead to brittle bone disease (at any age).

Antiaging Bonus: One cup of non-fat, fruit-flavored yogurt has about 150 calories and less than 2 grams of fat.

Vinegar Rx: When eating a fiber-rich baked potato, rather than sabotaging it with high-fat butter or margarine, try a dollop of plain yogurt with a splash of vinegar for a tasty and good-for-you treat.

10 **SMOOTH SKIN** Salmon, like oranges, is a great skin-nourishing food. Rich in fatty acids (essential omega-3s), salmon will help keep your skin moisturized, say nutritionists. That means silky hands, smooth thighs, and soft legs and feet.

Antiaging Bonus: With just 233 calories per 4.5-ounce serving, this tasty fish is a dieter's delight. Plus, it's fairly low in sodium and has just 3 grams of fat per 3-ounce serving.

Vinegar Rx: Try cooking salmon with red wine vinegar and olive oil, two super-powered antiaging wonders.

VINEGAR PLUS TESTS FOR A HEALTHY YOU

While using vinegar with health superfoods can certainly help keep you on the healthy track, taking precautions even though you may be feeling fine just may save your life in the long run. And since metabolic syndrome is not going anywhere soon (see Chapter 15, "The Liquid to Heart Health"), it's time to welcome little tests that can have a big impact on your overall wellness throughout your life. In other words, I repeat, vinegar isn't a miracle cure-all. You need to do more.

In Your 20s

At 20-something, you're at your physical peak. You'll want to get annual checkups, which should include a blood pressure measurement and body weight check. Keep in mind that even slim people can be obese. Above 28 percent body fat for women and above 23 percent body fat for men are red flags. Diet, exercise, and fat-fighting vinegar should be your first courses of action.

In Your 30s

In your 30s, like your 20s, your overall health is typically decent, provided your diet, exercise regimen, and lifestyle are healthy. You'll want to continue getting annual checkups (including a dental checkup twice a year—remember, vinegar is acidic, like citrus, which may cause problems for some people's teeth), and you should also start to consider getting some blood tests.

A complete cholesterol test—commonly called a "lipid profile"—is a blood test that will calculate your total cholesterol and triglyceride levels. Levels of 240 milligrams or higher, are considered high risk, and levels from 200 to 239 are considered borderline high risk, according to the American Heart Association (AHA). Levels below 200 milligrams are desirable and put you at a lower risk for heart disease, reports the AHA. The ideal is an HDL cholesterol (the "good" stuff) level over 40, an LDL cholesterol (the artery-clogging "bad" stuff) level below 100, and a triglyceride level below 150. If you have high cholesterol, your doctor will discuss lifestyle changes. Diet, exercise, and heart-healthy vinegar should be your first courses of action.

In Your 40s

In their 40s, women and men begin to enter middle age, and chronic diseases may begin to make their appearances. During your annual checkup, you should begin to request specific tests.

A fasting blood sugar test will identify whether you have diabetes (type 1 or 2) or pre-diabetes, a disease characterized by elevated levels of blood sugar, or glucose, which result from the body's inability to make enough insulin, a hormone.

When fasting, your blood sugar should be under 100. If it's between 100 and 125 you have pre-diabetes and should be counseled about the risks of diabetes. The good news is, most people with diabetes have type 2, not type 1, which requires daily insulin injections. And people with type 2 diabetes can usually control the disease with diet and lifestyle changes. Diet, exercise, and healthful vinegar should be your first courses of action.

In Your 50s and Beyond

If you are a menopausal or post-menopausal woman, doctors caution, your heart might experience some physical changes (due to loss of estrogen) that can lead to an increased risk of cardiovascular diseases. After your annual checkup, ask for one more must-have test.

An electrocardiogram (EKG) diagnoses silent heart disease or thickening of the heart muscle by checking the electrical activity of the heart. If any of these problems are found, you'll be advised about lifestyle changes (such as a heart-healthy diet and exercise) and/or prescribed the appropriate medication. Personally, I prefer diet, exercise, and vinegar to costly drugs with side effects. Diet, exercise, and heart-healthy vinegar should be your first courses of action.

Balsamic Honey Marinated Carrots and Parsnips

❖ ❖ ❖

½ pound carrots
½ pound parsnips
3 tablespoons olive oil
1½ tablespoons balsamic honey
   vinegar
zest of one lemon

juice of ½ lemon
½ tablespoon fresh chopped
   oregano
1 teaspoon crushed garlic
⅓ teaspoon salt
pinch of pepper

Peel and cut the carrots and parsnips into uniform pieces. Place in a pot with cold water and heat slowly, never boiling, until desired tenderness is achieved. In a bowl mix the remaining ingredients including oil, vinegar, lemon zest, lemon juice, oregano, garlic, salt, and pepper. Drain and cool the carrots and parsnips, pour the marinade over the cooked carrots and parsnips. Great side dish for any occasion. Note: ½ cup is one serving size.

(*Courtesy:* Honey Ridge Farms.)

VINEGARY HEALING HINTS TO PRESERVE

✓ Vinegar can be a great tool in the fight against hypertension, high cholesterol, diabetes, and obesity.
✓ Celebrities use vinegar for its touted health and longevity benefits.
✓ Health guru Patricia Bragg practices what she preaches and includes vinegar in her daily regimen.

✓ Teaming antiaging superfoods and a variety of vinegars may help you stay healthy and live longer.

✓ Must-have health tests are essential for long-term health, which can often be achieved with a healthy lifestyle, exercise, and vinegar.

Now that you know some of the ways to live longer, let me show you how to make your days, weeks, and years happier and healthier with simple and easy-to-use vinegar home cures.

PART 6

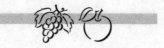

VINEGAR REMEDIES

1 8

Home Cures

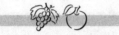

Nature opened the first drugstore.[1]
—D. C. Jarvis, M.D.

During my second treasured journey to Montreal, Quebec, an untimely mishap occurred and vinegar—not my soul mate with paws—was my best friend. On the first day I stayed close to the city knowing my trip to Quebec City was up next. I ended up at a large drugstore. A young French Canadian woman who waited on me wore catlike eye makeup that looked smoky, natural and beautiful. She gave me a one-on-one demo. Once back at my hotel room, I tried the tricks and it worked.

Two hours later, trouble paid me a visit. The eye makeup I used was not hypoallergenic. The skin around my eyes began to itch, turn red, and swell. I was miserable. I kept my nail appointment at the hotel. The manicurist removed the eye makeup and it burned badly. I ended up calling the hotel doctor once back at my room. He told me to use cold compresses. I ordered a dinner salad since I was too embarrassed to go out and be seen. Not to mention the pain of it all. So once my salad with a wine vinaigrette arrived, I dipped the washcloth that had been soaked in into the vinegar and put it under and around my eyes. I knew that red wine vinegar, like cider vinegar, has anti-inflammatory benefits. By four A.M. my eyes looked less red and puffy. Once in

Quebec City I found a pharmacy and a bilingual pharmacist said, "You need antihistaminique." The over-the-counter white tablets in a box with French words helped dry up my watery eyeballs. But so did the vinegar (on my irritated red eyelids), like a comforting canine (as it did its job of soothing the burn when I was in pain and away from home and creature comforts).

Chances are, apple cider, red wine, rice, and other vinegars—your everyday household products—contain even more extraordinary healing powers that you might not know about. The next time you need a natural remedy for a minor ailment, check this list first to see if a cure is as close as your kitchen cabinet or pantry.

I'll describe 55 common health ailments and cosmetic uses, from A to Z, and provide common at-home vinegar folk remedies. Some treatments can be used inside and others outside the body. Keep in mind, these are based on anecdotal evidence. There is a lack of clinical double-blind studies (but research may be done in the future) to back up their effectiveness and make it conclusive.

But first, just listen to real stories from real people, like you and me, who have medical uses for vinegar and vow that it can and really does work!

"IT WORKED FOR ME!"
REAL STORIES ABOUT VINEGAR

Personal stories often are even more convincing than statistics, studies, and even doctors' advice. Here, take a look at real-life people. You be the judge.

Bee Stings

I have a high regard for vinegar since it has come to my rescue more than once. I was stung on the hand by a bee while in the garden one day. The sting was very painful and frightening. I came running into the house, yelling to my husband that I'd been stung. I proceeded to tell him how painful it was.

I'm the nurse in the family so I should have known what to do, but sometimes when the injury is to yourself and you're in a lot of pain, you don't. My dear husband took over; he told me all about the vinegar book he was reading and how vinegar would take the pain away. I was quite leery. I knew that vinegar was acetic acid and I was afraid it would make it hurt more. My husband poured vinegar over my inflamed finger and within 15 seconds the pain was completely gone! The finger never swelled and the redness that had already started went away completely! I had no more pain and I was able to go on with my day and use my hand like nothing had ever happened![2]

—*Bonnie K. McMillen, R.N.*

Plantar Warts

The next time vinegar came to my rescue was for an ongoing problem I was having with plantar warts on the bottom of my foot. I contracted the pesky virus from the local Y's locker room floor. It was spreading and I was dreading going to the podiatrist because I knew it would involve money and pain. Instead, I luckily thought of vinegar . . . it had saved me before . . . could it get rid of plantar warts? I decided it was worth a try. I soaked my foot about three times a week. I should have done it every night but I just couldn't remember to do it every night. Nothing happened for about 2–3 weeks but I was determined to make life on my foot very uncomfortable for these warts. So after every soak I would rub my foot vigorously with a clean towel. Finally after about 2–3 weeks I noticed the nasty little black warts were loosening their grip on my foot and some were being toweled away!

This was incredible but it made perfect sense! Salicylic acid is the common ingredient in over-the-counter remedies for treating warts, and vinegar is acetic acid . . . still an acid but a much gentler treatment. I continued to soak my foot every night and within 5–6 weeks or so from the beginning of treatment the 15 or 20 warts were completely gone and have not recurred. I also learned to wear shower shoes at the gym and to never walk around a locker room or pool area in my bare feet.[3]

—*Bonnie K. McMillen, R.N.*

Sunburn

I remember getting the worst sunburn of my life on a Florida beach. I did not use sunscreen, but at the time I was taking Bactrim, and completely forgot about the warnings to avoid the sun while taking that medication. The result was a sunburn so painful and blistering that I could not even sit down comfortably. I took some acetaminophen and whined a lot. Then our neighbor suggested using white vinegar on the sunburn. I will never forget the relief that the vinegar provided.[4]

—*Carol Mulvihill*

Burns

In the spring of 1956, I was 18 years old and living in Sacramento with my parents. One evening after frying bacon, I was draining off the boiling grease when the handle on the frying pan broke and the grease spilled all over my right palm and fingers. Needless to say, it hurt a great deal. All the emergency room doctors could do was put some sort of cream on it and a bandage and suggest I immerse the hand in cold water to ease the pain. Big help that was! Took quite a while to heal.

Many years later, 1970 I think, while yet again frying bacon for my three sons and me, the handle on the frying pan broke loose and once again boiling grease flowed over my right palm and fingers. Oddly enough it was the same frying pan my father had put a new handle on, and up till then it worked fine. But this time I was prepared!

I had been delving into metaphysical healing, and of the many things I came across was using "apple cider vinegar" on burns. So I quickly and calmly poured the vinegar over my hand and intoned the prayer, "I am now perfectly healed in the name of Jesus Christ our Lord!" Immediately upon looking at both my palms, it was impossible to tell which one had been burned. The hand was perfect. To this day, we always use the vinegar and prayer for any burns of any kind, with the same healing results.

—*Mrs. Janice Oszust*

FIFTY-FIVE AMAZING VINEGAR REMEDIES

Did you know that vinegar is considered one of the top 20 home remedies, according to an article in the *New York Daily News*?[5] "Vinegar has been a trusted home remedy that your mother, your grandmother, and their grandmothers have known. It literally can be used from head to toe. Scalp problems such as dandruff, athlete's foot, yeast infections, even headaches, are no match for this remedy. It can also be used as a cosmetic, to help protect and beautify your skin," agrees Dr. Earl Mindell, author of *Dr. Earl Mindell's Amazing Apple Cider Vinegar*.

Well, if this surprises you, read on, and you'll see why it's an amazing remedy that you want to have in your home.

1 ACID REFLUX DISEASE (Zap the burn) This common ailment is simply an inflammation of the esophagus. It's also known as heartburn or GERD (gastroesophageal reflux disease). Simply put, "Hydrochloric acid from the stomach backs up into the esophagus. Drugs that combat acid reflux disease reduce the amount of acid produced by the stomach, but that is not necessarily the best way to treat the condition," says *Natural Cures* author Mary Ann Cooper.[6]

What Vinegar Remedy to Use: I recall one young woman who believed in natural remedies telling me that when she was pregnant, the only thing that would cure her acid reflux problem was vinegar. She said that she religiously took a tablespoon of apple cider vinegar in a glass of water to treat and prevent this pesky problem.

Why You'll Like It: If you don't like taking unnatural, yucky-tasting antacids or prescription medications for this annoying condition, all-natural vinegar may be just the natural cure for you.

2 ACNE (Good-bye to breakouts) Acne plagues not only teenagers, but adult women too. More than 17 million American women—in their twenties, thirties, and forties—suffering from postadolescent outbreaks of adult acne.

If you have acne, genetics may be the primary cause. Unfortunately, some of us are born with acne-prone pores. Yet if you're predisposed to mild acne, you can keep it under control with vinegar.

What Vinegar Remedy to Use: To get rid of acne, make a mixture of 2 teaspoons of plain or herbal apple cider vinegar in 1 cup of water and dab on blemishes several times a day after washing.

Why You'll Like It: If you already have acne, you know the physical pain and self-consciousness it can create. Instead of having to go out and buy acne medicine, you can go to your kitchen cabinet. Not only is ACV readily available but it costs pennies to use. The best part is, it can help dry up blemishes. One day, I noticed a red blemish on my nose. I quickly turned to ACV (I didn't have any alcohol). And you know what? The very next day, the blemish was gone. No kidding.

3 ANGINA (Baby your heart) Angina is usually caused by a lack of blood and oxygen supplied to the cells of your heart muscle, which occurs after an emotional upset. It can often be relieved by rest and relaxation. That's where vinegar and my favorite chamomile tea comes to the rescue.

What Vinegar Remedy to Use: Pour 1 cup of boiling water over 1 tablespoon of dried flower heads or 1 tea bag. Let the mixture steep for a few minutes, strain, and add 1 teaspoon of apple cider vinegar and honey to taste. Drink 1 cup. (See "Anxiety," below, to learn how ACV works to calm the chest pains and tightness that may occur when you are stressed-out or under pressure.)

Why You'll Like It: It beats going to the ER and spending thousands of dollars to be told by a doctor or nurse that you need to "decompress." Also, an improved, low-fat, low-cholesterol diet, an exercise regimen, and stress-reduction techniques are cardiologists' first courses of action for treatment of angina.

4 ANXIETY (Soothe your nerves) Want to chill from modern-day stressors? Vinegar can be used for calming and mild sedation. In fact, past research at Yale University showed that for some people, the aroma of spiced apples can stave off a panic attack and lower stress levels.

What Vinegar Remedy to Use: Make an anti-anxiety cocktail by putting 1 tablespoon of apple cider vinegar into 1 cup of boiling water and simmering it for a few minutes. Add a cinnamon stick and honey to taste. For an extra relaxing boost, drop a chamomile tea bag into the cup.

Why You'll Like It: On a hectic day or cold winter night, this wonderful smelling hot drink (or iced tea) will soothe your frazzled nerves and help you to chill out.

5 ARTHRITIS (Stop the pain) Folk medicine holds that ACV can help fight arthritis. While no scientific studies prove this to be true, and conventional doctors frown at the thought of vinegar as an antiarthritis remedy, testimony gives nutrient-rich apple cider vinegar kudos for providing relief for the debilitating disease.

What Vinegar Remedy to Use: The popular remedy is simple. Take 2 spoonfuls of apple cider vinegar and honey in a glass of water several times daily.

Why You'll Like It: If it works for you, you will be happy because it's natural, which means there will be no ill side effects from pain medications. Plus, it's low-cost and easy to apply.

6 ASTRINGENT (Freshen it up) An astringent can help close facial pores and refresh the skin. An ancient formula created by the gypsies in the 5th century was used by the Queen of Hungary.

What Vinegar Remedy to Use: Mix red wine vinegar, witch hazel extract, pure rose water, rosemary, and rose fragrance.

Why You'll Like It: Not only can this help perk up your skin, it can be used as an after-bath, after-wash, or after-shave, too.

7 ATHLETE'S FOOT (Treat your feet) Athlete's foot is a form of fungus infection of the feet. The fact is, athlete's foot doesn't happen among people who go barefoot. It's moisture, sweating, and lack of proper air of the feet that provide the ideal setting for athlete's foot to grow.

What Vinegar Remedy to Use: Rinse your feet several times a day with plain or herbal apple cider vinegar. I can personally attest that it burns, then soothes the skin between the toes and redness.

Why You'll Like It: Apple cider vinegar may relieve the itching of athlete's foot. Better yet, it can help prevent it, too. Its acid content helps stop fungus growth. A bonus: Apple cider vinegar is not as messy as prescription ointments. One ACV user praises its abilities: "After trying all kinds of over-the-counter stuff, I finally cured my athlete's foot by spraying regular white vinegar on my feet at night for about a week. I still swear by this—much cheaper and effective."

8 BLACK-AND-BLUE BRUISES (Heal the marks) Let's face it. Bruises hit everyone (at any age) sooner or later. A black-and-blue mark shows up when a bump to the body injures blood vessels, causing bleeding under the skin. If you get Humpty Dumpty bruises often, you might want to take a look at your diet. Is it well balanced? Are you getting enough vitamin B? Meanwhile, to make that bruise disappear, try vinegar.

What Vinegar Remedy to Use: A common method is to soak a cotton ball (gauze will work, too) and put it on the bruise for about 60 minutes. I suggest watching your favorite TV program to make the time pass faster. It's believed that the vinegar decreases the discoloration and the healing period.

Why You'll Like It: If you have an unsightly black-and-blue mark in an area that can be seen (for example, on your leg or arm), any remedy that speeds up the recovery process will make you more apt to wear that dress or blouse for the special occasion.

9 BURNS (Ease the pain) Ever burn yourself on the stovetop, iron, or fireplace? Ouch! Any burn that affects your body should be attended to ASAP. The reason: You'll want to keep inflammation and swelling at a minimum.

What Vinegar Remedy to Use: Apply apple cider vinegar, straight out of the bottle, to a burn on the surface of the body. Better still, apply ice cold vinegar right away for fast relief.

Why You'll Like It: It may help alleviate smarting and soreness and prevent blisters.

10 CANKER SORES (Baby the ouch) Uh-oh! If you have ever had those small, oh-so-painful, round ulcers inside your mouth, you know that you'd do anything for a cure that works. Sometimes a flare-up hits (and lasts for up to 10 days) when you're stressed-out, wearing dentures, eating hot food, or having an aggressive dental procedure—like I had.

What Vinegar Remedy to Use: Dab apple cider vinegar onto the canker sores using a cotton swab. Repeat four times daily.

Why You'll Like It: While some over-the-counter medications can help ease the pain, their taste isn't anything to write home to mom about. I tried salt water, green tea, ice—nothing worked. (I didn't know about ACV for this ailment, or I would have tried it.) If it works for you, you will be smiling sooner than later.

11 CHAPPED SKIN (Smooth it on) During the dry, cold winter months, dry skin can be a problem from head to toe. If you can't fly off to the Bahamas, what's the next best thing to do? Take a vinegar vacation.

What Vinegar Remedy to Use: Mix your best hand cream and vinegar. Apply this vinegar cream each time after you wash your hands.

Why You'll Like It: If your hand cream is made of natural ingredients, you will have a natural product that can soothe, smooth, and heal hands fast naturally.

12 COLD (Bye-bye sniffles) Got a runny nose, sore throat, cough, muscle aches, and pains? Poor baby, you've got a cold. Rose hips, a key staple in the diets of Native American tribes, may help boost immunity and provide relief from cold and cough symptoms. If you pair up this herbal wonder with vinegar, you might be able to say good riddance to your nasty bug. Or, you can turn to vinegar solo.

What Vinegar Remedy to Use: Mix ¼ cup of apple cider vinegar with ¼ cup of honey. Take 1 tablespoon six to eight times daily.

Why You'll Like It: Personally, when I have a cold, I don't like to turn to store-bought cold remedies, with all of their ingredients that I can't pronounce. I prefer a cold to run its course naturally. But I do turn to Mother Nature—drink plenty of liquids, including herbal teas; get bed rest; and, of course, "take" my vinegar. (I vow to do it next time.)

13 CONGESTION (Clear it up) When it comes to fighting colds and sinus congestion, apple cider vinegar comes to the rescue, according to folk medicine. Joann Korzenko of Ohio knows too well that her grandson gets terrible colds and congestion. "We make sure he has plenty of salad, and we get him to eat that with ACV on it. My daughter says she notices a difference right away. So I guess you wouldn't have to gargle with it," she points out. But there's one more way to get the anti-congestion effect, too.

What Vinegar Remedy to Use: To clear up clogged respiratory congestion, inhale a vapor mist from a steaming pot containing water and several spoonfuls of vinegar.

Why You'll Like It: It will help clear the air passages naturally, and you'll be breathing easy again.

14 CONSTIPATION (Stay super regular) Ugh! While irregularity tends to hit seniors who are inactive, it can strike people of any age, especially if you're stressed out, not drinking enough water, and not eating enough dietary fiber. Fiber-rich apple cider vinegar comes to the rescue.

What Vinegar Remedy to Use: To clear up a clogged system, try 2 tablespoons of apple cider vinegar in a glass of warm water upon rising in the morning. I remember a 52-year-old woman who lived in a Northern California coastal town. She was the epitome of health: lean, glowing, and energetic. And this is the remedy she used and recommended that I follow seven days a week like clockwork.

Why You'll Like It: Rather than be sluggish or turn to laxatives, try this all-natural and cost-effective remedy to help you stay regular, and you'll feel energized whether you're 22, 52, or 72.

15 CORNS (Say good riddance) Corns are the most common condition of the foot. Simply put, a corn is a thickening of the outer layer of skin—often at the tops of the toes.

What Vinegar Remedy to Use: Combine two slices of white bread and two onion slices with 1 cup of vinegar for one day. Put the bread on your corn, top with a slice of onion, and wrap with a bandage overnight.

Why You'll Like It: It is a creative folk remedy that can be fun and worth the time and effort if it works.

16 COUGH (Stop that tickle) Hack, hack, hack. Coughs come with everything from the common cold to acute bronchitis, which causes mucus in the throat and lungs. Not only is coughing annoying, but it can hurt your chest after a while, too. Soon you want something to make the symptom go away.

What Vinegar Remedy to Use: Mix $1/2$ cup of apple cider vinegar, $1/2$ cup of water, 1 teaspoon of cayenne pepper, and 4 teaspoons of honey. Take 1 tablespoon when your cough starts up. Take another at bedtime.

Why You'll Like It: Cough drops and syrups are available, but they can be costly. Plus, if you run out in the middle of the night, it's a hassle to have to go to the store. It would be nice to find an inexpensive, natural cure that you always have around the house, like vinegar, which works, right?

17 DANDRUFF (Lose the flakes) If you suffer from dry flakes and dry scalp, you are hardly alone. Skin complaints can be helped with external use of vinegar. It is thought that the vinegar kills the bacteria which is believed to be the cause.

What Vinegar Remedy to Use: Massage a small amount of apple cider vinegar directly into the washed scalp, leave on for up to 1 minute, then rinse. Repeat this regimen daily until the flakes are gone.

Why You'll Like It: Apple cider vinegar is a safe and nontoxic remedy, whereas many dandruff shampoos on the market are chock-full of toxic chemicals. Plus, vinegar costs much, much less.

18 DEPRESSION (Feel more upbeat) The blues, which can happen during the winter (when they are called seasonal affective disorder) or as a result of psychological woes, can often trigger overeating, say medical experts, and the fiber-rich carbohydrates of vinegar may affect brain chemicals in a positive way. Vinegar can be used as a home remedy for people whose eating problems have an emotional basis.

What Vinegar Remedy to Use: To boost your mood, drink a cup of hot water with a teaspoon of apple cider vinegar. It might make you feel better because it's a soothing beverage with natural vitamins and minerals.

Why You'll Like It: If you're feeling down and overeat, you will just feed your depression. Instead, have a healthful hot apple cider drink, which is considered a "happy food."

19 DIZZINESS (Start feeling grounded) Feeling dizzy can be attributed to many causes, from prescription meds to hormonal changes. The fact remains, dizziness is not fun, and if you have ever felt this unsettling feeling, you might be willing to try a natural remedy such as vinegar to help keep you grounded, so to speak.

What Vinegar Remedy to Use: Dr. Jarvis notes that Vermont folk medicine is successful in treating dizziness, which he claims is due to "an alkaline reaction of the urine." He recommends the apple cider treatment, with the timing and dosage similar to those used for other ailments.[7]

Why You'll Like It: If you have ever felt lightheaded or like your world is spinning, you'll love this apple cider treatment, which will keep your feet and head steady without any side effects.

20 DOUCHE (Clean down below) As a child of the fifties, I remember a pink douche bag hanging up on the towel rack in my mother's shower stall. In my twenties, buying ready-to-use disposable douching products (scented) was the trendy thing to do. And I did it.

But that was the seventies. Things have changed. Today, some experts believe frequent douching may endanger a woman's health. It may increase a woman's risk of a vaginal infection and even her risk of cervical cancer.

But if you have chronic vaginal infections, medical doctors believe that an occasional douche can be helpful. What's more, if you have trichomonas (a one-celled organism causing a vaginal infection) while pregnant, rather than taking the prescribed Flagyl, a vinegar and water douche is recommended.

What Vinegar Remedy to Use: Try 2 tablespoons of white vinegar to a quart of water. Vinegar changes the acid balance of the vagina, staving off pesky monilia.

Why You'll Like It: For your health's sake, bear in mind that infrequent douching—once a week or less—with a mild solution of vinegar is safer than other strong chemical preparations.

21 EARACHE (Stop the hurt) Since moving to the Sierra mountains, I have realized that every winter I get an earache thanks to the low humidity and the high altitude. In fact, one time I ended up enduring a perforated eardrum. Since vinegar fights infection, it makes sense that it can be used to fight an oncoming earache caused by bacteria.

What Vinegar Remedy to Use: Dab apple cider vinegar on sore areas surrounding the outer ear canals (like you would do when cleaning out your cat's or dog's ears).

Why You'll Like It: If your ear is throbbing and it's late at night or no doctor is around, vinegar is the next best thing to help you fight an infection without antibiotics, which can have side effects.

22 ENERGIZE (Boost your drive) Feeling tired, run-down, a lack of drive? You're hardly alone. According to Edward Conley, D.O., in Grand Blanc, Michigan, an estimated 80 percent of adults complain of fatigue at one time or another. It is believed by many health gurus that vinegar can help you to feel more alert and energized.

What Vinegar Remedy to Use: Take 1 tablespoon of the potassium-rich energizer three times a day, preferably in 1 cup of water each time.

Why You'll Like It: While coffee and sugar can give you an instant boost, they can also leave you feeling like you're on a roller coaster with their ups and downs, and they can wreak havoc with your bedtime bliss. Vinegar beats fatigue and leaves you energized without ill effects.

23 FIBROMYALGIA (Lessen flare-ups) If you've got aches and pains in your muscles, you may have fibromyalgia. It's marked by tenderness upon the application of pressure in 11 or more of 18 "tender points," which include the back of the neck, lower back, and lateral hips. Stress, anxiety, and cold-weather changes can trigger flare-ups.

What Vinegar Remedy to Use: Forgo sugary soft drinks, caffeine, and alcohol. Instead, turn to 2 teaspoons of apple cider vinegar in a glass of hot spring water three times per day.

Why You'll Like It: Not only can this give you an energy boost, but when you drink an ACV beverage, you might chill out naturally.

24 FLU (Blast the bug) Do you have muscle aches and pains, headaches, low back pain, fatigue, and fever? If you are a victim of the flu season—or don't want to be—drink plenty of fluids. Water, herbal teas, and other liquids can flush out any toxins that you might accumulate, notes Ray Sahelian, M.D., of Southern California. For instance, goldenseal makes a great immunity-boosting tea because it contains berberine, an antibiotic substance that is a great flu fighter.

What Vinegar to Use: Try 1 teaspoon of the ground root of goldenseal in 1 cup of boiling water. Steep for a few minutes, then strain.

Add 1 tablespoon of apple cider vinegar with honey or lemon. Repeat three times daily.

Why You'll Like It: Nobody likes getting the flu, but everybody likes to pamper themselves back to good health. This herbal tea–vinegar remedy can be a cure that you will find just as soothing as Mom's chicken soup (which isn't a bad idea either).

25 FRECKLES (Lighten up spots) Although some people like the freckle look, many women want to lighten up freckles on the body.

What Vinegar Remedy to Use: Popular folk medicine believers claim that you can lighten freckles from neck to toe (not your face) by applying horseradish vinegar.

Why You'll Like It: Rather than use a harsh facial product to remove freckles, a natural remedy, like vinegar, may do the trick without ill side effects.

26 HANGNAILS (Smooth rough skin) Yes, this can be a health problem. In dry climates, the face and hands can become as dry as a lizard's skin, especially in the winter. After a day of shoveling snow, bringing in firewood, making a fire, and washing dishes, my hands are dry. Often, I will pull the cuticles, and that can lead to open, painful sores.

What Vinegar Remedy to Use: Dab apple cider vinegar on a tissue, and blot your cuticles.

Why You'll Like It: I swear you'll love this "miracle" remedy because it really works, and it does the job fast. After a visit to a dermatologist who suggested I use vasoline, I decided to give ACV a try. I've applied it twice in a three- to four-hour span. The redness is gone, and my fingers feel as smooth as my face does when I splash it with ACV.

27 HEADACHE (Lose the ache) The most common type of headache is the tension headache. It feels like a rubber band is being tightened around your head. And let's face it, almost everyone has or will experience at least one whopper.

What Vinegar Remedy to Use: To get rid of a tension headache, dab an herbal vinegar on your temples and lie down. Or dampen a cloth with the vinegar and put it on your forehead.

For relieving migraines, Dr. Jarvis recommends a vinegar vapor. Mix equal parts of vinegar and water in a pan on the stove and bring it to a boil. Lean your head over the pan and inhale the fumes for 75 breaths.

Why You'll Like It: If you have ever endured a headache, you will appreciate any remedy that works. And if it's easily accessible, like vinegar, and without the side effects that aspirin can have, all the better.

28 HEMORRHOIDS (Pamper your bum) I remember my dad had hemorrhoids, which are swollen blood vessels in the rectum and anus. And in college, when I dealt with constipation woes, I, too, developed this painful condition. Pregnant women are also often plagued by hemorrhoids.

What Vinegar Remedy to Use: Drink 3 glasses of water per day with 1 tablespoon of apple cider vinegar in each one. While you're at it, drink at least 5 more 8-ounce glasses of water daily, too.

Why You'll Like It: A natural remedy such as vinegar and water is good for you and less of a pain than over-the-counter soothing lotions, which are just a temporary fix. Drinking more liquids is good for you, and the more you drink, the more regular you will be. And remember, when you feel the need to go, do so and don't strain.

29 HERPES (Calm the irritation) Any woman or man who has contracted genital herpes, an infection of the genitals, buttocks, or anal area caused by the herpes simplex virus (HSV), is not a happy camper. It has no cure. Outbreaks can last for several days to weeks. Read: tingling, itching, and painful little bumps on the private parts.

What Remedy to Use: For an outbreak, try blotting the region with apple cider vinegar for quick and long-lasting relief of itching and pain.

Why You'll Like It: Prescription antiviral medications are available to help you prevent future outbreaks. But with ACV, you will get relief immediately—and you won't have any drug side effects. Plus, if you're seeking a fast and soothing solution, vinegar might be your best friend.

30 HICCUPS (Stop the hic) When the diaphragm gets irritated, it pushes up and makes your breath come out abnormally—and you let out a "Hic!" The causes can vary from eating too fast or too much to over-excitement.

What Vinegar Remedy to Use: Sip a glass of warm water with 1 teaspoon of vinegar mixed in it. I suggest drinking from the far side of a glass for antihiccup double effect.

Why You'll Like It: It beats having someone jump out and scare you, and has fewer calories than putting sugar in a glass of water.

31 IMPETIGO (Heal the sore) This streptococcus infection of the skin is very, very contagious. I remember as a preteenager my girlfriend's best friend had impetigo on her chin. My mother was very wary and warned us to keep our hands to ourselves.

What Vinegar Remedy to Use: Apply apple cider vinegar straight from the bottle on each infected area of the skin.

Why You'll Like It: If the home remedy works, it prevents a doctor bill and will stop an impetigo epidemic in your neighborhood.

32 IMPOTENCE (Rev up libido) A diet rich in vegetables, fruits, and whole grains enhances good health, which can result in better sexual energy. While some afficionados claim apple cider vinegar is also a love potion due to its antioxidants boosting the libido, I don't believe this is possible. However, eating a healthful low-fat, high-fiber diet can help a man stave off obesity, heart disease, and the need to use medications, all of which can certainly put a damper on his sex drive.

What Vinegar Remedy to Use: Try 1 or 2 teaspoons of apple cider vinegar in a glass of spring water three times a day.

Why You'll Like It: Vinegar beats those little blue pills, which have potential side effects that can make any man or woman lose that loving feeling.

33 INSECT AND BEE STINGS (Swat the ouch) Ouch! Bug bites hurt first, itch later. And nobody likes to look at red bumps and lumps. Mosquitoes, bees, and ants, oh my! What's an outdoor and indoor human to do?

What Vinegar Remedy to Use: Make yourself more comfortable in a homemade paste made from vinegar and cornstarch. Apply it directly to the bumps and blisters.

Why You'll Like It: It soothes the itch and dries out blisters.

34 INSOMNIA (Savor sweet dreams) Your eyes are wide open. The fear of not getting a good night's sleep tonight haunts you like a spooky Stephen King nightmare. The neon numbers on the clock (2:00 A.M.) are a glowing reminder of the sleepless zombie you'll be tomorrow morning. You toss. You turn. Now it's 3:20 A.M. Still not asleep. Whether you've had too much caffeine, didn't say no to your nightcap, or didn't solve your problems during the daytime, it's time to try an old secret for sweet dreams.

What Vinegar Remedy to Use: Dr. Jarvis recommends making a mixture of 3 teaspoons of apple cider vinegar to 1 cup of honey, and keeping it on the night table in a wide-mouthed bottle or jar along with a teaspoon.

Why You'll Like It: The Vermont folk medicine doctor touts honey as the ideal remedy for getting shut-eye. While I personally prefer chamomile tea for sleepless nights, vinegar and honey is worth a try and a better option than both taking prescription sleeping pills, which come with a mixed bag of side effects, or being sleep-deprived, which can wreak havoc on your health.

35 IRRITABLE BOWEL SYNDROME (Get regular again) Ever have abdominal pain, bloating, gas, diarrhea, and constipation? Welcome to the world of irritable bowel syndrome (IBS). While these symptoms aren't life-threatening, they are a pain in the rear, so to speak. If you want to get back to a regular schedule, fiber-rich apple cider vinegar and water may be just the remedy you need.

What Vinegar Remedy to Use: Take 1 tablespoon of apple cider vinegar in a glass of water three times a day. Also, include an adequate amount of dietary fiber at least 25 to 35 grams in your daily diet. And note, do drink an additional 5 glasses of water each and every day. Learning how to chill out with de-stressing techniques such as exercise will also help relax your mind and stomach.

Why You'll Like It: Chances are, by teaming apple cider vinegar, water, dietary fiber, and exercise, you won't care if it's the vinegar or the combination of the home cure. But most likely, you will feel 100 percent better.

36 JELLY FISH STINGS (Rid the burn) I can personally attest that jelly fish stings are extremely painful. In my 20s, I was swimming in the warm Floridian ocean. Once stung, I was shocked and clueless about what to do for the red and swollen area on my leg.

What Vinegar Remedy to Use: Vinegar Man Lawrence Diggs recommends 2 liters (about 2 quarts) of vinegar applied over the skin.

Why You'll Like It: It may help release some of the throbbing venom and redness, and prevent you from crying out in excruciating pain.

37 LAMENESS (Walk the walk) Walking s-l-o-w can occur for many reasons, from too much exercise or not enough. Whatever the cause, lameness can be painful. But there is a liniment that may provide relief.

What Vinegar Remedy to Use: In his book, Dr. Jarvis recommends to beat up the yolk of one egg with 1 tablespoon of turpentine and 1 tablespoon of apple cider vinegar. Rub into the skin.[8]

Why You'll Like It: If it relieves lameness, you'll like it.

38 HOT FLASHES (Just chill out) Pesky hot flashes or temperature disturbances affect countless women going through "The Change." I was told by many women that if you get a hot flash, you'll know it. So my guess is that I didn't. But I did take soy religiously for one year. In Asian countries, where women consume plenty of soy, hot flashes are uncommon.

What Vinegar Remedy to Use: Try 1 tablespoon in one 8-ounce glass of spring water with ice cubes.

Why You'll Like It: While a hot beverage can be soothing, it can also trigger a warm sensation that may feel like a hot flash, according to some women. If you sip a cold, refreshing apple cider drink, you will keep those hot flashes at bay. (But don't forget soy, which also may ease menopausal discomfort.)

39 MORNING SICKNESS (Go away, blahs) Nausea and vomiting often in the A.M. are common in almost half of all pregnant women. Morning sickness starts the first month of pregnancy and can last until the fourteenth to sixteenth week. The cause is unknown; however, it may be due to hormones or lower blood sugar during pregnancy.

What Vinegar Remedy to Use: To relieve morning sickness, as soon as you rise drink a glass of water with a teaspoon of apple cider vinegar.

Why You'll Like It: Morning sickness sufferers will gladly use any remedy that has a chance of beating the A.M. blahs.

40 MUSCLE CRAMPS (Relax your body) Ever wake up in the middle of the night and cringe at that sharp, painful muscle cramp? They can strike the feet, legs, and even the stomach. What to do?

What Vinegar Remedy to Use: Doctors Patricia and Paul Bragg recommend taking 2 teaspoons apple cider vinegar and 1 teaspoon of honey in a glass of distilled water three times per day.

Why You'll Like It: It may work, claim the Braggs, by allowing the precipitated acid crystals in your circulatory system to enter into a solution and pass out of the body.

41 NIGHT SWEATS (Hello, dry sheets) Ever have a bad case of the flu? Sometimes before it hits, in the middle of the night, you'll wake up in the wee A.M. hours and your sheets will be drenched. Eek! Also, menopausal women may experience night sweats in between hot flashes (not something to look forward to).

What Vinegar Remedy to Use: Try a sponge bath of apple cider vinegar at bedtime.

Why You'll Like It: This Vermont folk medicine remedy offers you help in preventing night sweats.

42 POISON IVY, OAK, AND SUMAC (Stop the itch) These three Canadian plants—poison ivy, western poison oak, and poison sumac—contain a poisonous sap that causes dermatitis—a pesky skin disorder. Symptoms include severe itching of the skin and oozing sores. While most cases of poisoning go away in 7–10 days, you can find relief without going to the drugstore.

What Vinegar Remedy to Use: Neal Schultz, M.D., a dermatologist in New York, recommends two vinegar solutions: mix equal parts vinegar and rubbing alcohol and apply to rash. Be sure to wash—thoroughly—plus everything that came in contact with the plant. Or mix equal parts buttermilk, vinegar, and salt and apply.

Why You'll Like It: These homemade vinegar pastes have a chemical that draws out the poison—so it relieves the burning and itching of the skin like calamine lotion.

43 RASH (Relieve itchy spots) Common rashes can occur for a variety of reasons. However, if it's a mild itching (jock itch or a rash on your buttocks), a natural remedy might clear up this common ailment without a doctor's visit.

What Remedy to Use: Use a cotton ball to dab irritated and itchy areas of skin on your body with cider vinegar straight from the bottle.

Why You'll Like It: For one, it doesn't hurt your pocketbook. For another, if you're camping or in a place where you don't have a doctor or medication, vinegar can nip the itching in the bud—fast.

44 RINGWORM (Round up lesions) *Tinea corporis* is caused by your body's response to advancing fungi. Lesions appear in a circular shape—with a raised border. Worse, inflammation and itching sets in.

What Vinegar Remedy to Use: Dr. Jarvis recommends applying apple cider vinegar with your fingers to the ringworm area six times daily.

Why You'll Like It: Since apple cider vinegar is antiseptic, it may help treat ringworm.

45 SHINGLES (Stamp out pain) My neighbor had shingles. She sheepishly confessed to me how painful the skin area on her chest was where the shingles were located.

What Vinegar Remedy to Use: Dr. Jarvis recommends dabbing apple cider vinegar directly on the shingles. Repeat four times daily and three times during the night.

Why You'll Like It: You'll find instant relief of the itching and burning in the skin, and the shingles may heal faster.

46 SORE THROAT (Smooth the hoarseness) When you feel the sniffles or flu coming on, a sore throat is often a symptom. While healing foods like vitamin C–rich citrus juices can lessen the severity of an illness, vinegar may help relieve that scratchy, painful feeling in your throat that makes it so hard to swallow.

What Vinegar Remedy to Use: To get rid of a painful sore throat, gargle with a 50–50 solution of warm water and vinegar.

Why You'll Like It: It is easy to do, all-natural, and doesn't have the sugar or chemicals that many sore throat lozenges contain.

47 SUNBURN (Soothe the redness) Exposure to ultraviolet rays in sunlight is the primary cause of sunburn. Sunburns can cause short-term redness, pain, blistering, and fever. Long-term skin damage includes premature aging and skin cancer.
While we know sun exposure is unhealthy, sometimes a sunburn is inevitable. But vinegar comes to the rescue. Treatment includes applying cold compresses to the burned area.

What Vinegar Remedy to Use: Apply ice cold vinegar immediately for fast relief.

Why You'll Like It: It will prevent blisters. My mother put cold compresses of red wine vinegar and ice on my very red back and thighs after a bad burn at the beach. It did its job.

48 SWIMMER'S EAR (Protect your ears) A common ailment that I remember getting as a teenage competitive swimmer. You can develop this ailment by swimming and showering as well.

What Vinegar Remedy to Use: To protect against ear infections from swimming pools, a popular folk remedy to try is using a mixture of one part white vinegar to one part rubbing alcohol.

Why You'll Like It: Vinegar is a good preventive strategy that can help keep pesky swimmer's ear at bay, while you splash in the pool or indulge in long showers.

49 TOENAIL FUNGUS (Tackle the monsters) Geologist George Stancliffe may like eye-catching fissures and rocks in his work, but ugly toenail fungus was something he didn't want to look at on his own feet.

"I first bought a product from the store that I saw advertised in the paper. It was worthless. My doctor told me that there was no cure for toenail fungus except one expensive prescription medicine that even he wouldn't use on his own toenail fungus, because of the danger of liver damage."[9]

What Remedy to Use: Distilled vinegar is believed to prevent fungus from growing. Try soaking your toes in a solution of vinegar and water, using 1 part vinegar to 2 parts water, 15 minutes per day, recommends the Vinegar Institute.

Why You'll Like It: Vinegar is all natural, and you don't have to get blood tests like you do if you take the prescription drug that is available but offers only a low rate of success plus takes a long time to work. "I'm slowly curing my toenail fungus. Vinegar has killed it on one or two toes," says Stancliffe, who knows that finding a perfect cure for this hard-to-get-rid-of problem is a task.

50 TOOTHACHE (Get quick relief) While an aching tooth is a good sign that you need dental attention, sometimes temporary relief is necessary especially if the pain starts in the middle of the night or if you are out of town. That's where vinegar comes into play.

What Vinegar Remedy to Use: One popular remedy is to dab a cotton swab soaked in acacia vinegar.

Why You'll Like It: Like oil of cloves, this natural vinegar remedy may provide temporary relief. And you won't compound your misery with the ill side effects of pain medications.

51 THRUSH (Wash away coating) Years ago, when I was stressed-out and taking antibiotics, I developed thrush, which is a white coating in the mouth. I went to the doctor and was prescribed a mouth rinse, which worked. But I didn't know about all-natural vinegar.

What Remedy to Use: Try rinsing your mouth four times a day with a 50–50 mixture of apple cider vinegar and warm water.

Why You'll Like It: Not only will you save the time and money it takes to go to the doctor, but you will also spend less on the vinegar than on the prescription remedy.

52 VITAMIN DEFICIENCY (Rate your supplement) Ever wonder if your multivitamin is doing what it is supposed to do for your health? Evidently, one way to find out is to let vinegar tell you what's up.

What Vinegar Remedy to Use: Drop your vitamin into ½ cup of vinegar. Stir the solution a few times during the course of 20 minutes. If the vitamin separates into tiny pieces, it's good. If not, it may be time to look for a different brand, according to health experts at Prevention.com.

Why You'll Like It: I've been taking a popular all-natural multi-vitamin-and-mineral for women. When I tried this do-it-yourself rating system, it worked, so I felt that I got a quick thumbs-up for my choice of brand.

53 WARTS (Zap viral creepies) If you've ever had these small, hard lumps on your hands or feet, you know that they are unsightly and embarrassing. These little viral monsters can be spread through direct contact with another person, as well as through public showers and locker rooms, too.

What Remedy to Use: Mix one part apple cider vinegar to one part glycerin and apply the lotion daily to the wart until it dissolves.

Why You'll Like It: Over-the-counter products often don't work but cost a pretty penny. Also, making a doctor's appointment, and grinning and bearing it when they use painful remedies like dry ice isn't fun, nor does it always work. If this kinder vinegar remedy can nip warts in the bud, it will make your life easier. It did mine. One week before a book signing, an unsightly wart appeared on my right thumb. Instead of following my dermatologist's recommendation of cauterization, I applied apple cider vinegar several times a day. By the time of my signing a week later, the wart was completely gone.

54 VARICOSE VEINS (Welcome smoother legs) It's estimated that more than two-thirds of all American women and half of all men in the United States have swollen veins that appear near the surface of the skin. While they are unsightly, they can ache, too. Some natural remedies include: watch your weight, and avoid constipation. Perhaps that's why fiber-rich apple cider vinegar is the ticket to shrinking spider veins.

What Vinegar Remedy to Use: Dr. Jarvis reports that his patients taught him to apply apple cider vinegar straight to the varicose veins at morning and night. Plus, he recommends taking 2 teaspoons of vinegar in a glass of water twice a day.[10]

Why You'll Like It: Dr. Jarvis's patients got results, so mark your calendar. You, too, will notice shrinkage in 30 days.

55 WEIGHT (Gain some girth) While countless Americans struggle with obesity, there are a lot of people who want to put on the pounds. According to the Braggs, underweight people lack natural enzymes and food is not utilized by the body.

What Vinegar Remedy to Use: The good doctors suggest drinking 1 teaspoon apple cider vinegar and 1 teaspoon honey in a glass of distilled water upon rising. "Add to this 2 drops of liquid iodine made from seaweed, available in health stores. This adds natural iodine, which is so important to body health, and helps normalize body weight up or down as needed," they claim.

Why You'll Like It: Natural apple cider vinegar is healthier than loading up on high-fat fare. And it may be more palatable to you than caloric protein drinks and less costly!

A BONUS FOR GOOD MEASURE: YOUR UNIVERSAL EMERGENCY BARE ESSENTIAL Yes, disasters such as earthquakes, tornadoes, hurricanes, fires, and floods can and do happen. While you want to include medications that you, your family, and your pet are taking, you also want to have a first-aid kit and handbook.

What Remedy to Use: Pour apple cider vinegar into a large plastic container (or two), and store it with your emergency supplies.

Why You'll Like It: It is the medicine of the twenty-first century. Rather than trying to remember if you have every type of ailment remedy, with vinegar you will be covered whether you cut yourself, get a bruise, come down with a yeast infection, or run into anything healthwise that will irk you during a disaster.

Blueberry Vinegar Scones

❖ ❖ ❖

These scones are a perfect fall warming food. One September I experienced ten-degree mornings and pumpkins lined up in front of shops on cobbled streets greeted me as I walked up and down the streets in Quebec City. I admit a horse and carriage took me for the longer trek. It was all a sign that autumn—my favorite season at Lake Tahoe—was waiting for me as well as cooking and baking fall foods, especially breakfast fare.

When I was up by four A.M., and checked in at the Montreal-Pierre Elliott Trudeau International Airport and waiting to board the plane to take me back home, I ordered a latte and blueberry scone—a large, triangle-shaped, gem cake–like, semisweet quick bread (glazed or plain served with butter). It was in one of those big glass jars. The café owner told me, "Everyone loves them." The texture was a bittersweet surprise. Each bite was like a rich butter cookie, not cake-like or moist. It was sweet enough and big enough with an unexpected crunch. I, the California fussy scone girl, thought, "Ah, but she hasn't tasted my sweet scones." I vowed once back home snug in my cabin, inspired by the Canadian savory and sweet scone, I'd bake up a batch of fresh blueberry scones and match its look and taste.

3 cups all-purpose flour
3 tablespoons baking powder
¼ cup granulated white sugar
5 tablespoons European-style
  butter (cold cubes)
1 organic egg
⅔ cups buttermilk
1 tablespoon apple cider vinegar

1 teaspoon honey vanilla Greek
  yogurt
1 teaspoon vanilla extract
2 tablespoons fresh orange rind,
  grated
¾ to 1 cup dried blueberries
½ cup hazelnuts, chopped
raw sugar

Preheat oven to 350 degrees. In a bowl, mix flour, baking powder, and sugar. Add chunks of butter. In another bowl, combine egg, buttermilk, vinegar, yogurt, and vanilla and stir till mixed. Add rind, berries,

and nuts. Put into lightly greased round baking dish (I used my favorite white tart dish for an earthy look). Bake till golden brown,
about 30 minutes. Sprinkle with sugar. Cool. Cut in triangle shapes
like a pizza. Makes approximately 12. Serve with honey or cream
cheese. (For a special touch, make an orange glaze. Mix confectioners'
sugar with a bit of fresh orange juice and orange rind. Drizzle on tops
of scones.)

VINEGARY HEALING HINTS TO PRESERVE

If it doesn't specify which type of vinegar to use, go ahead and use
your own preference: an apple cider vinegar, a red wine vinegar, or a
white vinegar.

It's no surprise to discover surprising vinegar home cures—using a
variety of vinegars, not just apple cider—whether consumed or used
topically. Many of the remedies and results are anecdotal and some do
prove their worth by scientific research. You, like me, may agree that if
nature's therapies work, it doesn't matter if lab rats or your grandmother give it a stamp of approval. In Chapter 19, you'll find out how
the future of vinegar—all types—is here to stay in the United States
and around the world and why.

Ailment	Vinegar	What It May Do
✓ Acid reflux disease	Apple cider vinegar	Gets rid of heartburn
✓ Acne	Plain or herbal apple cider vinegar	Gets rid of blemishes
✓ Angina	Apple cider vinegar	Relieves chest pain
✓ Anxiety	Apple cider vinegar	Soothes frazzled nerves
✓ Arthritis	Apple cider vinegar	Relieves soreness
✓ Astringent	Red wine vinegar	Perks up skin
✓ Athlete's foot	Plain or herbal apple cider vinegar	Soothes burning
✓ Black-and-blue marks	Vinegar	May speed the healing process
✓ Skin burns	Apple cider vinegar	Lessens soreness
✓ Canker sores	Apple cider vinegar	Reduces the pain
✓ Chapped skin	Vinegar	Heals
✓ Colds	Apple cider vinegar	May speed recovery
✓ Congestion	Apple cider vinegar	Reduces mucus
✓ Constipation	Apple cider vinegar	Maintains regularity
✓ Corns	Vinegar	Gets rid of corns
✓ Cough	Apple cider vinegar	Controls coughing
✓ Dandruff	Apple cider vinegar	Fights flakes
✓ Depression	Apple cider vinegar	May lift the spirit
✓ Dizziness	Apple cider vinegar	Helps steady you

Ailment	Vinegar	What It May Do
✓ Douche	White vinegar	Mild, safe
✓ Earache	Apple cider vinegar	Staves off infection
✓ Fatigue	Apple cider vinegar	Acts like a pick-me-up
✓ Fibromyalgia	Apple cider vinegar	Helps reduce stress
✓ Flu	Apple cider vinegar	Relieves fever
✓ Freckles	Horseradish vinegar	Fades spots
✓ Hangnails	Apple cider vinegar	Gets rid of redness
✓ Headache	Herbal vinegar	Provides headache relief
✓ Hemorrhoids	Apple cider vinegar	Helps regularity
✓ Herpes	Apple cider vinegar	Soothes itching, pain
✓ Hiccups	Vinegar	Hiccups will stop
✓ Hot flashes	Apple cider vinegar	Helps to refresh
✓ Impetigo	Apple cider vinegar	Heals the skin
✓ Impotence	Apple cider vinegar	May enhance libido
✓ Insect and bee stings	Vinegar	Relieves pain and inflammation
✓ Insomnia	Apple cider vinegar	Aids sleep
✓ Irritable bowl syndrome	Apple cider vinegar	Improves well-being
✓ Jelly fish stings	Vinegar	Soothes the burn
✓ Lameness	Apple cider vinegar	Reduces pain and stiffness

Ailment	Vinegar	What It May Do
✓ Morning sickness	Apple cider vinegar	Subdues nausea
✓ Muscle cramps	Apple cider vinegar	It may excrete acid crystals
✓ Night sweats	Apple cider vinegar	Controls sweating
✓ Poison oak/ ivy/sumac	Vinegar	Relieves itching/ burning
✓ Rash	Apple cider vinegar	Soothes itching, pain
✓ Ringworm	Apple cider vinegar	Dries it up
✓ Shingles	Apple cider vinegar	Relieves burning/ itching
✓ Sore throat	Vinegar	Relieves soreness
✓ Sunburn	Red wine vinegar	Relieves pain
✓ Swimmer's ear	White vinegar	Prevents ear infection
✓ Thrush	Apple cider vinegar	Gets rid of infection
✓ Toenail fungus	Apple cider vinegar	Fights the infection
✓ Toothache	Acacia vinegar	Relieves pain temporarily
✓ Universal emergency	Apple cider vinegar	Acts as a cure-all medication
✓ Vitamin deficiency	Apple cider vinegar	Helps determine vitamin strength
✓ Warts	Apple cider vinegar	Dries up hard lumps
✓ Weight gain	Apple cider vinegar	Helps metabolism
✓ Varicose veins	Apple cider vinegar	Shrinks the veins

PART 7

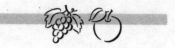

FUTURE VINEGAR

Vinegarmania: Using Vinegar for the Household, Beauty, Kids, and Pets

A poet that fails in writing becomes often a morose critic; the weak and insipid white wine makes at length an excellent vinegar.
—William Shenstone

After my trip to Quebec City, despite the eyes-gone-wrong saga, I wanted to see more of Canada. I craved another trip and yearned to taste another fruit-flavored balsamic vinegar. This time I was booked for a book signing in Bellevue, Washington, followed by a journey north to Vancouver. Being on the road is a youth-boosting adventure each time—and vinegar, despite the fact that I was researching tea-rooms, did greet me once again. It was like meeting an old friend in a new place.

On the Saturday night before my six A.M. Amtrak ride across the Canadian border, I left the book event with foraging healthy food on the brain. Room service wasn't on my list, but dining out felt right. I was leaving early in the morning for B.C., Canada, and a light dinner seemed in order. Someone suggested Joey's. I obliged. Once entering the full sports-type bar I felt I had aged decades. The music was loud and intense. The servers were bubbly and young.

I ordered a spinach salad. I wanted a baked potato, but for some odd reason they were nonexistent. I was served skinny fries. Also, I noticed that all the fresh greens were paired with fruit, not only vegetables.

Perhaps this is a Seattle trend. I felt my palate longing for home fries homemade in my home. In the Pacific Northwest salads come with fruit *and* vegetables drizzled with vinaigrettes.

My server was accommodating, but I was feeling like a fish out of water because baked potatoes, red wine vinegar, and baguettes like I learned to love in Quebec were MIA. The sweet fruit-flavored vinaigrette made me feel at home as I picked at the fruit pieces in my salad and savored the fresh greens as I would eat in California.

There's no doubt about it. Vinegar is hot these days. Not only can you find vinegar on the market and online, a variety of vinegar types are growing by leaps and bounds. What's more, while doctors use it, and plenty of people, like you and me, use it, even conventional associations are jumping on the vinegar wagon.

Sweet Vinegar Fact

Almost Everybody Does Vinegar: Who in the nation buys vinegar—and why? Ninety percent of American households use vinegar, although folks in the Pacific and mid-Atlantic states buy the most vinegar. Why? It may be due to the interest in salad and gourmet cooking in metropolitan areas. Also, during the late summer, vinegar sales soar because people buy gallons of vinegar for pickling and food preservation. The most popular food uses of vinegar are for salads, as a cooking ingredient, and for pickling and home canning.

(*Source:* Heinz.)

The American Dietetic Association (ADA) encouraged consumers to load up your pantry with a "variety of vinegars." The association released the slogan for 1999 National Nutrition Month: "Take a fresh look at nutrition." The ADA suggests flavoring foods with things other than salt and fat. That means filling up your pantry with quick-fix items, including rice, pasta, beans, and a variety of vinegars, herbs, and other flavorings. And there's more.

VINEGAR STATISTICS

Vinegar Sales Growth (21st Century)

According to ACNielsen, vinegar sales growth, at 15 percent, was stronger in 2000 through 2002 than the sales growth of most comparative categories, including meat marinades, Oriental sauces, Worcestershire sauce, and cooking wine and sherry. Stronger dollar sales appear to have contributed to this growth due to higher-end products in the category. According to supermarket sales, vinegar sales increased 29 percent from 1993 to 2003.

(*Source:* "2002 ACNielsen Data Presented at 2003 VI Annual Meeting.")

Reports vary, and demand for specialty vinegars is in vogue, but due to consumer demand, favorite vinegar flavors may change year by year, decade by decade. But these statistics are a good baseline to know:

Vinegar Retail Sales by Flavor (21st Century)

46% distilled white
22% cider
12% red wine
10% balsamic
5% rice
5% all other

(*Source:* ACNielsen, "Vinegar Unit Shares by Flavor, 2000–2002.")

Although bottled vinegar sold at retail makes up a large part of the vinegar market, vinegar is also a key ingredient in a number of familiar products. Vinegar adds flavor and zip to salad dressings, sauces, marinades, ketchup, mustard, pickles, tomato products, and more. Next time you're at the store, check out the ingredient statement on some of your favorite products—chances are vinegar makes the list.

21ST-CENTURY VINEGAR PURCHASING BEHAVIOR

- In 2002, 49 percent of U.S. households purchased vinegar at least once.
- In 2001, U.S. households spent an average of $3.79 per household on vinegar.
- According to ACNielsen, from 2001–2002, 53 million households bought vinegar and spent $4.07 per household on the category.
- Vinegar sales were somewhat seasonal, with a peak in the summer months and a secondary peak in April, most likely due to the Easter holiday and the use of vinegar in dying Easter eggs.
- Vinegar buyers like the 16- and 17-ounce sizes the best, followed by the 32- and 34-ounce sizes.

(*Sources: Progressive Grocer*, September 2001 and 2002; "2002 ACNielsen Data Presented at 2003 VI Annual Meeting.")

VINEGAR FLAVORS IN HOUSEHOLDS

In a 2003 report, ACNielsen noted that distilled white vinegar was still the mainstay of the category, although white and cider vinegars were giving way slowly to red wine, rice, and balsamic vinegars. Raspberry was an emerging flavor (with a 25 percent increase in sales since 2000), while garlic and tarragon decreased slightly. According to Information Resources, Inc. (IRI) information for 1994 through 1998, of the 48 percent of households that purchased vinegar, 5 percent purchased the growing balsamic type. (Specialty vinegars continue to cure foodies and chefs in the 21st century.)

(*Sources:* Information Resources, Inc., based on data for 1994–1998; "2002 ACNielsen Data Presented at 2003 VI Annual Meeting.")

Q. Where do consumers buy vinegar?

A. As the supermarket industry consolidates, other retail outlets such as mass merchandisers and drugstores are taking the opportunity to draw in consumers. According to ACNielsen, an increasing percentage of vinegar sales are moving through clubs and mass merchandisers. From 2000 to 2002, the percentage of sales in outlets other than supermarkets increased from 23 percent to 29 percent. The chart below provides insight into where vinegar is purchased in various retail outlets.

(*Source*: The Vinegar Institute.)

DETOXIFY YOUR WORLD

I remember as a little girl, my mother used white distilled vinegar to wash the windows inside and outside of our pink and white house in the suburbs. In my twenties, as a Denny's waitress, I remember using vinegar to wash out the coffeepots at the restaurant. In my thirties, as a college student, I used vinegar in the kitchen drain to get rid of odors. And today, I use vinegar for all those reasons—and more. Why?

We live in a very toxic world. And what better natural remedy to use for household purposes than natural vinegar? Science shows that many chemicals previously thought safe are not. The fact is, low levels of some common chemicals found in cleaning products can affect your immune and nervous systems.

I know firsthand how the body can be adversely affected by household chemicals. When I was in graduate school at San Francisco State University, I cleaned homes to pay for my tuition and living expenses. Three times a week (sometimes more) I'd clean houses for affluent people in Hillsborough and Palo Alto.

At first, even though I have always been a believer in natural foods, I didn't think twice about using harsh cleaning products. The oily furniture polish and strong-smelling shower cleaner got the job done.

As time passed, however, I began to experience some ill effects of those oh-so-powerful cleaning agents I valued. One time as I began to spray the shower, my employer grabbed her baby and dog and dashed for another room. I began to wonder, "If this cleaner is so toxic for infants and pets—what about me and my health?"

After a few bouts of coping with a runny nose or a sore throat, I wised up. I took a self-taught crash course on basic household cleaners. I began to read the labels of household cleaners (just like I read labels on food items). It was a wake-up call. But did you know that some chemical compounds in cleaning agents aren't even listed on the label?

The fact remains, there are toxic chemical compounds that are not safe for humans or animals. Here's some of the culprits:

ARE YOUR HOUSEHOLD CLEANERS MAKING YOU SICK?

Cleaning Chemical	Found In	Potential Side Effects
Ammonia	Glass cleaners, floor cleaners, furniture polishes	Irritates your eyes, nose, lungs; causes rashes, redness.
Bleach, mixed	Disinfectants, laundry bleaches, toilet bowl cleaner	Irritates the skin; when mixed with ammonia forms a toxic gas.
Formaldehyde	Disinfectants, furniture polishes, detergents	Nasal stuffiness, itchy red eyes, nausea, headache.
Glycols	Degreasers, dry-cleaning chemicals, floor cleaners	Irritates skin, eyes, nose, throat.
Lye	Tub and tile cleaners	Mixed with acids, lye can cause harmful vapors; splashed in eyes can cause blindness.
Napthalene	Air fresheners, carpet cleaners	Dangerous to breathe and can cause headaches, nausea, confusion.
Petroleum distillates	Oven cleaners, pesticides	Irritate the skin.

The good news is, I switched to the natural stuff. One by one, I spoke to my clientele. Many of the women (especially the teacher with allergies; the multicat household owner; and housewife with multiple chemical sensitivity) did not mind that I insisted on using the natural household cleaners. In fact, we would make a nonchemical household cleaner list together. And white and cider vinegars were on the grocery list.

Here are some things you can do by using the "Kitchen Magician" to detoxify *your* household and planet.

DETOX YOUR KITCHEN

- **Disposal Fresh as a Rose.** To help keep your garbage disposal clean and fresh-smelling, try vinegar cubes. Mix one cup of vinegar in a sufficient amount of water to fill an ice tray. Freeze the mixture and run the cubes through the disposal. After the grinding action has stopped, flush with cold water for a minute or so.
- **Dishwasher Fresh.** To help keep the drain line on your dishwasher clean and fresh-smelling, add one-half cup of white vinegar to the rinse cycle.
- **Fixtures That Sparkle Bright.** Remove soap and stain buildup on chrome and plastic fixtures by cleaning with a mixture of 1 teaspoon salt dissolved in 2 tablespoons of white vinegar.
- **Shine on Counters.** Clean formica tabletops and counters by rubbing with a cloth soaked in white vinegar. The finish will shine. (Trust me on this one.)
- **Stamp Out Grease.** Dampen your cleaning rag in vinegar and water and use it to wipe out your oven. It will prevent grease buildup.
- **Mr. Dishwashing Magic.** To remove chalky deposits left on dinnerware and glasses, place affected pieces in dishwasher. Place cup filled with vinegar on bottom rack. Run the machine for 5 minutes. Stop the machine and empty cup which is now filled with water. Refill with vinegar and complete cycle. Follow by a complete cycle with dishwasher detergent.

PERSONAL PROTECTION

- **Put Out Smoky Odors.** To remove smoky odors from clothes, fill a bathtub with hot water and add 1 cup of white vinegar. Hang the garments above the steaming bath water.
- **Freshen Up Baby!** Baby's clothes will be fresher if you add 1 cup of white vinegar to each load during the rinse cycle. Vinegar naturally breaks down uric acid and soapy residue in diapers, leaving the clothes soft and fresh.
- **Easy Wash Silks.** To wash silks at home, add a half capful of Woolite and 2 tablespoons of white vinegar to 2 quarts of very

cold water. Dunk clothes up and down in the mixture but do not soak. Dry just enough to iron by rolling in a Turkish towel and pressing while still damp. You may wish to test a particular item by dipping the tail of the blouse or detachable tie before doing the entire piece.

- **Sock It to the Suds.** Get rid of excess suds that billow up during hand laundry by adding a splash of vinegar to the second rinse. Then rinse again in plain water.
- **Gentle Hand Helper.** To restore moisture to hands when they have been in strong cleaning solutions, plaster, concrete, or powdered detergents, simply rub them with vinegar.
- **Cola Spots Fizzle.** To remove cola-based soft drink spots from 100% cotton, polyester and cotton blends, and permanent press cotton fabrics, sponge the stain within 24 hours. Apply undiluted vinegar directly to the stain and rub away the marks. Launder or dry clean according to the manufacturer's care tag instructions.
- **Good-bye Wine Stains.** To remove wine stains from 100% cotton, polyester and cotton blends, and permanent press fabrics, sponge the stain with full strength vinegar. Treat the stain within 24 hours and wash and dry as directed on the manufacturer's care tag instructions.
- **No More Catsup.** For catsup stains in 100% cotton, permanent press, and polyester cotton materials, sponge stain with undiluted vinegar within 24 hours. Wash immediately.
- **Lime Fighter.** Lawn and garden lime washes off the hands readily with a dousing of vinegar. Follow with a cold water rinse and apply skin lotion if desired.
- **Rub Out Deodorant Stains.** You can get rid of smelly deodorant and antiperspirant stains from your garments by gently rubbing them with distilled white vinegar before washing.
- **Remove Holes in Fabrics.** Ever notice how after you remove a hem or seam, you're welcomed by pesky holes in the fabric? Don't despair. You can remedy these unsightly dots by putting a cloth dampened with distilled white vinegar under the fabric and ironing the holes away.
- **Preserve Colored Clothes.** Love your black sweater, red blouse, and green pants? Keep their true colors longer by soaking these favorite threads in distilled white vinegar before you wash them.

- **Love Your Leather.** Yes, leather articles can be cleaned with a solution of distilled white vinegar and linseed oil. Gently rub this protector into your lovely leather items and rub gently with a cloth.
- **So Long, Scorch Marks.** Save a slightly scorched fabric item with a bit of distilled white vinegar. Dab on some vinegar, then gently rub the unsightly scorch marks away.

NONTOXIC FLOOR CLEANERS

- **No-Wax Linoleum.** To wash no-wax linoleum, add one-half cup of white vinegar to a half-gallon of warm water. Your floor will become sparkling clean.
- **Liven Up Carpet.** To bring up the color in rugs and carpets, brush them with a mixture of 1 cup of white vinegar to a gallon of water.

NATURAL BATHROOM CLEANUP

- **Good Riddance Bathtub Film.** To remove film buildup on bathtubs, wipe with vinegar and then soda. Rinse clean with water.
- **Natural Bowl Cleaner.** Got kids and pets so you're nervous about using bleach in the bowl? Clean it the natural way. Pour undiluted white vinegar into it. Let it stand for 5 minutes and then flush. Stubborn stains may be removed by spraying them with vinegar and brushing vigorously. (Works like a charm, really!)
- **Unclog Showerhead.** To remove corrosion from showerhead or faucet, soak them in diluted white vinegar overnight. For convenience, saturate a cloth in vinegar and wrap it around the faucet or showerhead.
- **Shower Curtain Clean.** Nothing is better than a brand-new shower curtain. After a while, though, it begins to look spotty with soap film. Toss your favorite plastic shower curtains in the washing machine with a bath towel. During the rinse cycle, add 1 cup of white vinegar. Then, tumble dry briefly. (I've put this on my To Do list.)

Miscellaneous Nontoxic Household Uses

- **Lose the Ants.** Ants are pesky. And using toxic chemicals to zap them is worse. Opt to wash countertops, cabinets, and floors with equal parts of vinegar and water to deter ant invasions the natural way. (Good idea. You don't want my Fido and Fluffy exposed to toxins.)
- **Chrome Polish Perfect.** To polish chrome and stainless steel, simply moisten a cloth with white vinegar and wipe clean.
- **Wood Paneling Delight.** Wood paneling is beautiful. To keep it looking good, mix 1 ounce of olive oil with 2 ounces of white vinegar and 1 quart of warm water. Dampen a soft cloth with the solution and wipe the paneling. Then wipe with a dry, soft cloth to remove yellowing from surface.
- **Meltdown Dust.** Got a stubborn ring resulting from wet glasses being placed on wood furniture (water or alcohol)? Don't despair. Rub with a mixture of equal parts olive oil and white vinegar. A bonus tip: Rub with the grain, then polish.
- **Fresh as a Daisy.** Everyone wants to keep fresh-cut flowers fresh longer. Just add 2 tablespoons of vinegar plus 3 tablespoons of sugar to each quart of warm water (100° F). Keep flower stems in 3–4 inches of water to allow constant flow of nourishment.
- **Rx for Wobbly Furniture.** Ready to toss out old chairs or tables? Instead apply vinegar with a small oil can. It will loosen old glue around rungs and joints.

Keep It Green Outside

- **Water Cleanup.** Can vinegar be used to clean contaminated water? According to a report from Albuquerque, New Mexico, vinegar was put to the test to clean up Albuquerque's South Valley water woes. As the story goes, a vegetable farm used too much fertilizer over time. The nitrates seeped into the ground and contaminated the water below, making it unusable for anything but watering plants. Scientists believe a mixture of bacteria and vinegar might neturalize the contamination by transforming the nitrates into "non-toxic, harmless nitrogen gas."[1]

- **Bye Bye Grass.** To kill grass on sidewalks and driveways, pour full-strength vinegar on it.
- **Natural Weed Killer.** Organic, vinegar-based weed killer may be a safe way to control unruly weeds, according to Eco-Safety Products, based in Arizona. The company boasts its product may zap a variety of weeds and grasses within an hour, not days.[2]
- **Melt Icy Roads.** Transit New Zealand is vouching for a solution of dolomite lime and vinegar to dry up icy roads. It seems that after a five-year trial, it found the vinegar mixture (calcium magnesium acetate) is less damaging to the environment than salt and doesn't harm vehicles.[3]
- **Fuel Forever.** To make gasoline or propane lantern mantles last longer, soak them for several hours in vinegar and allow them to dry before using. They'll burn brighter on the same amount of fuel.
- **Cut That Rust.** To free a rusted or corroded bolt, soak it in vinegar.

(*Source:* The Vinegar Institute.)

LIGHTEN UP WITH VINEGAR FENG SHUI

You may have heard about feng shui, an age-old practice that holds the idea of living in harmony and balance with our environment. Now think of Martha Stewart and her beautiful household tips. Then, think vinegar. That's right, vinegar. Infused vinegar, that is.

Feng shui is often used in homes, and can be very valuable when you place special objects in a room. Now take those flavored vinegars you made and line them along a windowsill to catch the sunlight. It will show off their healthful ingredients—parsley, sage, rosemary, and other herbs.

And remember, at the same time the seasonings infuse their flavor into vinegar and olive oil, to be used later for tasty recipes. Taking that special bottle (or two) of infused vinegar out of the shelf and placing it along a windowsill can make your living environment healthier and you may feel more connected to the life forces which surround us.

Show Your Stuff

- Flavored vinegars look great on kitchen countertops.
- Be creative when selecting containers.
- Choose ceramic or glass bottles with secure lids.
- Display herb vinegar in clear glass.
- Find elegantly detailed bottles at flea markets, garage sales, or antique stores, or order them from specialty catalogs or cookery stores.
- Prevent vinegar from clouding by sterilizing your containers first.

(*Source:* Heinz.)

VINEGAR BEAUTIFUL

The following healthful vinegar beauty recipes are all natural and without harsh toxic chemicals:

- **Recipe 1: Vinegar to Aid Oily Skin.** One pint apple cider vinegar, 1 cup each lavender petals, lemon rind, rose petals, and sage. Steep this in a sunny window in a dark, glass jar that's well sealed for 3 weeks. Shake daily, then strain and rebottle.
- **Recipe 2: Vinegar for Dry Skin.** The same as the first recipe but use chamomile, mint, parsley, and primrose petals instead.
- **Recipe 3: Astringent/Hair Rinse.** Use white wine vinegar to which you add 1 cup orange peel (and if possible a half-cup orange leaves). Follow same procedure.
- **Recipe 4: Alternative Astringent for Your Skin.** Use any type of vinegar to which 1 cup of chopped marigolds has been added. This will dry pimples and also help heal minor scrapes.

(*Courtesy:* Patricia Telesco, Amherst, New York.)

Martha Washington's Famous Facial

In 1754, during the French and Indian War, Martha Custis bewitched George Washington at a dance. The legend is, that from across the dance floor it was her radiant complexion that caught his eye—and won his heart. The two married four years later. So what was Martha's beauty secret that made a big statement? Vinegar, ladies. Here's the famous facial mask:

Beat 1 egg, separate, till frothy. Combine the egg, 1 teaspoon honey, and ¼ teaspoon apple cider vinegar. Apply to your face and neck. After 15–20 minutes, rinse with warm water and dry.[4]

SURPRISING BEAUTY TIPS WITH VERSATILE VINEGAR

- **Thick and Shiny Hair.** "Cider vinegar is proven not to only rehydrate hair that is structurally weak, dry, or unmanageable, it also will strengthen hair that has been permed, colored, highlighted, or subjected to single or double processing, and will assist in restoring hair's natural pH balance," explains hair expert Karen M. Shelton.

  A famous rinse contains 2 tablespoons apple cider vinegar to 2 cups warm water. This recipe is used as a final rinse in order to remove the residue left on hair by commercial shampoos. It also imparts magnificent shine.

- **Super Hair Rinse.** They say apple cider vinegar is perfect for beautiful Salma Hayek–like brunettes (dark brown). White vinegar is ideal for Meg Ryan–type blondes.

- **A Rosy Glow.** The fact is, as your circulation slows, your complexion may lose some of its rosiness. While eating vitamin A–rich foods and using a moisturizing sunscreen daily will help, during the cold and dry winter months, you may need to give your skin an extra lift.

  To brighten your complexion, I suggest using a gentle exfoliant to zap dead surface cells. I personally tried applying apple cider vinegar directly on my forehead, cheeks, and chin. Within minutes, my skin had a youthful glow and felt soft and radiant. And yes, I am now addicted to this super remedy.

- **Smooth Hands.** Age spots on your hands are part of the aging process. While my Brittany, Simon, a dog with orange and white spots, is adorable, you may find that an age spot fader that works may be both woman's and man's best friend.

  Try dabbing vinegar on those pesky age spots. Use it daily, and you may or may not see results. (Remember, apple cider vinegar works wonders as an exfoliant on facial skin, so it might lighten age spots, too.) But even if you don't lose the spots, you just may have softer hands.

- **Clean Dentures.** Of course, nobody plans on getting a partial denture—or full dentures. But sometimes, people don't have a choice. Dentists advise removing dentures overnight to allow the mouth to rest. Often, people will brush their dentures with a toothbrush to clean the surfaces.

  Soak dentures overnight in white vinegar, then brush off tartar with a toothbrush. This tip is good because it's natural and less costly than denture-cleaning solution.

- **Personal Hygiene.** Good grooming includes wearing deodorant, unless you do not perspire, which is unusual.

  After bathing, apply distilled white vinegar to each armpit. While this beauty remedy is inexpensive, it's also natural and, doesn't smell. And I can personally attest that yes, it works.

- **Fragrant Sweater.** Ever have a favorite wool sweater that ended up smelling like secondhand smoke? Ugh! Keep in mind that fragrance is part of good grooming. But don't despair.

  Simply wash that beloved garment in gentle soap, then rinse in equal parts vinegar and water to remove that ugly stench.

- **Sparkling Eyeglasses.** Accessories, including eyeglasses, should complete or complement your overall look, say image consultants. That means you want squeaky clean (not smudgy) eyewear, because this shows good grooming and that you take care of yourself.

  Mix a 50:50 solution of white vinegar and water. It's not harsh like window and glass cleaners, and you won't have to smell a chemical-like odor.

- **Pretty Nails.** There's nothing more frustrating than spending time giving yourself a perfect manicure and then having your clean, filed nails look sloppy because the polish becomes chipped. But there is a nail care tip.

  Simply rub vinegar on your nails before you use nail polish. Not only will your polish go on smoothly, but it will last longer, too.

- **Sexy Feet.** Joann, a devout vinegar lover, insists vinegar is great for dry feet. She half-fills a dishpan with warm water, adds about a cup of ACV (yes, 1 cup!), and soaks her feet for about 5 minutes. "You can go as long as you like, but that's all it takes. All the dead skin comes off, and your feet will be as soft as a baby's."

HEALTHY KID STUFF

- **Coloring Easter Eggs.** Here is a recipe my mom used for me when I was a kid. Mix 1 teaspoon vinegar with ½ cup hot water, then add food coloring. (If using a commercial egg-coloring product, check the box or insert for specific directions.) Vinegar keeps food dyes bright and prevents streaky, uneven coloring.

  Kids can be fussy eaters and may shun eggs. These days, however, nutritionists and medical doctors say we can eat fatty foods such as eggs, fish, and even chocolate, which contain "good" fats, along with our antioxidant-rich fruits, vegetables, and legumes. Eating these foods, as do heart-healthy people in the Mediterranean countries, can help your kids learn a healthful way of eating so they can avoid heart disease and obesity.

- **How to Create a Volcano 1-2-3.** Another vinegar-related recipe is not only fun for kids but a way for parents to explain what a volcano is and where they exist in the world. It also offers a perfect opportunity to discuss Mother Nature's earth changes and how to be prepared, not scared.

1. Make the cone of the volcano. Mix 6 cups flour, 2 cups salt, 4 tablespoons cooking oil, and 2 cups water. The resulting mixture should be smooth and firm (add more water, if necessary).
2. Stand a soft drink bottle in a baking pan and mold the dough around it into a volcano shape. Do not cover the bottle's hole or drop dough into it. Fill the bottle most of the way with warm water and add a few drops of red food coloring. (You can do this before sculpting if you do not take so long that the water gets cold.) Add 6 drops detergent and 2 tablespoons baking soda to the bottle.
3. Slowly pour vinegar into the bottle. Look out—it will erupt!

- **Berry Good for Your Ink and Quill Pens.** Ever think your kid is spending too much time at the computer and eating too much high-fat junk food? It's time to go back to nature and have your child make some all-natural ink and an old-fashioned pen. Then, go one step further and have your child write a poem or short story about nature—and nibble on a small bowl of some healthful low-cal, high-fiber, vitamin C–rich berries, too.

Berry ink:

½ *cup ripe berries (such as blueberries, cherries, blackberries, strawberries, elderberries, or raspberries)*
½ *teaspoon vinegar*
½ *teaspoon salt*

Fill a strainer with the berries and hold it over a bowl. Using the rounded back of a wooden spoon, crush the berries against the strainer so that the berry juice strains into the bowl. Keep crushing the berries until most of their juice has been strained out and only pulp remains. Add the vinegar and the salt to the berry juice. The vinegar helps the ink retain its color, and the salt keeps it from getting too moldy. If the berry ink is too thick, add a tablespoon of water. Store the ink in a baby food jar. Make only a small amount of berry ink at a time, and when not using it, keep it tightly covered.

Quill pen:

Craft knife
Large feather (find your own or purchase one from a craft store)
Berry ink
Paper toweling

Using the craft knife, cut the tip of the feather at an angle. Next, carefully cut a slit in the tip. To use the quill pen, dip it into the berry ink. Before writing on paper, dab the end on a paper towel to remove any excess ink. Now your child can write the way the pioneers did back in the good old days. (And note, adults, please supervise this project.)

(*Courtesy*: Vinegar Institute.)

PETS AND VINEGAR

1 **Here's to Good Pet Health** Even cats, dogs, and horses can benefit from vinegar. Holistic veterinarians such as Bob Goldstein, D.V.M., of Westport, Connecticut, believe organic apple cider vinegar is food for your pet's coat and for cleansing its body of toxins. "The natural acidity helps regulate digestion, and the pectin helps keep the intestines in good shape"[5]

What Vinegar Remedy to Use: Add 1 tablespoon apple cider vinegar to your cat's or dog's water bowl.

Why You'll Like It: Anything natural that can enhance your pets' good health and longevity will make them wag their tails, and you will wag yours, too.

2 **ACV Can Prevent Stones in Horses** Enteroliths, commonly known as stones, form in the large intestines of horses. Veterinarians at the University of California–Davis have seen many horses suffering from this health ailment. Removal of stones can cost more than $3,500, for surgery and postoperative care.

What Vinegar Remedy to Use: The good news is, diet can play a preventive role. According to Douglas L. Langer, D.V.M., oat hay and grass hay tend to be low in minerals and don't seem to maintain the high pH linked with alfalfa hay. Grain—and even apple cider vinegar—can also be good, since it promotes a lower intestinal pH. U.C. Davis vets recommend 1 to 2 cups of apple cider vinegar per day as a preventive measure.

Why You'll Like It: Use caution, since some horses do develop a loose stool from consuming vinegar. If this happens, discontinue the treatments, but after the stools are normal again, find the right vinegar solution that does not produce loose stools for your horse.[6]

3 **Fight Pesky Fleas and Ticks** Did you know that flea collars and sprays are full of poisons? Instead of using chemical insecticides, use natural and less toxic methods of flea control, such as vinegar.

What Vinegar Remedy to Use: Drop a teaspoon of distilled white vinegar into each bowl of drinking water for Fluffy or Fido. The ratio of 1 teaspoon to 1 quart is for a 40-pound animal, notes the Vinegar Institute.

Why You'll Like It: Pet lovers know how frustrating it can be to fight the battle of fleas and ticks. It's not fun to watch dogs and cats scratch and whine, nor is it fun to experience your household being infested by bugs. Plus, by using an all-natural flea product on your pet, you will put your mind and household at ease.

4 **Giving the Cat or Dog a Bath** Minnie, a 14-year-old-black-and-white feline, was flea infested last summer. After using flea products on her for a few months, JoAnn Korzenko of Ohio tried an alternative remedy.

What Vinegar Remedy to Use: Korzenko reports that after soaping up her cat with baby shampoo and using a handheld shower sprayer to rinse off the soap, she added about 2 tablespoons of apple cider vinegar to a pitcher of warm water, poured it over her cat, and watched the remaining soap come out as well as the dead fleas. "She now gets a monthly bath," says the happy cat lover.

Why You'll Like It: If you can't move to the mountains, where I can vouch that the high altitude and cold weather zaps fleas year round, the next best thing is to turn to vinegar to put annoying fleas in their place!

5 **Pet Accident** Oops! In the real animal world, pet lovers know that furry and feathery creatures can and do have accidents. Yes, furballs, urine, stools, and droppings can and do happen on our favorite furniture and carpets.

What Vinegar Remedy to Use: According to the Vinegar Institute, sprinkling distilled white vinegar over the fresh pet accident may be the antidote for that unsightly spot. Wait a few minutes and sponge from the center outward. Blot up with a dry cloth. Repeat as needed for stubborn stains.

Why You'll Like It: Anything natural is good for you and your animal friends. I have oriental rugs, which don't like harsh cleaners. Plus, if your guilty and sensitive cat or dog sniffs around its mess, you won't have to shout "No!" twice. Adds Kim Copél, a small-animal lover in Northern California: "It quickly eliminates odor and stains on everything from my parakeet's cage bottom to my rabbit's and guinea pigs' litter pans, and floor areas where they occasionally have accidents, and I don't have to worry about poisoning them with chemicals." (I tried it immediately after my puppy had an accident. No odor!)

6 **Bunny Litter Boxes** Want a must-have rule to follow with your oh-so-adorable and affectionate Peter Rabbit–or Peter Cottontail–type bunny with big red or brown soulful eyes, long whiskers, and floppy pink satin ears? For starters, for the sake of your bunny's health, be sure to empty all soiled litter every day, and completely clean his cage once a week.

What Vinegar Remedy to Use: "White vinegar is an inexpensive, safe way to clean your rabbit's litter pan. Spritz the litter pan with white vinegar to clean and deodorize. Let the pan soak if there is a urine buildup and then rinse clean," recommends Copél, the rabbit go-to person. Also, occasionally rinse the litter pan with distilled white vinegar to keep calcium residue down. Do not use chemicals! If your rabbit marks in an area, blot up the urine and dab on some vinegar. This will neutralize the smell and will discourage your rabbit from marking there again.

Why You'll Like It: Copél adds, "I'm one to save a penny whenever I can, and with white vinegar being so inexpensive, it is a natural for me to use it on all of my animals' living quarters, including litter pans."

7 **Cat Litter Box Deodorizing** Do you have a catfit when your feline uses the houseplants as his litter box? If the cat litter has

such a pungent odor that your cat must find a clothespin to clip on his nose, it's time to find the purr-fect solution.

What Vinegar Remedy to Use: To get rid of odor, clean the box at least every other day. I just discovered that using a splash or two of white vinegar and hot water nips that bad smell for good.

Why You'll Like It: It is easy to do and all-natural, and the best part is that it really does the trick. Not only will you be smiling, but your cat with the amazing olfactory powers will go back to doing his business in the litter box.

8 **Fat-Buster for Cats and Dogs** Like people, pets can pack on the pounds, especially if they don't get enough exercise and are fed fatty snacks, note veterinarians. Excess weight can also cause or aggravate health problems such as heart disease and diabetes in pets. But humans can help their furry friends to pare down with fat-busting supplements such as vinegar.

What Vinegar Remedy to Use: Try 1 teaspoon organic (and only organic) apple cider vinegar in drinking water twice a day to help dissolve fats.

Why You'll Like It: Vinegar is a great way to get your pet fit and trim gradually and safely. Never starve a dog or cat skinny, for its overall health's sake.

9 **Immune System–Boosting Vitamins** Like they do for humans, vitamins can do more than just maintain your dog or cat in its current state of health. Some vitamins and other supplements act as disease-fighting antioxidants in the bloodstream, providing antiaging effects and protecting the body from damaging toxins.

What Vinegar Remedy to Use: Holistic veterinarians suggest putting 1 tablespoon apple cider vinegar in your dog's or cat's water bowl. Research, in fact, shows the powerful vitamins in this natural remedy help undo the damage done by sunlight and pollutants, fight cancer and heart disease, and may even slow down the aging process.

Why You'll Like It: Rather than feeling powerless against the deadly diseases that can strike our pets, especially as they age, you can be proactive and feed both yourself and your pet a healthful, natural diet—including longevity-boosting apple cider vinegar.

10 **Getting a Squeaky Clean Fish Tank** Ever spend a lot of time siphoning the water from a 15-gallon (or larger) fish tank, scrubbing it out, and filling it up with new fish rock and water, just to find that the water isn't clear? Not fun. While I have had two hardy goldfish (Romeo and Juliet) for a few years, I want to be able to see both of them swimming happily in clear waters.

What Vinegar Remedy to Use: The remedy is easy. Take distilled white vinegar and mix it with water as you clean the tank. Rinse well and repeat.

Why You'll Like It: It beats using soap detergent or those chemicals that promise to keep your water from being cloudy. Also, you'll be able to enjoy a clear tank and healthy fish.

11 **Lose the Skunk Odor** Yes, skunks can and do spray other animals with their not-so-pleasant scent. In fact, one dog person told me that her Siberian husky, who is born to run, went AWOL one day in the mountains. One hour later, she had one skunk-sprayed pooch to deal with, and it wasn't fun.

What Vinegar Remedy to Use: Try rubbing vinegar on the coat of your furry friend, whether it's a wayward cat or a pooch on the run.

Why You'll Like It: Well, if you've ever had a close encounter with a skunk, you will be apt to reach for the fastest cure that works. Plus, if it's chemical-free, you may be more likely to feel good about using it on your "naughty" companion animal.

A DAY-IN-A-LIFE WITH VINEGAR

Vinegar can keep people (and pets) happy in countless ways. Take a look at my new, improved daily vinegar agenda.

8:30 A.M. Splash apple cider vinegar on my face to enjoy that healthy glow whether the sun is out or not.

9:00 A.M. Clean the litter box with distilled white vinegar to keep both my sensitive kitty and me happy.

10:00 A.M. Enjoy a hot cup of chamomile tea with a teaspoon of apple cider vinegar. (Well, this is on my list of things to do.)

1:00 P.M. Eat a salad chock-full of vegetables and white albacore tuna, and splash red wine vinegar on top for extra flavor.

3:00 P.M. Wash favorite black turtleneck sweater and use distilled white vinegar in the rinse cycle to preserve its bold color.

5:00 P.M. Make a vegetable stir-fry dish and include rice vinegar to enhance the flavor.

7:00 P.M. Blot apple cider vinegar on my fingernails before giving myself a manicure and a pedicure.

9:00 P.M. Savor a hot cup of chamomile tea with a teaspoon of apple cider vinegar. (I will do this, but I'm going to start with ½ teaspoon of vinegar and include ½ teaspoon of honey and a sprinkle of cinnamon on top.)

10:00 P.M. Indulge in one (or two) of those Vinegar Man cookies (I add healthful nuts and raisins).

11:00 P.M. Wipe out my dog's ear canals with apple cider vinegar because I don't like the chemical smell of the solution I purchased.

Midnight. Read *The Healing Powers of Vinegar* to discover new ways I can use versatile, all-natural vinegar to make my life easier, happier, and healthier.

CAN VINEGAR GO BAD?

So, how long does vinegar last, anyhow? Well, this question is a tricky one. First, people will tell you that it lasts a long time. The Vinegar Institute conducted studies to determine vinegar's longevity. And the fact remains that vinegar's shelf life is almost indefinite.

For one, because of its acidic nature, vinegar is self-preserving and doesn't need to be refrigerated. Distilled white vinegar will remain unchanged over a long period of time, but note that other vinegars may experience some changes, such as color alterations or development of a sediment. Still, evidently, the change is only in overall appearance.

If you're wondering about the shelf life of a vinegar product, it depends on a variety of things, such as storage time, temperature, age, and container. But note that the following guidelines are recommended by Heinz for vinegar products stored properly:

Apple cider vinegar, 18 months
Distilled white vinegar, salad vinegar, 42 months
Malt vinegar, 24 months
Tarragon vinegar, 30 months

And, of course, if a vinegar product has a "use-by date," all the better for peace of mind.

Mini Cheesecakes with Balsamic Berries

❖ ❖ ❖

Cheesecake comes in a variety of forms. Baked New York cheesecake includes sour cream, but is dense and dry. Premium cream cheese makes a creamy and light French cheesecake. No eggs are used in the unbaked (refrigerated) cheesecake, and it can be sweetened with sugar and topped with fruit drizzled with vinegar for more flavor.

Mini cheesecakes, like these, are easy to make, and tame a sweet tooth as well as feed your cravings. That means you can indulge without guilt. Also, berries paired with vinegar can help you fight fat by increasing your calorie-burning power. More berries, less cheesecake. They have a nice appeal to the palate and are fun to plate in many ways, incorporating other dieter's friends, like dark chocolate shavings or nuts. Not only are they perfect for one, they can also be a nice sophisticated dessert for family and friends.

GRAHAM CRACKER CRUST

7 graham crackers, ground very
   fine (use a blender)
¼ cup granulated white sugar

¼ cup European-style butter, melted
1 tablespoon Bragg Organic Raw
   Apple Cider Vinegar

In a bowl, mix cracker crumbs, sugar, butter, and vinegar. Press mixture firmly against the bottom and sides of 3 or 4 ramekin dishes. (You can also you can bake mini cheesecakes in cupcake pans with liners.) Bake 10 to 12 minutes in a 350-degree oven. Set aside. If there is extra, it makes a nice garnish.

FILLING

1 cup whipped cream cheese
½ cup sour cream
½ teaspoon pure vanilla extract
¼ cup granulated sugar (or less, if
   you prefer)
½ cup whipped cream

1 teaspoon Katz white wine
   vinegar
topping
1 cup strawberries, sliced
4 teaspoons balsamic honey
   vinegar

In a mixing bowl, blend cream cheese and sour cream. Add vanilla and sugar. Once there are no lumps, fold in whipped cream; add wine vinegar. Put into graham cracker–lined dishes. Place in refrigerator (I used the freezer) till firm for a few hours before serving. Take a knife and circle each cheesecake along the sides of the dishes. Place plate over top; turn back over onto dessert plates (graham cracker crust on the bottom). Top with strawberries drizzled with honey balsamic vinegar (any brand will work). Serves 3 or 4.

VINEGARY HEALING HINTS TO PRESERVE

✓ While vinegar is a known remedy for common health ailments, it is also used often for beauty, pets, and kids.
✓ Vinegar statistics prove that vinegar is more popular today than ever.
✓ Vinegar can clean and detox your entire house, naturally.

✓ By placing beautiful infused vinegar bottles in your household space, you can healthy up your mind and spirit.

✓ Natural vinegar can help beautify you from head to toe.

✓ Vinegar can be healthful for kids, whether it is added to their diet or used to teach them disaster preparedness for survival.

✓ Vinegar can help keep your pets healthy.

✓ Vinegar has a long shelf life, but the expiration dates for the different types and brands of vinegar may vary.

Throughout the pages in this book, I've displayed the versatile virtues of vinegar. It's not just for salads; however, it has been and will be a staple for salads. In Part 8, you'll be captivated by recipes and vinegars that'll whisk you away to different countries while you treat your palate and body to deliciousness.

Vinegar Is Not for Everyone: Some Sour Views

Of such vinegar aspect
That they'll not show their teeth by way of smile
Though Nestor swear the jest be laughable.
—William Shakespeare, *The Merchant of Venice*[1]

Vinegar is served in Northern California, Northeastern Canadian provinces, and the Pacific Northwest—all types—as I shared in the previous chapter. But the thing is, not everybody can or does embrace the remarkable remedy because it is not perfect.

Several years ago, in between writing books, I took a job (much like the character in *The Devil Wears Prada*) as a copywriter for a luxury real estate company. One cold, winter day a sophisticated English Realtor invited me to join her to look at a multimillion-dollar home at Tahoe on the Nevada side of the lake. Once inside the dwelling I was awestruck. I mumbled, "It's so warm." The Realtor replied, "Yes, the décor is marvelous." She was spot-on, but I meant the heated floors were inviting, as well as the gourmet kitchen.

It boasted a wide variety of artisanal vinegars and olive oils on the marble countertop next to the six-burner stove. Not to forget the living room boasting a panoramic view of the lake—a memorable feast for my eyes, with tribute to Ernest Hemingway's classic novel title, who got sensory details from head to feet. "I would love to cook and bake here," I said. "Look at all the vinegar!" I marveled at the array of bottles of balsamic and wine vinegars. "I don't like it," said the Realtor. "Vinegar is good for a salad, but nothing more." I smiled. I was speechless. A lot of folks, like the anti-vinegar Realtor, believe vinegar is good for washing windows and coloring Easter eggs. But despite her ignorance of Vinegar World, there are some real reasons why vinegar just isn't the right choice. Here's why.

Versatile vinegar can be used inside and outside your body. But internal use of different vinegars may not be ideal for some people, according to Susan M. Lark, M.D., of Los Altos, California. In her book *The Chemistry of Success*, she discusses the pH and alkaline mineral content of vinegar.

In Dr. Lark's clinical practice, she has found that consumption of certain acidic, low-pH foods such as different types of vinegar can be stressful to overly acidic people—despite vinegar's potential nutritional perks.

"The reason for this is that their highly acidic pH can trigger either immediate or slower-acting stress responses within the body," she reports. Also, adds Dr. Lark, many of her overly acidic patients have complained about vinegar causing unpleasant reactions such as canker sores, heartburn, bladder pain, and joint discomfort.[2]

"Other potentially nutritious but highly acidic foods like tomatoes, pineapple, raspberries, and wine can also cause similar symptoms. Repeated consumption of these low-pH foods tends to trigger chronic damage, inflammation, and overacidity in the affected tissues of sensitive people."[3]

CAN VINEGAR CURE ARTHRITIS?

Veteran international vinegar consultant Lawrence Diggs is also not convinced that vinegar is everything it's cracked up to be. "One of the persistent rumors about vinegar is that it will cure arthritis," he says. Some people believe apple cider vinegar thins body fluids. As a result, stiff joints are supposed to move easier so one won't be walking around like the Tin Man in the *Wizard of Oz*. "To date there is no scientific evidence that any kind of vinegar or vinegar cocktail will cure or relieve the pain of arthritis. I should mention also that it doesn't seem that scientists are all that interested in providing evidence either."[4]

Most doctors know it is not possible for apple cider vinegar to cure arthritis. However, because aches and pains can come and go, the healing vinegar may seem like it works wonders at times. But there is no scientific proof.

Meanwhile, if you have arthritis, watch your weight (heavy people are more at risk for osteoarthritis) by eating a low-fat diet, and get a move on. Keeping in shape can help strengthen your muscles.

NOT 100% TUMMY TERRIFIC

Other people vow that vinegar is a cure-all for an upset stomach. While Vinegar Man Lawrence Diggs claims he has used vinegar for himself "and it seems to have worked," he does not recommend it. "The stomach is always playing a balancing act to get the right acid and base balance. It usually doesn't get much help from us. The result is that sometimes the stomach is too base or alkaline and sometimes too acid. If it is too base, then adding an acid like vinegar could help. However, if it is too acid, the problem could be made worse."

He believes because the symptoms of both conditions feel similar, we don't know if vinegar, baking soda, or burnt toast will be the best Rx. "If I had to gamble, I'd put my money on the burnt toast, even though I am not nor ever have been a member of Burnt Toast Connoisseurs International."[5]

Vinegar Remedy Flushed down the Toilet?

On May 19, 1994, a court order resulted in the destruction of 13,320 half-gallon bottles of "Jogging in a Jug"—a concoction of grape and apple juices and vinegar—because the product became an unapproved new drug due to health claims made by promoters. Jack McWilliams, owner of Third Option Laboratories, Muscle Shoals, Alabama, claimed that his vinegar solution had helped him beat arthritis and heart disease, and could lower the risk of cancer. Third Option also paid the Federal Trade Commission $480,000 to settle charges of false advertising.[6]

A Trigger for Interstitial Cystitis

While some women claim vinegar can help stave off painful bladder infections, many people don't realize that the acidic wonder food may also trigger interstitial cystitis (IC), which is a chronic inflammatory condition of the bladder.

The symptoms include frequency of urination, urgency of urination, and pelvic pain, pressure, or discomfort.

"We know that many people with IC have symptom flares if they eat or drink something that is acidic. There has been little research into why certain foods and beverages tend to cause IC flares," explains Salin. "However, anecdotally over many, many years, and from our best source—people with IC—it is apparent that acidic (and other) things (whether or not they become alkaline in the GI tract) do cause IC flares. Vinegar in any form is one of these that many with IC symptoms say make their symptoms worse."

Adds Jill H. Osborne, president and founder of the Interstitial Cystitis Network (ICN), "There is a myth that vinegar or lemon juice can cure 'all' bladder problems. Wrong! For interstitial cystitis, foods high in vinegar and any other high-acid products can provoke urgency, frequency, and for some, agonizing pain. Why? Because IC patients have 'wounds' on their bladder. Pouring acid on those wounds will certainly create more inflammation and trigger the symptoms."

The good news is that staying clear of the dietary culprits—acidic foods—may lower the severity of IC symptoms. In a list of problem foods compiled by the ICN, vinegar is included in the category of seasonings and additives and called "usually problematic." But note, Prelief, an over-the-counter dietary supplement, may help IC patients better tolerate acid foods and beverages.[7]

By the way, vinegar is not on the list of the five "biggest misery makers" for people with IC. These potential troublemakers include cranberry juice, coffee, carbonated beverages, tomatoes, and tobacco.

Is ACV Taboo for Your Teeth?

Let's face it, acids can be bad news for dental enamel. Recently, when I had my teeth cleaned, I asked my dental hygienist if drinking orange juice late at night without brushing my teeth is a bad idea? My cat or dog occasionally awaken me, and when I tend to their needs, I often grab a piece of fruit or juice. She told me that I should definitely brush my teeth afterward, or at least rinse my mouth out with water. And vinegar is the same deal.

Dr. Earl Mindell once told me that carbonated diet drinks are not only bad for the bones, but also bad for the teeth. Again, vinegar is an acid food. But that doesn't mean you can't use it. Instead, use it with caution.

It's best to drink ACV with water, as advised throughout this book. (But folk doctor Jarvis often recommends taking an ACV remedy straight. In the twenty-first century, people tend to keep their teeth longer, if not for life. If that's your goal, please dilute the golden liquid.) Plus, rinse your mouth after drinking an ACV cocktail.

Also, I recall that when I had a tooth bonded, I didn't want it to be discolored, so I began drinking tea with a straw. It's not a bad idea to try this if you are concerned about ACV and its effect on your dental enamel.

VINEGAR—NOT FOR EVERYONE'S TASTE

In Chapter 1, I noted that many people turn up their nose at the idea of drinking the healthy brew solo. Remember Kris, who lowered her cholesterol levels and gave credit to apple cider vinegar? Well, she drank liquid organic ACV at first, until she found an alternative.

"I couldn't stand it—a tablespoon after every meal. Then I started taking the pills. They are pure dried apple cider vinegar. They also help with digestion and that bloated feeling. If I find my numbers are back up, I start taking it again, until I get them down," she explains.

"Three months is actually a very short time in which to get your cholesterol levels down. If they put a person on a cholesterol-lowering drug, they expect that it would take at least six months or more. So the ACV is much healthier and a quicker way to combat high cholesterol," she adds. "Yes, my doctor had no choice but to believe that the apple cider vinegar worked. The numbers were indisputable."

If you, like Kris or me (I still don't drink it solo), want the benefits of ACV but can't bear the smell or taste, the tablets are an alternative. ACV tablets are available online and at health food stores.

But on the flip side, vinegar connoisseurs like Lawrence Diggs say the pills are "junk." For starters, he asks, "Why? If somebody says 'I didn't like the taste,' well, the taste of which one? There's over three hundred and fifty, and that is just the tip of the iceberg. And there are many of them that if you don't tell people they are vinegar, they don't even know it."

KEEPING IT REAL AND SWEET

Countless vinegars are available on the market. There are also dozens of vinegar books that boast miracle benefits for the golden liquid. While I do believe that vinegar is one of the most natural, accessible, and inexpensive foods in the world, it's not a magic bullet.

Adds Vinegar Man Diggs, people who prefer the scientific process will always have a problem with books like this one. "Even using a scientific method, half of the stuff that we figure today is true we'll find is not true tomorrow." Diggs also notes that scientists' findings about vinegar and its health benefits don't always stand up to peer review. But he does caution that people should be wary of anecdotal evidence.

As a former diet and nutrition writer for women's magazines, I have to say that I have written about the nutritional perks of antioxidants, green tea, "good" fats, and fat-burning foods, which were often first noted in European countries by open-minded scientists. Today, many of these benefits are acknowledged by mainstream medicine.

So yes, incorporating versatile vinegar into your lifestyle (both externally and internally) certainly may help you to live a longer, healthier, and happier life. But when it comes down to the question of whether vinegar itself can be the cure-all to each and every common ailment and life-threatening disease, the answer is no. There is no magic bullet.

The bottom line: A healthy diet and exercise paired with vinegars of all types can enhance your health—and that is the real truth. Vinegar is healthful. Vinegar can do many amazing things. Vinegar is a good thing, as long as you remember that no one food can make you healthy. It's the combination of practicing a healthy lifestyle and using ancient remedies like vinegar that can give you remarkable results.

THE MOST UNFORGETTABLE
QUESTIONS ABOUT VINEGAR

Despite people's fervor for vinegar power, hype or hope is often the case. People of all ages actually want to know the real scoop on the virtues of vinegar, especially when a pesky ailment or potential threat of a disease is affecting their well-being. And when we do hear success stories, like how a woman lives to be more than a hundred years old and gives thanks to daily vinegar intake, we may ponder, "Why isn't it working?" or "Will it work for me?"

Ever wonder if apple cider vinegar might be the beginning of the end of your heart health scare? Do you know which vinegar is the best for *you* and your health challenges? As the author of *The Healing Powers of Vinegar*, first and second editions, I have been asked hundreds of questions—all types from run-of-the-mill to weird—from around the world via e-mail and radio talk show hosts and their call-in listeners. Here are some of my favorite questions and my down-to-earth responses (remember, I am a vinegar author, not a doc).

TELLTALE VINEGAR HEART HEALTH

Is vinegar *really* good for high blood pressure and cholesterol?

Yes and no. Apple cider vinegar, for one, seems to be helpful for a number of people, as I note in Chapter 15, "The Liquid to Heart Health." Folks continue to ask me if vinegar is a magic bullet to lower blood pressure and bad cholesterol numbers. True, apple cider vinegar is rich in potassium, which may help counterbalance sodium levels in your body and lower the risk of developing high blood pressure. Insoluble fiber in ACV reduces cholesterol by binding with fiber, which is eliminated by the body. But there's more.

I've noticed after talking to people who have been diagnosed with high numbers for blood pressure and/or cholesterol that they want a quick fix. Sure, vinegar can help you get heart healthy and if you look for miracle apple cider vinegar anecdotes you will find some. But I've discovered people who want a magical cure often may be struggling with body fat and unwanted pounds and/or have pre-diabetes. If they overindulge in salt, sugar, and alcohol and are sedentary, will apple cider vinegar be the key to heart health? It may be, but in reality using it in conjunction with lifestyle changes is going to give results—not just a quickie tonic daily fix.

Are fruits bad for you when you have high triglycerides and can vinegar be good for you and help lower those off-the-chart numbers?

High triglycerides (fats that circulate in the bloodstream) put you at risk for heart disease. A triglyceride level of less than 150 is what you should be aiming for to get the odds in your heart health favor. Insoluble fiber in apple cider vinegar and fruits (I discuss this in Chapters 4 and 5) can help reduce cholesterol by binding with fiber, which is eliminated by the body.

As you know, the Mediteranean diet—the underlying theme in the Healing Powers series—includes a variety of fruits. People in European countries consume many servings daily of heart-healthy antioxidant-rich fruits, which can also help stave off high levels of "bad" cholesterol and up "good" cholesterol. But why stop at vinegar and fruit? Also include protein (fish and eggs in moderation), whole grains, and exercise regularly to help get those triglyceride numbers down and you feeling up about it.

One more thing: Don't forget olive oil. In my book *The Healing Powers of Olive Oil*, I dish on how this heart-healthy fat can help you take charge of unwanted fat in your body. So yes, enjoy consuming fresh fruit salads with apple cider dressings, and an apple cider vinegar cocktail with honey (another heart healer) can help you to lower those triglyceride numbers. But first and foremost, take a serious look at your diet and lifestyle before you open a bottle of apple cider vinegar.

VINEGAR DETOX TO THE RESCUE

Can red wine vinegar be used as a detox like apple cider vinegar?

In Part 3, "Red Wine Vinegar," I chat it up with Lawrence Diggs, the Vinegar Man. Both of us, as well as medical doctors and researchers, agree that red wine vinegar contains good-for-you disease-fighting antioxidants that may help lower your risk of developing cancer, diabetes, and even stroke.

Apple cider proponents, however, will tell you apple cider vinegar with its potassium is the best detox vinegar to use. Personally, if I had a choice I'd choose apple cider vinegar for a serious detox regimen. Red wine vinegar is fine for a semi-detox diet. In other words, use it plain or paired with extra virgin olive oil on leafy greens or drizzled on raw vegetables. The water-dense produce with vinegar and oil (both have anti-bacterial and anti-inflammatory properties) will help flush out toxins in your body.

While on a detox diet, will apple cider vinegar lose any of its healing properties when used in cooking?

For starters, as you will read in *The Healing Powers of Vinegar*, disease-fighting, antioxidant-rich red wine vinegar is a more common choice for vinegars when you turn to cooking vegetables, poultry, meat, and casseroles. Both apple cider and red wine vinegars are used in vinaigrettes teamed with raw salads. Now that we have that topic off the table, I believe vinegar—any kind—will lose some of its healing compounds during the cooking process on the stovetop or in the oven or microwave.

Apple cider vinegar is often used in a variety of ways for internal use. Countless folks use the popular folk remedy by taking vinegar shots (a tablespoon or two daily) to help detox the body. What's more, when you do cook foods such as vegetables it is possible to lose some of the essential vitamins and minerals during the heating process so the same is probably true with vinegars. Processed food is not as healthful as fresh eats. Whenever possible eat raw, fresh foods, especially vegetables, fruits—and vinegar. And note, when you do cook with vinegar, cook lightly. Think nutrient-dense clean foods like stir-fry dishes—do not overcook your vegetables—and drizzle vinegar on top to enjoy the most healing benefits.

HELP ME, VINEGAR!

Can apple cider vinegar reduce the effects after a stroke?

Before I cut to the chase and say "yes" or "no"—let's take a look at what causes a stroke. Simply put, cardiologists will tell you it can be a narrowing of a blood vessel in the brain or a blood clot. Doctors will tell you the way to help prevent a stroke is to keep your blood pressure down, get essential fatty acids in your diet, keep your weight in check, exercise regularly, don't smoke, and stay calm.

So, if you follow doctors' orders, apple cider vinegar may actually help you to recover as well as lower the risk of having another stroke. But vinegar is not a miracle worker that will give you results overnight. Still, the potent elixir does contain disease-fighting ingredients, including potassium, and that may help lower high blood pressure and slash artery plaque. Some research points to plaque buildup in arteries causing strokes by blocking blood flow to the heart and brain.

Also, red wine vinegar contains potential disease-fighting compounds that may help prevent stroke, too. But note, consuming vinegars alone without adopting a healthful diet and making positive lifestyle changes most likely cannot prevent a stroke from reoccurring or reverse dramatic effects. However, teaming vinegar and olive oil along with a Mediteranean diet and lifestyle (as I include in the Healing Powers series) may help you to lower the odds of having another stroke and put you on the road to a faster recovery.

VINEGAR SMARTS, I NEED ASSISTANCE, PLEASE

I'm confused about white vinegar. Can you cook and bake with it?

Here's the real scoop. White vinegar and commonly named distilled white vinegar are the same thing. It is used more for cleaning (such as a coffeepot and windows). However, some recipes do call for white vinegar (like pie crust and potato salad). It has a sharp flavor, not as tart and fruity as apple cider vinegar or syrupy like balsamic vinegar. If you don't have it, you can substitute white wine vinegar, rice vinegar or even apple cider vinegar. And yes, if you don't have apple cider vinegar, but need vinegar to soothe irritated skin, some dermatologists will recommend white vinegar as a natural home remedy. A bonus: I used white vinegar with sea salt to soak my favorite silver necklace. Two hours later: It was sparkling clean.

So, what vinegar is the most popular?

The answer may surprise you as it did me. There are many organizations that do claim which vinegars are in demand. I created a quickie vinegar poll on a social media network. Twenty-five people (anonymous from around the United States) responded to what their favorite vinegar choice is.

The results: White vinegar led the pack, balsamic followed, apple cider third, and red wine vinegar placed fourth. Rice, herbal, and fruit-flavored vinegars were only noted by a couple of people. So there you have it. Are you surprised? I am.

Is apple cider vinegar safe to take during pregnancy?

Apple cider vinegar proponents will tell you it is safe to consume during and after being with child. However, as I always say—"moderation" is key. You do not want to overindulge in anything, whether it be herbs or superfoods. Balance is important for good health and well-being.

I'm allergic to wheat products, so what vinegars are gluten-free?

This question is interesting and has a variety of answers. The good news is, apple cider vinegar is gluten-free. Wine vinegars made from red and white wine are also gluten-free. Now, balsamic vinegar is tricky. Since it's aged in wooden casks, a problem (wheat or rye flour) could exist due to paste used to seal the containers and that could affect the gluten-free potential of this vinegar. Rice is on the okay list if it's not combined with other grains. Forget and forego malt vinegar (no Rachael Ray Malt Vinegar Oven Fries for you) because it's made from barley. Flavored vinegars, such as tarragon, also can contain barley. To be on the safe side of gluten, call the manufacturer and ask if the vinegar is gluten-free.

Where do I find apple cider vinegar?

You don't have to go far to get a bottle of this potent elixir. Bragg's Apple Cider Vinegar is a favorite of mine and is easily located at major grocery stores and health food stores. There are other brands, too, though. I have tried many different ones and for topical use I personally feel one works as well as another.

When a recipe includes white vinegar, I'm confused. Do I use distilled or what type?

White vinegar comes in different varieties, including distilled and wine. You can use white distilled vinegar for baking, beauty, and cleaning recipes. White wine vinegar, however, has more flavor and is used more for cooking.

GOING WITH THE FLOW FOR HEALTH'S SAKE

Does apple cider vinegar affect the urine flow in people?

Good question. While some apple cider vinegar book authors claim vinegar can help stave off painful bladder infections, many people don't realize that the acidic wonder, especially when consumed by the tablespoon or in a glass of water, may trigger a flare-up of interstitial cystitis (IC), which is a chronic inflammatory condition of the bladder. (Refer to this chapter.) Other vinegars, like other acidic culprits including citrus, can irritate tissue for some people (whether it be the esophagus, tummy, skin or bladder). The more you consume of the trigger food, the more you may find yourself going to the bathroom.

Plus, if you are consuming more vinegar drinks—store-bought or homemade—you are getting more liquid in your system and this in itself can cause an increase in urine flow. Men are less likely to be IC sufferers, but they are not immune. So, it's trial and error. If you discover symptoms, including frequency or urgency of urination, it may be time to switch to another superfood. May I recommend olive oil? The odds are, you'll get the same health perks from *The Healing Powers of Olive Oil* book as vinegar.

BALSAMIC BLUES

I read that balsamic vinegar can contain sulfites (used in foods as a preservative that can cause an allergic reaction). Is this true and is there anything I can do so I can have my vinegar and eat it too?

The good news is not all balsamic vinegars contain sulfites, but some less pricey ones do. Your best bet is to look at the nutritional label before you buy and indulge. Or, if you are eating at a restaurant, it couldn't hurt to ask your server about the preservatives in a balsamic vinegar that is used.

HOW MUCH IS TOO MUCH VINEGAR?

I love salty foods dipped in all types of vinegar. Is my vinegar addiction harmful to my health?

If you are consuming vinegar, less is more in my book (pun intended). Whether it is apple cider vinegar or olive oil, you must realize one is acidic, which can cause some problems in some people; the other is high in calories and fat. Moderation is key. The premise behind *The Healing Powers of Vinegar* is to use the versatile remedy in a variety of ways—not to drink it like it's water and you're a camel.

Pairing vinegars—all kinds—with fresh fruits, vegetables, whole grains, fish, and even in wholesome sweets can provide a host of health perks. In recipes the vinegar amount is often small, but offers big flavor to healthful food. But I'm not saying drink cups of vinegar each day and cook with it too.

Versatile vinegar can also be used topically for problems ranging from blemishes to burns (you may want to use it more than once a day). Go back to Chapter 18 and check out the wide variety of vinegar uses for home cures. So, can you drink too much vinegar? My answer is yes. Same goes for using it on your body. The key is moderation even with nature's remarkable remedy.

I've been using apple cider vinegar a couple times a day on an empty stomach. It has helped lessen my arthritis, but now my tongue aches and has spots on it. Is vinegar to blame?

Vinegar is acidic and can cause tummy woes, especially on an empty stomach. I haven't heard of apple cider vinegar causing a sore tongue. Ouch! I do know thrush (a growth of yeast in the mouth) can cause an inflamed and white-colored tongue. These symptoms can be due to lack of vitamins in your diet, antibiotics, or even a reaction after eating acidic foods.

Consult with the Academy of Nutrition and Dietetics to find out if your diet is balanced and you're getting essential nutrients. If your tongue doesn't get back to normal, walk fast, don't skip to your doctor to see what is causing that achy tongue of yours. Congrats on controlling arthritic woes; apple cider vinegar advocates would likely give credit to nature's remarkable remedy.

Also, if you continue using apple cider vinegar I recommend diluting it with water as well as taking the cure with food just as you would do with a cup of coffee or glass of orange juice. If you find that you're still having problems, may I suggest switching to olive oil or coffee—two more superfoods with amazing powers and abilities to help you lessen arthritic aches and pains.

Is drinking apple cider vinegar dangerous for bone health?

So many people e-mail with questions about the ill effects of vinegar and they confess to me that they're drinking a gallon of apple cider vinegar per day (well, I'm exaggerating, but the amount does seem a bit excessive). That said, I feel compelled to mention the word *moderation* with vinegar just like when drinking coffee or indulging in chocolate. If you go overboard and consume flavored-vinegar drinks 24/7, I suppose anything is possible, but bone loss from vinegar? Not years ago, my neighbor slipped and fell. She had a fractured hip, the result of osteoporosis (bone loss)—not vinegar usage.

If you want to lower your risk of preventing bone loss, watch out for the common bone robbers that can steal essential minerals and vitamins from you. They include: excess protein, salt, sugar, and lifestyle culprits, such as smoking and too much alcohol. I do not recall vinegar as a big culprit for causing osteoporosis.

I read using apple cider vinegar is a great way to get whiter teeth. Is this remedy a good one to try?

I'm surprised each time I see someone claiming to brush your teeth with vinegar—it's acidic like orange juice and Coke—the beverages that wear down your tooth enamel—something you can never get back, warn dentists. So why in the Vinegar World would you even think of trying such a home remedy?

I recommend that when you consume homemade vinegar cocktails, flavored-fruit vinegars, or vinegar dressings, rinse your mouth with water and if possible brush your teeth as you would after drinking orange juice. I recall an octogenarian friend who, late at night, would sip on orange juice as she watched television until she fell asleep. One night at a restaurant she told me about her dental appointment earlier in the afternoon. "I have four cavities on my front teeth. The dentist believes it's from the OJ." The bottom line: Try another whitening method advised by your dental hygienist or dentist.

VINEGARY HEALING HINTS TO PRESERVE

✓ Vinegar, like carbonated beverages, can be a trigger for interstitial cystitis flare-ups because of its acidic nature.

✓ Since vinegar is acidic, be sure to brush your teeth after enjoying a vinegar drink or using it on your food.
✓ If you want to get the potential health benefits of apple cider vinegar but don't like the taste, consider apple cider vinegar tablets.

Washing of Greens

❖ ❖ ❖

cold water; ice   *greens, picked through*
white vinegar   *perforated pan*
Kosher salt   *salad spinner*

For every gallon of water add 1 capful of vinegar and 1 tablespoon of salt. Add in a few handfuls of ice; if too much, you'll have to pick it out of the greens. Add your greens making sure there is enough room for them to move around freely. Let stand for 20 minutes. Carefully remove from the cold water and lay greens into a perforated pan. From there you can spin them. (Note: Past research shows vinegar can rid produce of bacteria. This isn't news, but it's a good thing its being put to use today when store-bought lettuce often has unwanted bacteria on it.)

(*Courtesy:* Chef Skelding of The Greenbrier.)

Finally, in Part 8 "Vinegar Recipes," you'll enter the world of more vinegary recipes and the Mediterranean diet for good flavor and good health.

PART 8

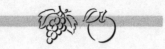

VINEGAR RECIPES

Vinegar Bon Appétit!

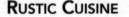

RUSTIC CUISINE

If you've gotten this far, it doesn't take a rocket scientist or psychic to tell you that the recipes woven throughout the pages for cooking and baking, beauty, household, and pet care are simple and chock-full of comfort superfoods.

All of my life was spent living in California—Southern California by the sea, Central California in the valley, and Northern California in the city and mountains. We are the Golden State known for its fresh flavors, coastal-inspired dishes, ocean fish, and super salads, not to forget its olive oil and vinegars that all lend themselves to rustic recipes.

My rustic roots, inspired by my mother's travels to Europe, were expanded by me following in her footsteps to Canadian provinces and getting my fill of both sophisticated and unsophisticated foods. When I wrote the first edition of *The Healing Powers of Vinegar*, I fell into the Mediteranean diet, which I'd been using all along. I had come full circle. As you will see, in the seasonal recipes and recipes section, there is a common theme: healthful food fit for a peasant or princess—and if you give it your heart, it can feed royalty anywhere around the globe.

FOUR SEASONS FOR SUPERFOODS
WITH HEALING VINEGARS

Winter: Superfoods during this season pair well with a variety of vinegars. My favorites, though, are red wine vinegar for hearty soups, and balsamic vinegar for drizzling on baked goodies, like scones and muffins.

Apricot Current Scones with
Balsamic Honey Glaze

❖ ❖ ❖

2 cups all-purpose flour
1 tablespoon baking powder
¼ cup confectioners' sugar
5 tablespoons European-style
  butter (cold cubes)
1 organic egg
⅔ to 1 cup buttermilk
1 teaspoon apple cider vinegar

1 teaspoon vanilla extract
2 tablespoons fresh orange rind,
  grated
¾ to 1 cup currants
½ cup dried apricots, chopped
raw sugar
¼ cup Honey Ridge Farms
Balsamic Honey Vinegar

Preheat oven to 350 degrees. In a bowl, mix flour, baking powder, and sugar. Add chunks of butter. In another bowl, combine egg, buttermilk, and vanilla. Stir till mixed. Add rind, currants, and apricots. Put into lightly greased round baking dish (I used my favorite what tart dish for a rustic look. Bake till golden brown, about 30 minutes. Sprinkle with sugar. Cool. Cut in triangle shapes like a pizza. Makes approximately 12. Serve with honey or cream cheese. For a special touch drizzle with honey balsamic vinegar.

Blackberry Balsamic Vinegar French Toast

❖ ❖ ❖

French toast had me at "hello" back when I was a kid growing up in the San Francisco Bay Area. In the twentieth century, my mom made it with white bread, white eggs, and whole milk. We drizzled the crispy bread with warmed up store-bought syrup and teamed it with bacon and homemade squeezed orange juice. It was a special treat that I liked in the past, but now I love it with a more sophisticated appeal.

French toast, also called "eggy bread," is a popular breakfast of bread dipped in an egg mixture and fried on a skillet. In the twenty-first century, my recipe includes a healthier redo with fresh fruit—like strawberries with balsamic vinegar (a pairing food goddess Ina Garten touts) for romance in February—organic dairy, wheat bread, spices, and a bit of earthy balsamic vinegar.

2 brown organic eggs, beaten
1 cup 2 percent low-fat organic milk
1 teaspoon each cinnamon and nutmeg
1 teaspoon pure vanilla extract (optional)
4 slices wheat sourdough bread

2 tablespoons European-style butter
1 cup fresh sliced strawberries
2 tablespoons Honey Ridge Farms all-natural maple syrup
confectioners' sugar
whipped cream

In a bowl, mix eggs, milk, spices, and vanilla. Melt butter on medium heat in large frying pan. Dip bread in egg-milk mixture. Cook till golden brown. Serve on plates and top French toast with strawberries. Drizzle with vinegar and syrup, dust with sugar, and add a dollop of whipped cream. Serves 2.

Spring: After winter it's a time for renewal and rejuvenation. Apple cider vinegar comes to mind because of its detoxifying benefits. Also, medicinal rice vinegar, fruit-flavored vinegars, and vinegar drinks help boost the immune system especially as we go through the transitional period of weather, from cold to hot, and are more prone to flus and colds as well as seasonal allergies.

Rice Pudding with a Tart Twist

❖ ❖ ❖

The first week of May is time to feast on more fresh fruits and vegetables, but my palate and mood takes a while to warm up to the seasonal change. This recipe of mine—with savory and sweet flavors of honey, apples (budget-friendly before summer produce is available), citrus, and vinegar(s) gives it a springtime touch. Created from rice combined with milk and other year-round ingredients, like raisins and cinnamon, it can be wholesome cold or hot. Since the temperatures are still erratic in the California Sierra, I baked the casserole-type wonder in the morning and it brought back bittersweet memories of budget-friendly comfort food during graduate school days.

1¼ cups cooked brown rice
2 brown organic eggs, beaten
2½ cups half-and-half, organic
¼ cup granulated white sugar
2 teaspoons honey
1 tablespoon each Bragg's Organic
   Raw Apple Cider Vinegar
   and Nakano Rice Vinegar
1 teaspoon vanilla extract
1 cup Granny Smith apples,
   chopped

1 cup golden raisins
European-style butter (to grease
   baking dish)
1 tablespoon cinnamon
1 teaspoon nutmeg
lemon and orange slices,
   cinnamon sticks, mint for
   garnish (optional)

In a bowl, combine rice, eggs, half-and-half, sugar, honey, vinegars, vanilla, apples, and raisins. Lightly grease butter on an 8 x 8 baking dish (or use ramekins). Bake at 325 degrees in a pan of water (about 2 or 3 inches) for 1 to 1½ hours and until golden brown. Top immediately with cinnamon and nutmeg. Serve warm. Garnish with citrus slices or cinnamon sticks. Makes 6–8 servings.

Fruit Crisp with Honey Vinegar

◆ ◆ ◆

This naturally sweet and tart comforting crisp is colorful like the promise of springtime flowers. The tang from blueberry vinegar makes it extra special. During the spring in the Sierra Nevada it can rain or snow through May, so this rustic dish is ideal on a cool night. It is good to eat warm with cold whipped cream. Baking and serving a crisp, like this one, in cute ramekins is easy on the eyes and yields a perfect portion size. It pairs well with a cup of hot black tea. This healthful treat is a foolproof fruity recipe (that will give you a taste of blueberries to come in the summer) that'll put a smile on your face and warm your spirit during springtime blues.

2 cups Granny Smith apples,
   quartered, cored, and chopped
½ cup strawberries, fresh

⅛ cup dark brown sugar
1 tablespoon all-purpose flour
½ teaspoon ground cinnamon

TOPPING

½ cup quick oats, uncooked
¼ cup dark brown sugar
1 tablespoon all-purpose flour
¼ teaspoon ground cinnamon
2–3 tablespoons European-style
   butter, small squares

sugar in the raw
whipped cream or Greek yogurt
4 tablespoons Honey Ridge Farms
   Balsamic Honey Vinegar

Preheat oven to 375 degrees. In a medium-sized bowl combine fruit, sugar, flour, and cinnamon. Place in 6-ounce ramekins. In another bowl, mix all the dry topping ingredients and butter together. Top onto fruit. Sprinkle each with raw sugar (for a nice crunch). Place dishes in a rectangular baking pan half filled with water. Bake for approximately 40 minutes or till fruit is bubbly and topping is golden brown. Turn up the heat to 400 degrees for a few minutes to get extra crisp. Cool. Serve with a dollop of whipped cream or yogurt. Drizzle with balsamic honey vinegar. Serves 4 to 6.

Summer: Summer is a time for iced tea—all types—with honey and a bit of apple cider vinegar for fresh fruit salads to help with energy and keeping slim. Also, savoring vinegar drinks—made of fruit, sugar, and vinegar—seems appropriate and cooling for this season of sun, frolic, and longer days. Not to ignore red wine seasoned vinegar to be teamed with oils in cold salads with fish or poultry, vegetables and fruits.

Avocado and Cheese Quesadilla

❖ ❖ ❖

It's a pretty dish, perfect for an appetizer, lunch, or even a light dinner. The chunky red salsa and sour cream add the perfect touch and textures to each wedge. I was going to make guacamole dip and chips, but the Avocado & Cheese Quesadilla took on a life of its own. And I'm glad it did. This is definitely a repeat recipe (you can add corn, chicken, or beans) in the warmer spring days.

1–2 tablespoons European-style butter or olive oil
4 whole-grain flour tortillas

4 slices cheese (cheddar or Swiss)
1 small avocado, cut into thin slices

TOMATO SALSA

2 small Roma tomatoes, diced
¼ cup red onion, diced
½ chili pepper, diced
1 tablespoon Heinz Red Wine Vinegar

1 cup lettuce (any dark green kind)

In a bowl, mix ingredients. Let set in fridge for a few hours for better flavor. Place a tortilla in a skillet with butter and sauté on medium heat. Top with cheese and avocado. Cover with other tortilla. Cook till cheese is melted and tortilla is golden brown. Cut into four wedges. Garnish with Tomato Salsa, sour cream and lettuce Serves 2.

Chocolate Mousse with Vinegary Fruit

❖ ❖ ❖

Mirabelle Restaurant, a French gem at Lake Tahoe, is the inspiration for my creating a twist on this decadent recipe. I often fantasized about flying away to Europe with its old charm. Once out of curiosity I called the owner/chef and I listened to him describe his restaurant, a mental escape for me. I was wowed by the current menu's Pot de Chocolate. I chose the eggless, no-cook method. Instead of dark chocolate (my preference), by accident I purchased milk chocolate. It made the mousse sweet enough for a limited palate as well as the sophisticated food critics. I used heavy whipping cream—not the creamy, ready-made fluff in the plastic container. The extra effort of whipping it is worth the time and trouble.

1 cup premium all-natural milk
   chocolate chips, 31 percent
   cacao
½ cup half-and-half
2 tablespoons European-style
   butter
1 teaspoon cinnamon
1 cup heavy whipping cream

1 capful pure vanilla extract
¼ cup confectioners' sugar
extra-whipped cream (for topping)
chocolate shavings (grated dark or
   milk chocolate chips)
2 cups fresh strawberries, sliced
Honey Ridge Farms Balsamic
   Honey Vinegar to taste

In a bowl pour one cup of chocolate chips. Place in microwave and melt. (Keep a close watch on it. Do not overcook. Stir until smooth.) Set aside. In another bowl, combine half-and-half and butter. Microwave until butter is melted. Cool. Mix into chocolate. (At first it will look lumpy, but stir it and it will turn creamy and smooth.) Sprinkle with cinnamon. Set aside. In a chilled mixing bowl pour whipping cream. Mix on high until it is a thick, creamy texture. (Warning: This can take a while.) Add vanilla and sugar (it does need the sweet flavor). Fold ½ cup into chocolate. Add the rest and stir until it's a superb chocolate creamy mousse. Pour into ramekins or small glasses. Place in refrigerator for 3 hours to firm. Garnish which chocolate shavings and berries. Drizzle with vinegar. Serves approximately 4.

This easy but elegant chocolate mousse is a keeper. The first bite is rich, creamy, and chocolaty. Cinnamon adds a nice savory taste married with the white whipped cream topping. Summer strawberries add a nice natural sweet freshness. This cool dessert (in moderation) is perfect for family, friends, or solo. It does its job on the hill any day of the week, rain or shine.

Fall: Red wine vinegar for soups as temperatures drop, fish salads, and herbal vinegars for casseroles and pasta plates are good for autumn. Balsamic vinegar, too, to complete poultry dishes is a must-have in every kitchen or restaurant.

And dessert doesn't have to be fruit at its worst. Dressing up an apple with good-for-you nuts, healthy honey, and a bit of a sugary treat is a taste of deliciousness. These apples, found year-round (even around the lake) are on-a-stick and the caramel is often hard. Preparing it at home, adding a few ingredients to the caramel and slicing apples, makes it softer for kids and adults.

Italian Tuna Sandwich with RWV

❖ ❖ ❖

1 6-ounce can albacore tuna in spring water, drained and flaked

2 tablespoons olive oil mayonnaise dressing

1 teaspoon European-style butter

2 sourdough sandwich French rolls

1 teaspoon Heinz Red Wine Vinegar

¼ cup red onion, chopped

¼ cup tomatoes, chopped

1 teaspoon herbs (your choice), preferably fresh

2 slices Jarlsberg cheese

¼ cup lettuce, chopped

2 tablespoons olive oil

1–2 teaspoons red wine vinegar (your preference)

Mix tuna and mayo. Spread butter on rolls, toast in a 450-degree oven. Remove and top with tuna mixture. Add onion, tomatoes, herbs, and cheese. Place face side up in oven until the tops are toasted. Fold and slice in half. Put lettuce tossed with olive oil and red wine vinegar mixture on side of sandwich (or serve on top). Serves 2.

Sea-Salted Caramel Apples

❖ ❖ ❖

20 *caramels, unwrapped*
2 *tablespoons raw honey*
1 *tablespoon Heinz Apple Cider*
  Vinegar
3 *tablespoons organic half-and-*
  half

2 *apples, Fuji or Granny Smith*
½ *cup pecans, chopped fine or*
  leave in chunks

Put caramels in a bowl and place in the microwave until melted. Add honey and half-and-half. Put back into the microwave until melted. Add vinegar. Roll apples in caramel mixture. Then roll caramel apple into nuts. Place apples on a plate and put in fridge for about an hour or till firm. Cut apple into slices. Serves two.

The recipes that follow—more than 100 mouthwatering delights—are full of nutritious fruits, vegetables, lean meats, fish, and poultry. Our tasty dishes, provided by chefs from around the country, contain a variety of vinegars—apple cider, red wine, balsamic, rice, and herbal vinegar. Plus, healthful garlic, onions, and olive oil are often part of the recipes, too.

For best results, use the vinegar brand mentioned in each recipe. However, feel free to use your own brand or a brand without sodium if so desired (because some herbal vinegars have a high sodium content).

Before you get started, I want you to first check out some must-have cooking-with-vinegar tips and pickling favorites. See how vinegars of all types can enhance immune-boosting, nutrient-rich foods. Not only will you be eating a heart-healthy, anticancer-type Mediterranean-style diet, you'll be enjoying more gusto in your meals.

VINEGAR PIZZAZZ!

Vinegar	Flavor	Uses
Apple cider vinegar	Sweet, tangy flavor	Adds golden color to sauces and marinades.
Balsamic vinegar	Sweet and flavorful	Use for special sauces, marinades or salad dressings, vanilla ice cream, fresh fruit and pasta.
Champagne vinegar	Smooth	In sauces with poultry or seafood.
Chinese black rice vinegar	Smoky flavor	Stir-fries and salad dressings.
Garlic-flavored red wine vinegar	Zest and added zip	Excellent marinade for meats.
Malt vinegar	Hearty, deep-flavored, made from barley malt extract	Excellent on fish 'n' chips, potato salad and cole slaw, spice pickles, chutneys, relishes, in mint sauce for lamb.
Plum vinegar	Salty, citrus flavor	Salad dressings, sauces, stews, soups, and steamed vegetables.
Raspberry vinegar	Fruit flavor	Salads, vegetable dishes, marinade for chicken, blended with vanilla yogurt to make dressings for fruit salad, mixed with jam for sweet and sour sauce.
Red wine vinegar	Low-sodium, robust	Marinating dark meats, red pasta sauces, grilled steak, salad dressings.
Red wine vinegar with Italian seasoning	Flavored with oregano, garlic, onion, red pep-	Salads, pasta sauces.

Vinegar	Flavor	Uses
Rice vinegar	Mild, slightly sweet	As dip for fried foods and steamed shellfish, in soups, stews, noodle dishes.
Seasoned rice vinegar	Light and zesty	Grilled chicken, cooked vegetables, green leaf salad dressing, pasta salads, quick marinade.
Sherry vinegar	Nutty flavor with a sweet aftertaste	Marinades, salad dressings, poultry dishes and tomato-based soups and sauces.
Tarragon-flavored white wine vinegar	Tasty, added zip	Excellent marinade for chicken; stir a tablespoon or so into veal recipes.
White distilled vinegar	Harsh, coarse flavor	All-purpose vinegar that can be used for a variety of kitchen and other household needs; pickling.
White rice vinegar	Pale golden color	Enhances sweet and sour dishes.
White wine vinegar	A good salt substitute	Excellent in marinades, mild salad dressings, sauces, and fish and chicken dishes.

(Source: Based on information provided by Mizkan Americas, Inc., and other sources.)

Healthful Marinating Tips

- Use red wine vinegar to marinate beef, pork, and lamb; white wine vinegar for poultry, seafood, and vegetables. Be experimental. Try tarragon white vinegar for fish; English-style malt vinegar to marinate beef or pork.
- Marinate in a nonmetallic container such as a plastic bowl, glass baking dish, or heavy-duty plastic bag.
- Marinate meat, poultry, and seafood in the refrigerator, not at room temperature.
- Pierce beef and pork several times with a fork so the marinade can seep into the meat and help tenderize it.
- *Always discard* leftover marinade used for meat, poultry, and seafood. If you want to serve some marinade on the side, it's best to make extra marinade *just* for serving.

  (*Source:* Mizkan Americas, Inc.)

Ways to Use Vinegar

1. **Vegetables.** Liven up slightly wilted vegetables by soaking them in cold water and vinegar.

2. **Cabbage.** Add vinegar to the cooking water of boiling cabbage to prevent the odor from permeating the house.

3. **Meat.** A marinade of ½ cup of your favorite vinegar and a cup of liquid bouillon makes an effective meat tenderizer.

4. **Rice.** A tablespoon of vinegar added to the water of boiling rice makes it fluffy and white.

5. **Fish.** Reduce fishy odors by rubbing fish down with white distilled vinegar before using it.

6. **Cheese.** Keep cheese moist and fresh by wrapping it in a cloth that has been dampened with vinegar and sealing it in an airtight wrap or container.

7. **Eggs.** To produce better-formed egg whites, add a tablespoon of your favorite vinegar to the water. When boiling eggs, add some vinegar to the water to prevent the white from leaking out of a cracked egg. When poaching eggs, add a teaspoon of vinegar to the water to prevent separation.

8. **Onion Odors.** Quickly remove the odor of onions from your hands by rubbing them with distilled vinegar.

9. **Thirst Quenchers.** Mix a tablespoon of strawberry or orange vinegar in a glass filled with eight ounces of club soda and ice. It makes a delightfully cooling drink.

10. **Pickling.** Cider, red wine, balsamic, and other dark vinegars are very good for pickling, but may discolor lighter-colored pickles such as pears, onions, or cauliflowers. In this case, a distilled or white vinegar is preferred.

(*Source*: Mizkan Americas, Inc., with support from the Vinegar Institute.)

MORE VINEGAR MOXIE IN THE KITCHEN

- Use vinegar to clean your microwave, cutting board and other kitchen equipment, and areas where you prepare food.
- Recipe calls for wine? Substitute red wine vinegar. Dilute one part of vinegar with three parts wine.
- Reduce salt. All Heinz vinegars are sodium-free, but a splash of vinegar replaces some of the salt in a recipe.
- When a recipe calls for 1 cup of buttermilk and you want a substitute, add a tablespoon of distilled white vinegar to a cup of milk instead.
- To remove pesticides from fruits and vegetables, just wash food with a mixture of 2–3 tablespoons of distilled white vinegar per quart of water.
- To keep cheese fresh and mold-free, wrap it in a cloth saturated with distilled white vinegar and store airtight in the refrigerator.
- Want gelatin recipes to hold firmer longer? Add a teaspoon of distilled white vinegar per box of gelatin to your favorite recipes.
    (*Source*: Heinz.)

PICKLING PASSION

The Chinese invented the art of pickling, but it's the Pennsylvania Dutch who have been credited with popularizing pickling in America. Pickling is the addition of vinegar and salt—often with spices and sugar—to vegetables and fruit.

Most important, to pickle properly, vinegar is necessary to preserve food by inhibiting the growth of food-spoilage bacteria. Vinegars should be "pickling strength" (5 percent acidity), which will ensure that they are at an acidity level that is ideal for safe home preservation of foods.

According to the U.S. Department of Agriculture, the boiling-water bath method is best because it helps to kill bacteria, molds, yeast, and enzymes that spoil food.

The following hints will help you get ready for pickling and canning:

- **To Prepare:** Get a cutting board, a paring knife, standard measuring cups and spoons, a strainer or colander, and a blender, food chopper, grinder, or processor.
- **To Fill:** You'll need metal and rubber spatulas, a jar lifter, a wide-mouth funnel, a ladle with a lip, potholders, and a clean, damp cloth for wiping the jar rims before adjusting caps.
- **To Process:** You'll need a water-bath canner or a large kettle with a tight-fitting lid. The container must be deep enough for the jars to be placed on a wire rack and covered with at least 1 inch of water. Allow for enough heat space so that water doesn't boil over.
- **To Store:** Label jars with the name of the recipe and date. Store the jars in a dark, dry, cool place where they can't freeze. Beware that freezing may crack jars or break the seals, allowing bacteria to enter, which may cause spoilage.

Ten Tips for Preserving Healthy Produce

1. Select slightly underripe fruits.

2. Do not use cucumbers with a waxy surface for pickling. For best flavor and texture, pickling cucumbers should be used within 24 hours of picking.

3. Avoid soaking produce.

4. Use pure granulated pickling salt. The iodine and additives in table salt may make the pickling liquid cloudy or cause discoloration.

5. Select standard canning jars and lids. (Jars from commercially packed foods are not suitable.) Be sure jars and closures are free from nicks, chips, or cracks.

6. Never reuse canning lids; canning jars, however, may be used again.

7. Don't use copper, brass, iron, or galvanized utensils when cooking pickles. These may react with the acid and salt in the liquid and cause undesirable changes or form hazardous compounds.

8. Many recipes call for distilled white vinegar. If you prefer a fruit flavor, you may substitute apple cider vinegar.

9. Follow directions exactly; never double or triple recipes. The ratio of ingredients to vinegar may be altered, which will affect flavor and texture and may cause spoilage.

10. Use fresh spices, either whole or ground. Old spices impart a musty taste to preserved food. Cheesecloth and string work best for a "spice bag."

(*Source:* Heinz.)

Ten Pickling Family Favorites

Here are 10 superb recipes—perfect for the season that fits. (*Courtesy*: from Heinz.)

Apple Chutney

❖ ❖ ❖

4 pounds tart red cooking apples,
cored, chopped
2 medium onions, chopped
2 cups golden raisins
1½ cups firmly packed brown sugar
1 cup Heinz Apple Cider or Apple
Cider Flavored Vinegar

2 tablespoons grated fresh gingerroot
½ teaspoon ground mace or
nutmeg
½ teaspoon salt

In a 6- to 8-quart saucepan, combine all ingredients. Bring to a boil. Reduce heat and simmer for 30–35 minutes or until thickened, stirring frequently. Immediately fill hot pint jars with mixture, leaving ½-inch headspace. Carefully run a nonmetallic utensil down side of jars to remove trapped air bubbles. Wipe jar tops and threads clean. Place hot lids on jars and screw bands on firmly. Process in boiling water canner for 10 minutes. Serve as an accompaniment to curries or beef, pork, chicken, or turkey main dishes or sandwiches. Makes 4–5 pints.

Cantaloupe Pickles

❖ ❖ ❖

4 cantaloupes (9–10 pounds),
quartered, seeds and rind removed
3 cups granulated sugar
3 cups Heinz Apple Cider or Apple
Cider Flavored Vinegar

1½ cups apple juice
6 (3-inch) cinnamon sticks, broken
2 tablespoons whole cloves
5 thin slices fresh gingerroot

Cut cantaloupe into 1-inch cubes. In a 6- to 8-quart saucepan, combine sugar, vinegar, and apple juice. Bring to a boil, stirring occasionally. Tie spices in spice bag or cheesecloth. Add spice bag to syrup and boil for 10 minutes. Add melon, reduce heat, and simmer for 15 minutes, stirring occasionally. Remove spice bag. Immediately fill hot, sterilized pint or half-pint jars with mixture, leaving ½-inch head-space. Carefully run a nonmetallic utensil down inside of jars to remove trapped air bubbles. Wipe jar tops and threads clean. Place hot lids on jars and screw bands on firmly. Process in boiling water canner—10 minutes for pints and 5 minutes for half-pints. Makes 6–7 pints or 12–14 half-pints.

Cranberry Chutney

❖ ❖ ❖

6 cups fresh cranberries (about
   1½ pounds)
1½ cups Heinz Apple Cider or
   Apple Cider Flavored Vinegar
½ cup cranberry juice cocktail
1 cup granulated sugar
1 cup firmly packed brown sugar
1 cup golden raisins
2 tart apples, peeled, cored,
   coarsely chopped

1 orange with peel, seeded,
   coarsely chopped
1 medium onion, chopped
1 tablespoon chopped
   crystallized ginger (optional)
2 teaspoons salt
1½ teaspoons salt
½ teaspoon ground cloves or
   allspice
½ teaspoon red pepper

In a 6- to 8-quart saucepan, combine all ingredients. Bring to a boil. Reduce heat and simmer for 45 minutes to 1 hour or until thick. Stir occasionally at the beginning of cooking and constantly at the end of cooking. Immediately fill half-pint jars with mixture, leaving ½-inch headspace. Carefully run a nonmetallic utensil down inside of jars to remove trapped air bubbles. Wipe jar tops and threads clean. Place hot lids on jars and screw bands on firmly. Process in boiling water canner for 10 minutes. Serve as an accompaniment to curries for chicken, turkey, wild game, lamb, or beef dishes. Makes about 8 half-pints.

Cucumber Dill Relish

❖ ❖ ❖

1 tablespoon mixed pickling
   spice
4 pounds pickling cucumbers,
   chopped
2 medium onions, chopped
1 small head cabbage, chopped
3 cloves garlic, minced

2 cups Heinz Apple Cider or
   Apple Cider Flavored Vinegar
½ cup granulated sugar
2 tablespoons snipped fresh dill
   weed
1 tablespoon pickling salt
5–10 sprigs fresh dill weed

Tie pickling spice in a spice bag or cheesecloth. In a 6- to 8-quart saucepan, combine spice bag and remaining ingredients except dill sprigs. Mix well. Bring to a boil over medium-high heat, stirring occasionally. Reduce heat to medium and cook for 15 minutes, stirring frequently. Remove spice bag. Immediately fill hot pint or half-pint jars with mixture, leaving ½-inch headspace. Place 1–2 sprigs of dill weed on top of mixture. Carefully run a nonmetallic utensil down side of jars to remove trapped air bubbles. Wipe jar tops and threads clean. Place hot lids on jars and screw bands on firmly. Process pints or half-pints in boiling water canner 15 minutes. Makes 5–6 pints or 10–12 half-pints.

Green Tomato Relish

❖ ❖ ❖

6 pounds green tomatoes, chopped
2 large red bell peppers (about 1
   pound), chopped
2 large green bell peppers (about 1
   pound), chopped
2 medium onions, chopped
¼ cup pickling salt

2 tablespoons mustard seed
2 tablespoons celery seed
1 tablespoon mixed pickling spice
4 cups Heinz Apple Cider or Apple
   Cider Flavored Vinegar
2 cups firmly packed brown sugar

In a large bowl, combine tomatoes, peppers, and onions. Sprinkle with pickling salt and mix well. Cover and chill overnight. Drain well. Tie mustard seed, celery seed, and pickling spice in a spice bag or cheesecloth. In a 6- to 8-quart saucepan, combine vegetables, vinegar, sugar, and spice bag. Bring to a boil over medium heat, stirring occasionally. Reduce heat and simmer for 30 minutes, stirring often to prevent sticking. Remove spice bag. Immediately fill hot pint or half-pint jars with mixture, leaving 1/2-inch headspace. Carefully run a nonmetallic utensil down inside of jars to remove trapped air bubbles. Wipe jar tops and threads clean. Place hot lids on jars and screw bands on firmly. Process pints or half-pints in boiling water canner for 15 minutes. Makes 6–7 pints or 12–14 half-pints.

End-of-the Garden Pickles

❖ ❖ ❖

6 cups Heinz Distilled White
   Vinegar
4 cups granulated sugar
1 1/2 cups water
3 tablespoons mixed pickling
   spice
2 tablespoons pickling salt
3 cups broccoli flowerets
3 cups cauliflowerets

3 cups carrot pieces (about 1-inch)
3 cups cubed unpeeled cucumber
   (about 1-inch)
3 cups zucchini chunks (about
   1-inch)
2 cups red or green bell pepper
   squares (about 1-inch)
2 medium onions, each cut into
   eight wedges

In an 8- to 10-quart saucepan, combine vinegar, sugar, water, pickling spice, and salt. Bring to a boil, stirring occasionally. Boil for 4 minutes. Add vegetables, reduce heat, and simmer until vegetables are hot, about 5 minutes. Immediately fill hot quart jars with mixture, leaving 1/2-inch headspace. Carefully run a nonmetallic utensil down side of jars to remove trapped air bubbles. Wipe jar tops and threads clean. Place hot lids on jars and screw bands on firmly. Process in boiling water canner for 15 minutes. Makes about 4 quarts.

Garlic Dill Pickles

❖ ❖ ❖

4 pounds (3- to 4-inch) pickling
   cucumbers
6 cups water
4½ cups Heinz Apple Cider or
   Apple Cider Flavored Vinegar

6 tablespoons pickling salt
¾ teaspoon of crushed red pepper
   (optional)
16 cloves garlic, split
16 heads fresh dill

Wash cucumbers and remove ¹⁄₁₆-inch from the blossom end. In a 3-quart saucepan, combine water, vinegar, salt, and red pepper. Bring to a boil. Meanwhile, place 2 pieces of garlic and 1 head of dill in each hot pint jar. Firmly pack cucumbers upright in jars, leaving ½-inch headspace. Place 2 additional pieces of garlic and 1 head of dill in each hot pint jar. Immediately pour hot vinegar mixture over cucumbers, leaving ½-inch headspace. Carefully run a nonmetallic utensil down side of jars to remove trapped air bubbles. Wipe jar tops and threads clean. Place hot lids on jars and screw bands on firmly. Process in boiling water canner for 10 minutes. Makes about 7–8 pints.

Pineapple Raisin Sauce

❖ ❖ ❖

4 cans (20 ounces each) crushed
   pineapple in unsweetened juice,
   undrained
3 cups firmly packed brown sugar
2 cups Heinz Apple Cider or Apple
   Cider Flavored Vinegar

2 cups raisins
1 cup chopped onions
3 tablespoons grated orange peel
3 tablespoons Dijon-style mustard
2 tablespoons soy sauce

In a 6-quart saucepan, combine all ingredients. Bring to a boil, stirring occasionally. Reduce heat and simmer about 45 minutes or until there is just a small amount of liquid remaining. Immediately fill hot pint jars with mixture, leaving ½-inch headspace. Carefully run a nonmetallic utensil down inside of jars to remove trapped air bubbles. Wipe jar tops and threads clean. Place hot lids on jars and screw bands on firmly. Process in boiling water canner for 10 minutes. Serve as an accompaniment to pork, ham, turkey, or chicken main dishes or sandwiches. Makes about 6 pints.

Summer Squash Relish

❖ ❖ ❖

*10 cups chopped zucchini and
yellow summer squash (about
10–12 medium)*
1 medium onion, chopped
*1 medium red bell pepper,
chopped*
*1 medium green bell pepper,
chopped*

*2 cups Heinz Apple Cider or
Apple Cider Flavored Vinegar*
2½ cups granulated sugar
2 teaspoons mustard seed
2 teaspoons celery seed
2 teaspoons ground cinnamon
2 teaspoons tumeric
1 teaspoon pickling salt

In a 6- to 8-quart saucepan, combine all ingredients. Bring to a boil over medium-high heat, stirring occasionally. Reduce heat and simmer for 10 minutes or until thickened, stirring frequently. Immediately fill hot pint or half-pint jars with mixture, leaving ½-inch headspace. Carefully run a nonmetallic utensil down inside of jars to remove trapped air bubbles. Wipe jar tops and threads clean. Place lids on jars and screw bands on firmly. Process pints or half-pints in boiling water canner for 15 minutes. Makes 5–6 pints or 10–12 half-pints.

Zucchini Pickles

❖ ❖ ❖

2 pounds zucchini
¼ cup pickling salt
6 cups water
1 package (16 ounces) frozen
pearl onions, thawed
3 cups Heinz Apple Cider or Apple
Cider Flavored Vinegar

2 cups firmly packed brown sugar
1 tablespoon mustard seed
1 tablespoon tumeric
1½ teaspoons ground ginger

Wash zucchini and cut into 3x½-inch pieces. In a large bowl, combine zucchini, salt, and water. Mix well. Cover and let stand for 2 hours. Drain and rinse well. In a 6- to 8-quart saucepan, combine zucchini, onions, and remaining ingredients. Bring to a boil over medium-high heat, stirring occasionally. Boil for 5 minutes, stirring constantly. Immediately fill hot pint jars with zucchini and onions, leaving ½-inch headspace. Immediately pour hot vinegar mixture over zucchini, maintaining ½-inch headspace. Carefully run a nonmetallic utensil down inside of jars to remove trapped air bubbles. Wipe jar tops and threads clean. Place hot lids on jars and screw bands on firmly. Process in boiling water canner for 15 minutes. Makes about 4–5 pints.

Sweet Vinegar Fact

Most vinegars will last for at least one or two years—if unopened. However, fruit vinegars do not keep as long as other vinegars.

Vinegar Substitutions

Although our chefs suggest specific flavored vinegars in some of these recipes, if you are on a low-sodium diet, try the dish with a plain vinegar such as apple cider, red wine, rice, or balsamic. Also, if you don't have the brand of vinegar or olive oil called for in these recipes, substitute a similar type for best results.

The Vinegar Health-Boosting
Five-Day Menu Plan

* Recipes appear in the previous chapters and following food categories. Or use your own spin-off recipe with the vinegar of choice.

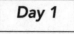

Day 1

Breakfast
    1 tablespoon each of vinegar
        and honey in 6-ounce glass of water (optional)
        (apple cider vinegar)
    Blackberry Balsamic Vinegar French Toast*
    1 cup fresh-squeezed orange juice

Lunch
    Peasant Salad with Red Wine Vinegar* (red wine vinegar)
    1 cup skim milk

Snack
    1 bowl Gazpacho* (red wine vinegar)
    4 low-sodium whole wheat crackers

Dinner
    Chili
    1 serving Steamed Artichokes with Yogurt
        and Buttermilk Dressing* (seasoned rice vinegar with basil and
        oregano)
    Cornbread with 1 teaspoon honey

Snack
    1 cup Melon Sorbet* (white wine vinegar)

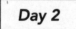

Day 2

Breakfast
    1 tablespoon *each* of vinegar
        and honey in 6-ounce glass of water (optional)
        (apple cider vinegar)
    1 serving Strawberries with Orange and Balsamic
        Vinegar* (balsamic vinegar)

⅔ cup oatmeal and ½ teaspoon nutmeg
½ cup skim milk

Lunch
1 fresh apple
1 cup skim milk

Snack
Chicken Bite Appetizers* (red wine vinegar)

Dinner
Simple Salmon* (red wine vinegar)
Asparagus
Focaccia dipped in olive oil

Snack
Fresh fruit (mango vinegar)

Day 3

Breakfast
2–3 tablespoons Nonfat Yogurt Cheese* (apple cider vinegar)
    spread on 1 cinnamon-raisin bagel
¾ cup bran flakes with ½ cup skim milk
½ pink grapefruit

Lunch
Cobb Salad* (apple cider vinegar)
Fresh bakery sourdough bread dipped in olive oil
1 cup skim milk

Snack
1 cup Mediterranean Vegetable Soup* (red wine vinegar)

Dinner
Baked Chicken
Baked Sweet Potatoes with
    Plantain and Citrus Chutney* (rice vinegar)
Tossed green salad (balsamic vinaigrette)

Snack
1 piece Old-Fashioned Raisin Pie* (vinegar)

Day 4

Breakfast

1 tablespoon *each* of vinegar and honey in 6 ounces water
(optional) (apple cider vinegar)
Scrambled eggs
2 slices whole wheat toast
6 ounces unsweetened grapefruit juice

Lunch

Greek Salad (red wine vinegar)
Herbal tea
1 slice sourdough bread dipped in olive oil

Snack

1 orange

Dinner

Mediterranean Beef Stew* (seasoned rice vinegar)
Tossed green salad with Vinaigrette*

Snack

Pound cake topped with fresh berries (peach vinegar)

Day 5

Breakfast

Whole wheat pancakes with blueberry syrup
Fresh-squeezed orange juice
Herbal tea

Lunch

Venetian Pasta Salad* (red wine vinegar)

Snack

Red grapes

Dinner

Tapa-style Mussels* (rice vinegar)
Marinated Green Vegetables* (red wine vinegar)

Snack

Vanilla ice cream with 1 tablespoon of vinegar drizzled on top
(balsamic vinegar)

Breakfast

Mixing apple cider vinegar with a glass of water before breakfast is one way to get your energy boost for the day. You may be thinking, "Vinegar for breakfast? I'll pass." But think again. Flavorful vinegars can add a punch to breakfast dishes, including pancakes or waffles with fresh seasonal berries. I love pancakes all year round. During December, pre-winter, and on a rainy day, flapjacks—a round cake made from a batter and cooked in a frying pan—are comfort food. What's more, you can infuse vinegar in breakfast muffins or with fresh fruit and serve it in a variety of ways. Vinegar for breakfast, anyone? Yes, please.

Chocolate Chip Pancakes with Balsamic Vinegar Berries
Pumpkin Muffins with ACV Cream Cheese Frosting

Chocolate Chip Pancakes with Balsamic Vinegar Berries
❖ ❖ ❖

Years ago traveling through Northern California en route to Canada I hitched a ride with a man and his son. They lived on the outskirts of Lake Tahoe. He invited me and my dog to sleep in the guest room at their large cabin. I felt safe and did just that. In the early morning there was a knock on the door. I opened it slowly and looked down on the floor. I was served pancakes, berries, and fresh-squeezed orange juice. A tray with the breakfast was left outside the door of my room. I was moved by the gesture; the breakfast was scrumptious. I never got to say thank you because when I got ready to go back on the road both son and father were at work. I dedicate this recipe to the boys who took care of me and made us feel welcome.

1 cup all-purpose flour
1 teaspoon baking powder
¾ cup organic 2 percent reduced-
    fat buttermilk
1 teaspoon apple cider vinegar
1½ tablespoons European-style
    butter
1 organic brown egg

1 capful pure vanilla extract
½ cup chocolate chips (dark or
    milk)
confectioners' sugar (optional)
1 cup fresh berries
1 tablespoon Honey Ridge Farms
    Balsamic Honey Vinegar

In a bowl, mix flour, baking powder, milk, butter, egg, and apple cider vinegar. Add vanilla and chocolate chips. On medium heat, pour batter (⅓–½ cup ice-cream-scoop size) into frying pan. When the pancakes bubble, flip. Serve with a small pat of butter, confectioners' sugar, balsamic honey vinegar and berries. Serves approximately 5–6 small pancakes.

I used to make pancakes from the store-bought box, the one that claims all you need to add is water. It is easy, but so is making pancakes from scratch, like my mother used to do it. Premium ingredients, like milk, eggs, syrup, butter, and chocolate are worth the extra effort. These pancakes hit the spot, are pretty to plate, and can appease anyone, anytime. Pay it forward this month, the time of giving.

Pumpkin Muffins with ACV Cream Cheese Frosting

❖ ❖ ❖

It's soothing to bake and eat healthful fall edibles, and often healthier than purchasing store-bought brands with their list of artificial ingredients that requires a translator. Come with me. Enter Pumpkinfest with a taste of apple cider vinegar. Enjoy the earthy aroma, presentation, originality, and flavor of pumpkin muffins.

1¾ cups all-natural whole wheat
    flour
¼ teaspoon baking soda
1½ teaspoons baking powder

2 eggs, brown
½ cup organic brown sugar
1 tablespoon clover honey
½ cup low-fat half-and-half

⅓ cup sour cream
1 cup of canned pumpkin purée
2 teaspoons apple cider vinegar
1 teaspoon pure vanilla extract

2 teaspoons pumpkin pie spice
1 teaspoon allspice
raw sugar (optional)

In a bowl, combine flour, baking soda, and baking powder. In another bowl, mix beaten eggs with sugar, honey, half-and-half, sour cream, pumpkin, apple cider vinegar, and vanilla. Add spices. Pour batter into cupcake tins. Bake at 350 for about 25 minutes or till golden brown and firm. Top with sugar and cool.

For a festive treat: Mix 1½ cups confectioners' sugar, ¼ cup half-and-half , 2 tablespoons apple cider vinegar, and ½ teaspoon pure vanilla extract. Frost cooled muffins. Makes 12.

These muffins are moist with a capital M, thanks to sour cream and pumpkin pie filling (low-fat and rich in fiber and vitamin A). Unlike a drier muffin, this recipe yields a cupcake-like muffin. No butter or honey is needed. Sweet pumpkin muffins and spicy lattes can still be part of your autumn in the Sierra (despite the economic crunch), complete with a crackling fire, human and furry friends, and our first snowfall. These things are unforgettable and priceless and can be enjoyed year-round.

Soups

As a kid, teen, and young adult, soup was usually the canned kind and used only for tackling a cold and something I put in a mental lock box until I'd be eighty. These days, after trying Gold Cold Soup with balsamic vinegar and Gazpacho with red wine vinegar, I have a new outlook on the world of soups. When I tried the vinegary concoctions I thought out loud, "Wow! My taste buds have grown up."

It's smart to go for good nutrition and filling, low-fat satisfaction. And these healthful soups offer just that, especially infused with vinegar.

Studies show that soup is particularly effective in filling you up, so a bowl of soup before a meal can take the edge off your appetite. And because it's eaten spoonful by spoonful, you'll eat it slowly, which gives your brain time to register that you're getting full.

Cold Gold Soup
Court Bouillon
Gazpacho
Hot and Sour Soup

Cold Gold Soup

❖ ❖ ❖

3 large peaches, ripe	*white pepper*
2 teaspoons honey	*1 tablespoon balsamic vinegar*
½ cup orange juice, fresh	*1 tablespoon mint, finely*
squeezed	*chopped*
2 drops Tabasco sauce	*orange peel*

Peel peaches and cut into small chunks. Add honey and orange juice. Blend until smooth. Stir in Tabasco and white pepper, cover, and chill at least 1 hour.

Stir in vinegar and chopped mint, then ladle soup into chilled bowls. Garnish with fresh whole mint leaves and zests of orange peel. Serves 3.

(*Courtesy: Amazing Apple Cider Vinegar* by Earl L. Mindell with Larry M. Johns.)

Court Bouillon

❖ ❖ ❖

Court bouillon is a very nice liquid for poaching fish and/or vegetables. It is very simple to make and will keep nicely in the refrigerator for 10 days.

2½ quarts cold water	8 ounces onions, sliced
5 ounces apple cider vinegar or white wine vinegar	pinch thyme, whole, dried
	3 or 4 parsley stems
1 teaspoon salt	2 bay leaves
6 ounces carrots, sliced	¼ ounce peppercorns, whole

Combine all ingredients except peppercorns and simmer for 45 minutes. Add the peppercorns and simmer for 15 more minutes. Cool and refrigerate for later use. This recipe makes ½ gallon.

(*Courtesy:* Chef Salvatore J. Campagna.)

Gazpacho
(COLD FRESH VEGETABLE SOUP)

❖ ❖ ❖

1 pound tomato concasse (recipe below)	3 ounces red wine vinegar
	Juice of 2 lemons
8 ounces onions, peeled, sliced	3 ounces olive oil
8 ounces red bell peppers, seeded, quartered	Juice of 2 limes
	1 teaspoon salt
8 ounces cucumbers, seeded, quartered	Tabasco, habanero (new) to taste
1 tablespoon garlic, minced	16 ounces tomato juice

Tomato Concasse

Cut out the stems of 4 tomatoes (1 pound) and cut a small "x" on the bottom of each one. Place tomatoes in boiling water for 15–30 seconds, depending on ripeness. Remove tomatoes with slotted spoon and immediately plunge into ice water and gently pull away the skin. Cut tomatoes in half and squeeze out the seeds and dice. For added flavor, sauté diced tomatoes in 2 ounces of olive oil with a teaspoon of chopped garlic. Set aside to cool.

Purée all ingredients except the tomato juice. Adjust the consistency and flavor with the tomato juice (or consommé). Adjust seasoning with salt and pepper and garnish with a very small dice of red and green bell pepper, cucumber, and tomato along with small seasoned croutons. A teaspoon of the diced vegetables and a few croutons are ideal. Makes ½ gallon.

(*Courtesy*: Chef Salvatore J. Campagna.)

Hot and Sour Soup

❖ ❖ ❖

1 (32-ounce) carton chicken broth or 4 cups homemade or canned chicken broth

3 tablespoons Nakano Natural Rice Vinegar or Nakano Seasoned Rice Vinegar—Original

2 tablespoons lite or regular soy sauce

¼ teaspoon crushed red pepper flakes or 1 teaspoon hot chile oil

4 ounces firm silken tofu,* well drained

1 (15-ounce) can stir-fry mushrooms or 2 jars (7 ounces each) straw mushrooms, drained

½ cup julienned canned bamboo shoots

3 tablespoons water

2 tablespoons cornstarch

1 egg white, slightly beaten

¼ cup thinly sliced green onions

2 teaspoons dark roasted sesame oil

Combine broth, vinegar, soy sauce, and pepper flakes in a large saucepan; bring to a boil over high heat. Reduce heat to medium; simmer 2 minutes. Stir in tofu, mushrooms, and bamboo shoots; heat through. Combine water and cornstarch, mixing until smooth. Stir into soup; cook until soup boils and thickens, about 5 minutes, stirring frequently. Turn off heat under saucepan. Stirring soup constantly in one direction, slowly pour egg white in a thin stream into soup. Stir in green onions and sesame oil. Ladle into soup bowls. Serves 4 (makes about 5½ cups).

*Tip: Look for silken tofu in the produce section of your supermarket. If it is not available, you may use 1 cup diced cooked chicken or pork.

(*Courtesy*: Mizkan Americas, Inc.)

Salads

My journey to Montreal, Quebec, the second time around, included salads and vinegars. In my hotel room overlooking the heart of downtown, the room service menu had me at *"Petites Salades"*: *Salades melangees et vinaigrette*, mixed greens with raspberry apple cider vinaigrette, made me feel cozy, as though I were at home despite the grueling jet lag at noon, all alone in a foreign city.

A salad should have plenty of fresh vegetables and fruits. To enhance its flavor and its nutrients, what better way than to top it off with vinegar. Whether it's apple cider, red wine, rice, balsamic or herbal vinegars, you can count on a salad being a healthful side dish or complete meal.

Combine olive oil, garlic, and onions—which many of these salads contain—and you've got a wholesome, nutritious dish.

Cactus Salad
Chickpea Salad
Five-Bean Salad
Green Bean and Mushroom Salad
Greek Salad with Spiced Onions
Indian Summer Potato Salad
Santa Fe Rice Salad
Tropical Fruit Salad with Fruit Vinaigrette

Cactus Salad

❖ ❖ ❖

This recipe captivated my interest. After my trip to the Pacific Northwest and salad adventures, it made me rethink my building salads at home. Instead of simple vegetable concoctions, it's healthier and more fun to combine fruit and vegetables—even better using different vinegars. No doubt, the creator of this recipe was ahead of her time or I am still a late bloomer.

½ pound fresh trimmed cactus
   pads (nopales)
½ pound spinach leaves
2 green onions, sliced thin
salt and pepper to taste
½ teaspoon chili powder or
   paprika
1 cucumber, sliced thin
⅓ cup Marsala Olive Fruit Oil
⅓ cup white wine vinegar

⅓ cup fresh basil or cilantro,
   chopped
2 mild yellow chilies, minced
4 garlic cloves, minced
2 yellow or red tomatoes, cut into
   wedges
2 or 3 cactus pears, peeled and
   sliced
¾ cup goat, feta, farmer or
   Gorgonzola cheese, crumbled

Remove any thorns or spines from cactus pads. Cut into about 2 x ½ inch strips. In saucepan add water, bring to a boil. Blanch nopalitos for 3 minutes. Do not overcook or they will turn grayish green. Drain well, set aside. Line serving platter with spinach leaves. In mixing bowl combine remaining ingredients except cheese, tomatoes and cactus pears. Arrange cactus mixture over spinach evenly. Garnish with tomatoes and cactus pear slices. Sprinkle with crumbled cheese. Serves 6 to 8.

(*Source: Cooking with California Olive Oil: Treasured Family Recipes,* by Gemma Sanita Sciabica.)

Chickpea Salad

❖ ❖ ❖

DRESSING

⅓ cup Marsala olive oil

2 tablespoons balsamic vinegar

1 teaspoon oregano

sea salt and white pepper to taste

1 tablespoon mustard

SALAD

4 cups Roma tomatoes, diced

2 carrots shredded

¼ head red cabbage, shredded

2 cups canned chickpeas
(garbanzos), drained and rinsed

½ cup olives, chopped

In a large bowl, whisk together dressing ingredients, including oil, vinegar, spices, and mustard. Add salad ingredients (tomatoes, carrots, cabbage, chickpeas, and olives) to dressing, toss gently to coat. Refrigerate about one hour before serving.

(*Source: Cooking with California Olive Oil: Recipes from the Heart for the Heart*, by Gemma Sanita Sciabica.)

Five-Bean Salad

❖ ❖ ❖

16-ounce can (2 cups) green and
wax cut beans, drained (fresh
beans may be substituted—1
cup each)

8-ounce can (1 cup) garbanzo
beans, drained and rinsed

8-ounce can (1 cup) pinto beans,
drained and rinsed

½ cup Nakano Seasoned Rice
Vinegar with Red Pepper

½ cup chopped green pepper

¼ cup chopped red onion

Combine all ingredients in large salad bowl. Refrigerate 1 hour or longer, stirring several times to blend flavors. Serves 9.

Green Bean and Mushroom Salad

❖ ❖ ❖

1½ pounds green beans, fresh
1¼ pounds button mushrooms,
   fresh
4 ounces extra virgin olive oil
2 ounces red wine vinegar

salt to taste
freshly ground pepper to taste
1 large head romaine lettuce
2 large tomatoes, ripe

Wash and clean green beans. Boil in 2 quarts of salted water until tender and immediately immerse in an ice bath. When cool, cut beans into 2- to 3-inch lengths. Set aside to dry on paper towels. Wash button mushrooms gently under cold running water. Cut into ¼-inch slices. Marinate mushroom slices in large bowl with two ounces of oil and 1 ounce of red wine vinegar with a little salt and pepper. Wash and dry romaine lettuce leaves. Discard outer leaves, saving lighter green leaves. Break into small bite-size pieces and place in large salad bowl. Add green beans to mushroom bowl and toss lightly. Pour marinade from green beans and mushrooms onto lettuce and toss. Add a little more oil if necessary. Now add 2 ounces of oil and 1 ounce of vinegar to green beans and mushrooms and toss. Taste for salt and pepper and adjust if necessary. Cut each tomato into 6 wedges. Place 2 wedges of tomato and a portion of lettuce on a cold plate. Place the marinated green beans and mushrooms on top of the lettuce and serve immediately. Serves 6.

(*Courtesy*: Chef Salvatore J. Campagna.)

Indian Summer Potato Salad

❖ ❖ ❖

1 pound red potatoes, cooked
½ cup chopped onions
¼ cup Nakano Seasoned Rice
    Vinegar
½ teaspoon salt
½ teaspoon dill weed

⅛ teaspoon white pepper
⅓ cup light mayonnaise
1 teaspoon mustard
½ cup frozen peas
1 cup sliced celery
1 cup tart red apple wedges

Peel potatoes while still warm and cut into wedges; place in large bowl with onions. (For milder flavor, cook onions with potatoes the last 2 minutes.) Pour vinegar, salt, dill weed, and pepper over potatoes to marinate until cool. Blend mayonnaise with mustard; mix with potatoes. Rinse peas in boiling water. Fold peas, celery, and apples into salad. Refrigerate salad for at least an hour. Best served same day. Makes eight ½-cup servings.

Santa Fe Rice Salad

❖ ❖ ❖

2 cups chilled cooked white rice
¾ cup rinsed and drained canned
    black beans or kidney beans
1 large tomato, seeded, diced
¾ cup diced sharp Cheddar cheese
⅓ cup sliced green onions
⅓ cup vegetable oil
¼ cup Nakano Seasoned Rice
    Vinegar with Roasted Garlic or
    Nakano Seasoned Rice
    Vinegar—Original

1 tablespoon minced canned chipotle
    chilies in adobo sauce or bottled or
    fresh minced jalapeño peppers*
½ teaspoon sugar
1 small ripe avocado, peeled,
    seeded, diced

In a large bowl, combine rice, beans, tomato, cheese, and green onions; mix well. In a small bowl, combine remaining ingredients except avocado; mix well. Pour over rice mixture; mix well. Cover and refrigerate at least 30 minutes or up to 24 hours before serving. Just before serving, stir in avocado. Serve chilled or at room temperature. Makes about 5 cups. Serves 6.

*Tip: Look for bottled minced jalapeño chili peppers in the produce section of your supermarket next to the bottled minced garlic.

Tropical Fruit Salad with Fruit Vinaigrette

❖ ❖ ❖

1 ripe papaya, seeded, peeled, and diced
1 ripe mango, peeled, pitted, and diced
2 kiwi fruit, peeled and sliced
2 cups diced fresh pineapple
¾ cup Nakano Seasoned Rice Vinegar
2 tablespoons chopped red onion

1 tablespoon honey
¼ teaspoon allspice
½ cup vegetable oil
salt and ground white pepper to taste
1 ripe medium banana
1 cup sliced strawberries
2 teaspoons chopped fresh mint leaves
¼ cup shredded sweetened coconut, toasted (optional)

Place half of papaya, mango, kiwi fruit, and pineapple in a small nonaluminum saucepan. Combine remaining papaya, mango, kiwi fruit, and pineapple in a medium bowl; cover and refrigerate. Add vinegar to fruit in saucepan; cook over medium heat 5 minutes or until fruit is softened. Transfer to refrigerator; chill 30 minutes. Pour vinegar mixture into a food processor or blender; add onion, honey, and allspice. Process until mixture is smooth. With motor running, pour oil through feed tube in a steady stream. Process just until well blended. Season with salt and pepper. Add banana, strawberries, and mint to reserved fruit; toss lightly. Add ½ cup dressing, toss again. Spoon into serving dishes; sprinkle with toasted coconut, if desired. Serves 6.

Remaining dressing may be refrigerated up to 1 week. Use as a marinade for chicken or pork or as a dressing on a mixed green salad with sliced ripe avocado and grapefruit sections.

(*Courtesy*: Mizkan Americas, Inc.)

Dressings—Sauces—Spreads

Dressings and sauces to accompany healing foods can be just more healthful ingredients—especially when they include vinegar, olive oil, and herbs. Not only will you enjoy the nutritious benefits of these recipes, but the Mediterranean flair and flavor are a health bonus.

Cool Fruit Salad Dressing
Honey Sherry Dressing
Make-Your-Own Salsa
Nonfat Yogurt Cheese
Silken Tofu Tartare Sauce

Cool Fruit Salad Dressing

❖ ❖ ❖

2 tablespoons Pompeian Pure or Extra Light Olive Oil
2 tablespoons Pompeian Red Wine Vinegar
1 teaspoon sugar
2 tablespoons mint leaves, chopped

½ cup sour cream (or light substitute
1 tablespoon lemon juice
1 tablespoon ground cumin
2 tablespoons fresh cilantro, chopped

Combine all ingredients, mix well, and chill thoroughly. Toss with your favorite seasonal salad ingredients such as apples, bananas, and citrus. Serve at once.

(*Courtesy*: Pompeian.)

Honey Sherry Dressing

❖ ❖ ❖

¾ cup oil
¼ cup wine vinegar
⅓ cup honey
1 teaspoon dry mustard

½ teaspoon paprika
½ teaspoon celery seed
1 clove garlic
1 cup sherry

Combine all ingredients in a jar or bowl. Shake or beat until well blended. Store, covered, in the refrigerator until needed, then shake or beat again before using. Garlic may be removed once its flavor has permeated the dressing. Excellent on fruits. Yield: about 1½–2 cups.
(*Courtesy:* Mizkan Americas, Inc.)

Make-Your-Own Salsa

❖ ❖ ❖

½ cup chopped red onion
¼ cup chopped green pepper
1 clove garlic, minced
1 tablespoon light olive oil
3 cups chopped very ripe fresh
   tomatoes
½ teaspoon oregano

3 tablespoons canned jalapeño
   peppers
2½ tablespoons Nakano Natural
   Rice Vinegar
2 tablespoons chopped fresh cilantro
¾ teaspoon salt
pepper as desired

Microwave onion, green pepper, garlic, and oil 1 minute on high, covered. Add tomatoes and oregano; microwave 2 minutes on high. Stir in remaining ingredients. Refrigerate an hour or overnight to blend flavor. Keeps for a week or freezes well. Makes about 3 cups sauce for 8–10 servings.
(*Courtesy:* Mizkan Americas, Inc.)

Nonfat Yogurt Cheese

❖ ❖ ❖

1 quart nonfat yogurt
4 tablespoons powdered sugar

2 teaspoons vanilla extract
1 tablespoon apple cider vinegar

Combine all above ingredients in a bowl. Whisk together until runny. Place strainer in a container that will hold it upright and also collect the liquid from the yogurt. Line strainer with double layer of cheesecloth. Pour in yogurt mixture. Leave overnight in refrigerator. Liquid will strain through. Remove from cheesecloth and store in refrigerator until ready to serve. A spread for bagels or toast. Makes about 1¼ cups of yogurt cheese. Serves 8.

(*Courtesy:* Chef Michel Stroot of the Golden Door Spa.)

Silken Tofu Tartare Sauce

❖ ❖ ❖

10 ounces silken soft tofu
¼ apple cider vinegar
1 tablespoon shallots, coarsely chopped
1 tablespoon Dijon mustard
2 teaspoons prepared horseradish, creamed
1 teaspoon finely ground black pepper

½ cup (Kosher) dill pickle, coarsely chopped
1 tablespoon capers
½ cup fresh parsley, coarsely chopped
2 teaspoons fresh tarragon, coarsely chopped
2 teaspoons fresh dill weed, or 1 teaspoon dried dill weed

In a blender, combine soft tofu, vinegar, shallots, Dijon mustard, horseradish, and black pepper and process until smooth. Add Kosher pickle, capers, parsley, tarragon, and dill to the blender. "Pulse" 5 to 6 times to keep the sauce "chunky." Makes about 2½ cups or forty 1-tablespoon servings. Serves 40.

(*Courtesy:* Chef Michel Stroot of the Golden Door Spa.)

Pasta

Adding red wine and balsamic vinegars to pasta infuses good-for-you, disease-fighting, anti-aging antioxidants and extra flavor—a win-win for this Italian cuisine. Pasta, one of my favorite foods, is one I serve to unnerving guests because of its foolproof record. I once cooked dinner for a friend's friend whom I wanted to impress. I felt like an orphan before she met the fairy godmother. I turned to store-bought marinara sauce (I added fresh zucchini, garlic, and onions) and used generic spaghetti. At dinner, the woman said, "I never have time to cook homemade dinners like this. I feel special." I was pleasantly surprised, especially since I didn't have name brand fancy pots and pan or kitchen tools like I loved to view in culinary magazines and department stores. I'd like to go back in time . . . make a different sauce with vinegar, fresh herbs and spices, and use whole grain penne and shavings of fresh Parmesan for a dish with more elegance.

Vegetables, fruits, and some grains make up a big part of the Mediterranean diet. Pasta with vinegar, garlic, onions, and olive oil is a healthy meal.

What is it about pasta that makes it such a diet-friendly choice? Simple: It's low in fat and sodium and has just about 200 calories per 2-ounce serving (about 1 cup).

Pasta's also a good source of fiber, so it's extra-filling. And if you switch to whole wheat pasta, which contains more bulk, you'll feel even more satisfied. In addition, fiber can stabilize blood sugar levels, say nutritionists, which keeps your appetite at bay.

Pasta is also high in nutrition, containing calcium, iron, niacin, magnesium, and protein. What more could a health-conscious pasta lover want?

Orzo and Vegetable Salad
Pesto Pasta
French Baguettes
Stuffed Shells with Cheese, Spinach,
and Balsamic Vinegar

Orzo and Vegetable Salad

❖ ❖ ❖

1 cup orzo (rice-shaped pasta)
¼ cup Heinz Apple Cider Vinegar
¼ cup vegetable oil
1 teaspoon Dijon-style mustard
½ teaspoon dried basil leaves
¼ teaspoon salt

⅛ teaspoon pepper
1 cup frozen green peas, thawed
4 green onions, sliced
½ cup chopped red bell pepper
lettuce cups
tomato wedges

Cook orzo according to package directions; cool. Combine vinegar and next 5 ingredients in jar. Cover and shake vigorously. Chill to blend flavors. Combine orzo, peas, onions, and bell pepper in large bowl. Pour dressing over and toss. Cover, and chill several hours or overnight. Serve in lettuce cups; garnish with tomato. Makes 4 servings (about 5 cups).

(*Courtesy:* Heinz.)

Pesto Pasta

❖ ❖ ❖

½ cup all-natural pesto sauce
  (store-bought)
2½ cups whole grain rotini pasta,
  cooked
½ cup black olives, sliced
½ cup fresh grape tomatoes,
  chopped

2 tablespoons sun-dried tomatoes
  (optional)
black pepper to taste
½ cup Parmesan cheese
¼ cup pine nuts
basil, fresh (garnish)

In a bowl mix pesto and hot pasta until blended. Add olives, tomatoes, pepper, and cheese. Chill in fridge for an hour or two. Serve hot (heat in the microwave) or cold. Sprinkle with extra cheese and pine nuts. Garnish with basil. Serves 4–6.

FRENCH BAGUETTES

½ *fresh baguette*   *fresh garlic, grated*
2 *tablespoons European-style*
  butter

Slice baguette in half and slice again into strips. Put on a foil-lined pan. Spread with butter and top with garlic. Bake in a 400-degree oven for about 10–15 minutes, till crispy and light golden brown. Serve warm. Serves 4.

Black olives and tomatoes (sun-dried boast a distinct flavor) give this dish a delectable taste that you can enjoy at home without going to an Italian deli or Mediterranean country. The Parmesan cheese adds an earthy texture, and the crunch of pine nuts is perfect. Making your own pesto sauce is easy, too, but during warmer days I'd rather be walking my dogs or swimming. Taking a semi-homemade shortcut for pesto pasta works and leaves you with more time to play. It's ideal for a side dish salad at an outdoor picnic or dinner wherever you are.

Stuffed Shells with Cheese, Spinach, and Balsamic Vinegar

❖ ❖ ❖

Eggplant parmigiana, pizza, and pasta shells stuffed with cheese. Ah, Italian food can be superb and an ultra-comfort food on a chilly night. Jumbo shells stuffed with cheese (and other foods) can be good for you and taste good, too. Meatless pasta with marinara sauce can be filled with cheese and nutrient-rich vegetables and boasts a bit of decadent deliciousness. And you don't have to book a plane to Tuscany, Italy, to enjoy. Just make this dish in the comfort of your home—like I did—and you'll feel like you're abroad with each bit of pasta and the deliciousness of vinegar.

½ of a 12-ounce package pasta jumbo shells
2 cups ricotta cheese
3 cups mozzarella cheese, shredded; save half for topping
1½ cups fresh baby spinach, chopped
¼ cup fresh basil, chopped
2 teaspoons fresh herbs
⅛ teaspoon black pepper to taste

1 tablespoon extra virgin olive oil for greasing pan
1 jar all-natural marinara sauce with olive oil and garlic
2 tablespoons Honey Ridge Farms Balsamic Honey Vinegar
Optional: Add boiled chopped eggs, mushrooms, lean poultry or meat. You can sprinkle with Parmesan cheese.

Boil pasta shells for about 10 minutes. Drain. Set aside. In a bowl, combine cheeses, spinach, basil, herbs, and pepper. Stuff into shells. Lightly grease a baking dish. (I used two: my favorite 8 x 8 inch red rustic one and a white tart dish.) Pour half sauce infused with all of the vinegar on the bottom of dish. Arrange shells. Pour the rest of sauce over shells. Top with remaining half of mozzarella cheese. Cover with foil. Bake at 375 or 400 degrees for about 25–30 minutes till shells are light golden brown. Optional: You can drizzle balsamic vinegar on top of hot stuffed shells. Makes about 12 servings.

Vegetables/Vegetarian

Meatless meals are becoming more popular in the twenty-first century. But I must warn you: People will often look at you like you're from another planet. On a plane from Salt Lake City to Atlanta, Georgia, en route to Montreal, Canada, for instance, meals were served for the long afternoon flight. I smelled some sort of mystery meat sandwiches and tried to remain calm (and the rough air didn't help). After I said, "No thank you. I'm a vegetarian," the flight attendant looked at me with sympathetic eyes and said, "Is there anything I can get for you?" Within minutes, like a cat trying to please its owner, she brought me gifts: a large bunch of fresh purple grapes, whole wheat crackers, and a green salad with vinaigrette. I was flying and munching on food to my taste.

Mediterranean Tostada

❖ ❖ ❖

I've experienced a returning Mediterranean-linked dream hundreds of times, which is based on my real life back in San Carlos on the San Francisco Bay Area peninsula in a Spanish-style bungalow. One night at my Italian restaurant of choice, I ordered black tea (as folks in Ireland do), and nibbled on French bread dipped in olive oil (like Italians do). The entrée was a shrimp salad that I munched on as I listened to tales of my constant dining companion, a former harpist who traveled abroad to work. It was her gift of storytelling and secrets—and after dinner purchasing a much-needed computer and printer for me and my budding writing career—that made this dinner unforgettable and left me longing to visit Europe.

It's no surprise that my last book tour took me back to San Carlos and the eatery; it was closed. The fourteen bungalows (once filled with European tenants) were replaced by a condo building. My friend, almost a hundred, had passed. I returned to Lake Tahoe with bittersweet thoughts knowing she was a link to me being an author of a book series based on a European diet and lifestyle. This quick and easy dish was inspired by the woman behind this book. (She wanted me to be a romance author, but a twist of fate had me write about my affairs with food and the exotic world of vinegars.)

TOSTADA SHELLS
2 large flour tortillas
extra virgin olive oil

SALAD

1½ cups organic mixed baby
  greens, washed
½ cup tomatoes, sliced
⅛ cup red onion, diced
½ cup feta, crumbled, or
  provolone cheese, shredded
½ cup black olives, sliced
6 ounces albacore tuna or cooked
  shrimp (you can substitute with
  beans or lean meat)

extra virgin olive oil and Heinz
  red wine seasoned vinegar with
  pepper to taste
black pepper and sea salt to taste
lime or lemon (for garnish)

Place tortillas snug on top of an upside-down cupcake tin. Brush lightly with olive oil. Bake at 400 degrees for several minutes till golden brown. Remove shaped tortilla "bowls" from oven; set aside. In a large bowl, combine lettuce, tomatoes, onion, cheese, olives, and fish. Drizzle oil and vinegar, pepper on top, mix. Place salad mixture in tostadas and plate. Garnish with citrus slices. Serves two. (Double recipe for four.)

Vegetables are also an excellent source of complex carbohydrates. Complex carbs raise the brain's levels of serotonin, a chemical that works to diminish hunger.

Another big benefit: Vegetables are chock-full of the antioxidant vitamins C, E, and beta-carotene (which converts into vitamin A). According to the American Cancer Society, studies show that a diet high in vegetables can lower cancer risk.

In these recipes you can pair vegetables with apple cider, red wine, and herbal vinegars, then toss in garlic, onions, and olive oil. The result? You've got a powerhouse of health-enhancing food and mouthwatering dishes to savor.

Baked Sweet Potatoes with Plantain and Citrus Chutney
Caponata
Marinated Green Vegetables
Steamed Artichokes with Yogurt and Buttermilk Dressing
White Bean and Fennel Sauté

Baked Sweet Potatoes with Plantain and Citrus Chutney

❖ ❖ ❖

4 medium sweet potatoes, washed
   and pierced with a fork
2 tablespoons peanut or vegetable oil
1 ripe plantain, peeled, cut into
   ½-inch cubes
2 teaspoons water
2 tablespoons diced red onion
2 tablespoons Nakano Natural
   Rice Vinegar
2 tablespoons orange juice

1 tablespoon lime juice
2 tablespoons brown sugar
1 teaspoon grated lime zest
dash of nutmeg
dash of ground cloves
1 tablespoon butter
1 large naval orange, peeled,
   separated into sections,
   sections halved

Preheat oven to 425°. Place potatoes on a cookie sheet lined with foil and bake until cooked through, 40–45 minutes. Meanwhile, heat oil in a nonstick skillet over medium heat. Add plantain, cover, and cook 3–4 minutes or until golden brown, stirring once. Add water, cover, and cook an additional 2 minutes or until liquid is absorbed. Add onion, cook 1 minute. Combine vinegar, orange and lime juices, brown sugar, zest, nutmeg, and cloves, mixing until sugar dissolves. Add to the pan; simmer over medium-high heat until sauce thickens. Stir in butter and orange sections; heat through. When potatoes are finished baking, split them open and top with orange mixture. Serves 4.

(*Courtesy:* Mizkan Americas, Inc.)

Caponata
(SICILIAN EGGPLANT APPETIZER)

❖ ❖ ❖

2½ pounds eggplant
salt
6–8 stalks of celery (11 to 12
  ounces, green parts only)
canola oil and olive oil
1 onion, chopped
3 or 4 cloves garlic, chopped fine
2¼ cups tomato sauce or 3 large
  tomatoes, peeled, seeded, and
  diced

½ cup parsley, chopped
8 ounces green olives, pitted and
  halved
3 ounces small capers, drained
  and rinsed
freshly ground black pepper to taste
1 cup red wine vinegar
2 tablespoons sugar

Peel or partially peel the eggplant and cut into ¾-inch cubes. Rinse and sprinkle with salt and drain in a colander while slicing celery into ½-inch pieces. Parboil celery for 5 minutes. Drain and set aside. In a large skillet, pour canola oil and olive oil (canola oil has a higher smoking point than olive oil, making it better for frying) about a half-inch deep over medium heat. After drying the eggplant, add it to hot oil mixture and brown all sides. Remove with slotted spoon and drain on paper towels and cover and pat with more paper towels. In another skillet, sauté onion and garlic in olive oil. Cook slowly, until the onions are golden (10 or 12 minutes). Do not brown. Add tomato sauce, parsley, olives, capers, and salt and pepper to taste. Stir together and bring to a boil. Stir in the red wine vinegar and sugar. Reduce heat and simmer for 15 minutes. Remove from heat and spoon in the eggplant, stirring to mix thoroughly. Taste to adjust seasoning. Remove as much liquid as possible and serve or cool for later service. Caponata will last for a week when refrigerated. It is usually served cold. Serves 8–10.

(*Courtesy:* Chef Salvatore J. Campagna.)

Marinated Green Vegetables

1 pound broccoli florets
1 pound asparagus, fresh spears
1 pound zucchini, fresh and firm
½ cup extra virgin olive oil
1 large yellow onion, sliced thin
4 garlic cloves, finely chopped

2 fresh basil leaves, chopped
  into ¼-inch strips
2 fresh sage leaves, chopped
  into ¼-inch strips
pinch of salt
1 cup red wine vinegar

Blanch broccoli in salted boiling water for 2 minutes. Remove and set aside. Blanch asparagus spears in same water for 1 minute or less. Set aside. Wash zucchini in cold water and cut into ¼-inch strips about 3 inches long. Heat 2 tablespoons of the olive oil in a skillet and sauté the zucchini strips over high heat until a little color is attained. Do not cook until limp. Use as little oil as possible. Remove while still al dente (firm to the bite). Set aside. In the same skillet, add more oil if needed and sauté the sliced onion until brown. Add the garlic, chopped basil, chopped sage, and pinch of salt. Before the garlic turns brown, add the vinegar, bring to a boil, and then reduce until there is just a little liquid left in the pan. Combine the set-aside green vegetables and pour the onion, garlic, and vinegar mixture over them. Toss to flavor all pieces. Serve at room temperature or save for later service. Serves 8 to 10.

(*Courtesy*: Chef Salvatore J. Campagna.)

Steamed Artichokes with Yogurt
and Buttermilk Dressing

❖ ❖ ❖

½ cup low-fat buttermilk
⅓ cup low-fat plain yogurt
2 tablespoons Nakano Seasoned
  Rice Vinegar with Basil &
  Oregano or Nakano Seasoned
  Rice Vinegar with Red Pepper

1 clove garlic, minced
  (optional)
2 teaspoons sugar
1 teaspoon Dijon-style mustard
⅛ teaspoon salt
⅛ teaspoon oregano

2 tablespoons lite or regular
  mayonnaise
2 tablespoons chopped fresh or 2
  teaspoons dried basil

⅛ teaspoon freshly ground black
  pepper, or to taste
4 fresh artichokes (about 6 ounces
  each), stems and leaves trimmed

Combine all ingredients except artichokes in a small bowl; mix well. Cover and refrigerate at least 1 hour. Steam artichokes 25–35 minutes or until leaves pull out easily. Serve hot or cold with dressing. Serves 4.
  (*Courtesy:* Mizkan Americas, Inc.)

White Bean and Fennel Sauté

❖ ❖ ❖

1 large fennel bulb, about 10 ounces
1 tablespoon olive oil
1 small onion, thinly sliced
2 cloves garlic, minced
½ cup diced yellow bell pepper
3 tablespoons Nakano Seasoned Rice
  Vinegar with Roasted Garlic or
  Nakano Seasoned Rice
  Vinegar—Original

¼ teaspoon salt, or to taste
⅛ teaspoon freshly ground black
  pepper
1 (10-ounce) can cannellini
  beans, rinsed and drained

Trim off stems of fennel bulb. If desired, chop enough feathery fennel fronds to measure 2 tablespoons; set aside. Thinly slice fennel bulb. In a medium skillet, heat olive oil over medium-high heat. Add sliced fennel, onion, and garlic; cook until soft and fragrant, about 4 minutes, stirring occasionally. Add bell pepper, vinegar, salt, and pepper; mix well and cook 1 minute. Add beans; heat through. Serve warm, at room temperature, or chilled. Serves 4.
  (*Courtesy:* Mizkan Americas, Inc.)

Seafood

It was my plan to visit the Space Needle in Seattle the last night I was there after a trip to British Columbia. Since Pacific Northwest cuisine includes fabulous fish—all kinds—it would be a mistake if I didn't order salmon or crab for dinner. The early spring weather was remembered—not the fish. While I was upgraded to a twenty-eighth-floor suite complete with a panoramic view of Elliott Bay surrounded by mountains and a cityscape, weathering the wind and rain for a pricey fish plate was scratched from my bucket list. Instead, I ordered a vegetarian pizza with anchovies—an oily Pacific Ocean fish—and dark leafy greens on top drizzled with red wine vinegar and olive oil. It was my way of doing things differently, but it was still unforgettable. Back at home, in my living room on the fireplace mantel is a picture-perfect photo of the hotel room with a view, amid the comfort of my home in the Sierra with my aquarium stocked with goldfish and a beloved pleco. The fish recipes I share with you are ones I enjoy too.

Fish contains the omega-3 fatty acids (which are found in salmon, swordfish, and tuna), potassium, and only a small amount of sodium. And it's these ingredients that help you have lower blood pressure and cholesterol levels. That means you'll be less prone to heart attacks and strokes.

What's more, when you include heart-healthy vinegar, garlic, onions, and olive oil with fish, as in our tantalizing fish recipes, you'll be on track to keeping a healthy heart.

Classic Seviche
Crab Cakes with Nakano Vinegar Mayonnaise
Sesame Fish with Sautéed Spinach
Roast Salmon with Balsamic Glaze
Simple Salmon
Tapas-Style Mussels

Classic Seviche

❖ ❖ ❖

1 pound bay scallops or firm white
   fish fillets, cut into 1-inch cubes
¼ cup fresh lime juice*
½ cup Nakano Seasoned Rice
   Vinegar with Red Pepper or
   Nakano Seasoned Rice
   Vinegar—Original
¾ cup diced red and/or green bell
   pepper

⅓ cup chopped red onion
1 clove garlic, minced
½ teaspoon hot pepper sauce, or
   1 jalapeño pepper, minced
assorted crackers, melba toast,
   or large corn tortilla chips

Place scallops in a shallow 1½-quart casserole dish. Pour lime juice over scallops; mix well and press into an even layer. In a small bowl, combine remaining ingredients; pour over scallops. Cover and refrigerate at least 24 hours or until scallops are opaque. Transfer mixture with a slotted spoon to a serving bowl. Discard marinade. Serve with crackers. Serves 5.

   *Fresh lime juice and vinegar "cook" the scallops as they marinate overnight.

   (*Courtesy:* Mizkan Americas, Inc.)

Crab Cakes with Nakano Vinegar Mayonnaise

❖ ❖ ❖

½ pound lump crab meat or 2
   (6-ounce) cans crab meat,
   rinsed, drained
1 egg
1 green onion, chopped
½ teaspoon seasoned salt
⅛ teaspoon cayenne pepper
2½ tablespoons plus ¼ cup dry
   bread crumbs

1 tablespoon vegetable oil
¾ cup lite or regular mayonnaise
3 tablespoons Nakano Seasoned
   Rice Vinegar with Red Pepper
   or Nakano Seasoned Rice
   Vinegar—Original
2 teaspoons Dijon-style mustard

Pick over crab meat, discarding any bits of shell. In a medium bowl, combine crab meat, egg, green onion, salt, and cayenne pepper. Add

2½ tablespoons bread crumbs. Mix well; shape into four patties about 3 inches wide and ½-inch thick. (Note: At this point, crab cakes may be covered and refrigerated up to 4 hours before cooking.) Place remaining ¼ cup bread crumbs on a shallow plate. Dip crab cakes in bread crumbs, patting to coat lightly. Heat oil in a large nonstick skillet over medium heat. Add crab cakes; cook about 4 minutes per side or until golden brown. Meanwhile, combine mayonnaise, vinegar, and mustard; mix well. Serve crab cakes with mayonnaise. Serves 4.

(*Courtesy*: Mizkan Americas, Inc.)

Sesame Fish with Sautéed Spinach

❖ ❖ ❖

3 tablespoons Nakano Seasoned Rice Vinegar—Original or Nakano Seasoned Rice Vinegar with Red Pepper

2 tablespoons lite or regular teriyaki sauce

1 tablespoon vegetable oil

2 teaspoons dark roasted sesame oil

1 teaspoon bottled or fresh minced ginger

¼ teaspoon crushed red pepper flakes

4 (4–5-ounces) skinless halibut, red snapper, or orange roughy fish fillets

1 (10-ounce) package washed spinach leaves, stems discarded

2 teaspoons sesame seeds, toasted (optional)

Combine vinegar, teriyaki sauce, vegetable oil, sesame oil, ginger, and pepper flakes; mix well. Set aside half of mixture. Place fish on a shallow plate; drizzle remaining vinegar mixture evenly over fish. Turn fish to coat both sides. Let stand at room temperature 20 minutes. Place fish on rack of broiler pan or on grid over medium coals. Brush fish with any remaining marinade from dish. Broil fish 4–5 inches from heat source 5 minutes. Turn; continue to broil 4–5 minutes, or until fish is opaque. While fish is cooking, heat remaining vinegar mixture in a large deep skillet over medium-high heat. Add spinach; cover and simmer 1–2 minutes or until spinach is wilted. Transfer with tongs to four serving plates. Arrange fish over spinach; drizzle with any remaining vinegar mixture from skillet. Sprinkle with sesame seeds, if desired. Serves 4.

(*Courtesy*: Mizkan Americas, Inc.)

Roast Salmon with Balsamic Glaze

❖ ❖ ❖

5-pound whole salmon center, bone removed
1 tablespoon grated lemon rind
2 cloves garlic, finely chopped
2 tablespoons chopped fresh thyme
3 tablespoons olive oil

½ cup balsamic vinegar
½ cup red wine
1 teaspoon granulated sugar
¼ cup butter
lemon slices

Preheat oven to 350°. Place salmon in baking dish. Chop together lemon rind, garlic, and thyme. Brush oil over salmon and inside cavity. Rub herb mixture over. (Prepare up to 24 hours ahead of time.) Roast 40 minutes or until white juices appear on top. Meanwhile, combine balsamic vinegar, wine, and sugar in a skillet. Bring to boil and reduce until syrupy. Turn heat to low and whisk in butter. Remove skin from salmon. Serve with sauce and lemon slices. Serves 8–10.

(*Courtesy:* The Vinegar Institute.)

Simple Salmon
(MARINATE AND BAKE THE SALMON IN THE SAME PAN)

❖ ❖ ❖

6 filets, 6 ounces each
1 tomato, peeled, seeded, and diced
4 ounces yellow onion, sliced
2 ounces carrots, sliced
1 lemon, sliced into rounds
2 cloves garlic, sliced
8 ounces vegetable broth

2 ounces olive oil
2 ounces red wine vinegar
2 ounces dry red wine
2 bay leaves
3 fresh thyme sprigs
4 fresh tarragon leaves
salt and pepper to taste

Place the 6 salmon filets in an oven-proof glass pan. Add all the other ingredients. Marinate for 1 hour in the refrigerator. In the same glass pan, cover salmon loosely with a piece of foil and bake for 15 minutes at 350°. When salmon is done, remove to a service plate. Strain liquid from baking pan and reduce to less than a cup using a whisk. Adjust seasoning and pour over salmon. Serves 6.

(*Courtesy:* Chef Salvatore J. Campagna.)

Tapas-style Mussels

❖ ❖ ❖

24 *large live mussels, scrubbed*
½ *cup water*
¼ *cup finely chopped red bell pepper*
¼ *cup finely chopped yellow bell pepper*
¼ *cup finely chopped pitted calamata or ripe olives*

2 *tablespoons Nakano Seasoned Rice Vinegar with Basil & Oregano or Nakano Seasoned Rice Vinegar—Original*
2 *tablespoons extra virgin olive oil*
1 *clove garlic, minced*

Combine mussels and water in a large deep skillet or Dutch oven. Cover; bring to a boil over high heat. Reduce heat to medium; continue to cook until mussels open, 4–5 minutes. Discard any mussels that do not open. Drain mussels; cool to room temperature. Meanwhile, combine remaining ingredients; mix well. Remove and discard one side of each mussel shell, leaving mussel in remaining shell. Arrange mussels on a serving platter. Spoon about 1 teaspoon vinegar mixture over each mussel. Serve at room temperature or chilled. Serves 8–12.

Tip: Most mussels are now farm-raised and contain very little sand and grit, but if the mussels are harvested from the ocean, soak them in cold water with a tablespoon of cornmeal and rinse them well before scrubbing.

(*Courtesy*: Mizkan Americas, Inc.)

Poultry

Protein helps you shed weight by decreasing your body's production of insulin. This is important because insulin locks fat in your fat cells, according to nutritionists.

You can keep insulin levels low by increasing your intake of protein-rich foods like skinless chicken and lean turkey meat.

Protein has just 4 calories per gram—about half the number of calories fat has. Says Columbus, Georgia, weight-loss specialist Jan McBarron, M.D., "Protein is digested slowly, so it helps curb your appetite." And protein-rich poultry is also rich in other nutrients.

And remember, season your food with spices such as garlic, pepper, and oregano. Lemon juice, vinegar, and hot sauce add zest without adding fat.

Chicken Bite Appetizers
Polynesian Chicken
Spinach and Chicken Wraps
Sweet and Sour Chicken
Turkey Wraps

Chicken Bite Appetizers

❖ ❖ ❖

2 whole chicken breasts (boned and skinned)
paprika, salt, and pepper

1 tablespoon Pompeian Red Wine Vinegar
⅓ cup Pompeian Extra Virgin Olive Oil

Cut chicken into bite-sized pieces, sprinkle with paprika, salt, and pepper. Add vinegar and stir well to coat all the pieces. Marinate in refrigerator for at least 1 hour. Heat olive oil in skillet to 320°. Add chicken and sauté both sides until golden brown (about 3 minutes). Serve immediately on wooden toothpicks.

(*Courtesy*: Pompeian.)

Polynesian Chicken

❖ ❖ ❖

1 pound skinless, boneless chicken breasts
1 medium green bell pepper, cut into 1-inch chunks
2 tablespoons butter or margarine
¼ teaspoon salt
dash pepper
2 cans (8 ounces each) pineapple chunks

½ cup water
⅓ cup Heinz Apple Cider Vinegar
2 tablespoons brown sugar
2 tablespoons soy sauce
1 teaspoon ginger
2½ tablespoons cornstarch
2½ tablespoons water
hot cooked rice
toasted slivered almonds

Cut chicken into strips about 2 inches long. In large skillet, sauté chicken and green pepper in butter just until chicken changes color. Season with salt and pepper. Stir in pineapple, pineapple liquid, and next 5 ingredients. Cover; simmer 10–12 minutes or until chicken is cooked. Combine cornstarch and 2½ tablespoons water; stir into chicken mixture. Cook until sauce is thickened, stirring constantly. Serve over rice; garnish with almonds. Makes 4 servings (about 4½ cups).

(*Courtesy*: Heinz.)

Spinach and Chicken Wraps

❖ ❖ ❖

¾ pound skinless chicken breasts, cooked
¼ cup Marsala olive oil
½ cup Yellow Delicious apple, sliced thin
½ cup green onions, chopped
¼ cup apple cider vinegar
¼ cup apple jelly

1 tablespoon Dijon mustard
1 cup almonds, slivered, toasted
2 slices lean ham, chopped
1 teaspoon Cajun spice mix
6 cups baby spinach leaves
¼ cup goat cheese (or feta cheese)
4 flour tortillas, 10 inches
4 cups salad of your choice

Slice chicken lengthwise into 12 pieces. In skillet add olive oil, apples, and onions; cook until soft. Add vinegar, jelly, and mustard. Cook 2 or 3 minutes on low heat. Add cooked chicken. Stir in almonds, ham, spice mix, spinach, and cheese. Heat tortillas according to package directions. Assemble wraps by arranging a cup of salad on each tortilla, top with chicken mixture. Roll tightly, secure with toothpick, and serve immediately. Serves 4.

(*Source: Cooking with California Olive Oil: Recipes from the Heart for the Heart*, Gemma Sanita Sciabica.)

Sweet and Sour Chicken

❖ ❖ ❖

1½ cups Marsala wine
1 large onion, chopped fine
3 whole cloves
3 cloves garlic, chopped
1 large bay leaf
6 chicken breasts, 7 ounces each, skin on

flour seasoned with salt and pepper
3 ounces olive oil
10 ounces chicken broth
3 tablespoons sugar
6 ounces red or white wine vinegar
¼ cup raisins (optional)
¼ cup pine nuts (optional)

In a saucepan, heat the Marsala wine, onion, cloves, garlic, and bay leaf. Just before it comes to a boil, pour over the chicken breasts in a shallow glass baking dish. Cover and refrigerate overnight or for at least 6 hours. Remove breasts from marinade, dredge in seasoned flour, and sauté in large skillet for 3 or 4 minutes on each side. Set aside on a plate. Pour off any excess oil from skillet. After discarding cloves and bay leaf from marinade, add this liquid to the skillet. Simmer for 5 minutes, then return breasts to the skillet, spooning sauce over the breasts. Add broth, stir, cover, and cook for 15 minutes, turning once or more. While chicken is simmering, heat sugar in a small saucepan until it melts to an amber color. Carefully stir in vinegar and, if you wish, the raisins and pine nuts. Pour this mixture over the breasts 2 or 3 minutes before they are done. Serves 6.

(*Courtesy:* Chef Salvatore J. Campagna.)

Turkey Wraps

❖ ❖ ❖

½ cup lite or regular mayonnaise
2 tablespoons Nakano Seasoned
   Rice Vinegar with Red Pepper or
   Nakano Seasoned Rice Vinegar
   with Roasted Garlic
⅛ teaspoon cayenne pepper
⅛ teaspoon ground cumin
⅛ teaspoon salt
4 (8-inch) flour tortillas or seasoned
   whole wheat tortillas, warmed if
   desired

4 leaves red leaf or romaine lettuce
⅓ pound deli slice turkey breast or
   smoked turkey breast
¾ cup julienned jicama (optional)
⅓ cup julienned carrot
1 cup shredded Monterey Jack cheese
alfalfa sprouts (optional)

In a small bowl, combine mayonnaise, vinegar, cayenne pepper, cumin, and salt. Spread half of mayonnaise mixture over each tortilla; top with lettuce and turkey. Spread remaining mayonnaise mixture over turkey; top with jicama, carrots, cheese, and, if desired, sprouts. Fold bottom of tortilla over filling; roll up burrito-style. Serves 4.

(*Courtesy:* Mizkan Americas, Inc.)

Main Meat Dishes

Beef, pork, and liver. What do these foods have in common? Even though fat is their common thread, they're packed with protein that health-conscious Americans can feel good about eating.

Researchers in Australia pitted a vegetarian diet (that included milk and eggs) against an equal-fat diet containing lean meat. In result, both diets lowered blood pressure and cholesterol.[1]

Both cuts of meat contain plenty of animal protein, B vitamins for better immunity, and blood-building iron. And when you team meat recipes with garlic, onions, olive oil—and vinegar—it becomes a healthy, mouthwatering dish that is great for you!

Sauerbrauten
Sweet and Sour Meatballs
Tropical Glazed Ribs

Sauerbraten

❖ ❖ ❖

MARINADE

1¼ cups dry red wine
1¼ cups red wine vinegar
2 quarts water
2 onions, sliced

8 black peppercorns, whole
10 juniper berries
3 bay leaves
2 cloves, whole

4 pounds beef bottom round
salt to taste
4 ounces vegetable oil
8 ounces onions, diced
4 ounces carrots, diced

4 ounces celery, diced
4 ounces tomato paste
2 ounces all-purpose flour
3 quarts beef broth
gingersnaps to taste

Combine all ingredients for the marinade and bring to a boil, then cool to room temperature. Remove all fat, gristle, and any membrane covering the meat. Season the beef round with salt and put it in the marinade. Refrigerate in a nonaluminum container for 3–5 days, turning 2 or 3 times daily. Remove meat from marinade. Strain and reserve marinade and reserve the onions and herbs separately. Bring the marinade to a boil (off center from heat) and skim off scum. Heat the oil in a braising pan, sear beef on all sides, remove, and reserve. Add diced vegetables and reserved onion-herb mixture. Brown lightly. Whisk in tomato paste then deglaze pan with reserved marinade and reduce this mixture by half. Sprinkle the flour into the reduced liquid and whisk thoroughly. Add the beef broth and whisk out any lumps. Bring to a simmer, place the beef round back in the braising pan, cover, and cook in a 300° oven until fork tender. Remove the meat and reduce the sauce. Remove any visible fat. Add the gingersnaps and cook sauce for 10 to 12 minutes or until the gingersnaps dissolve. Strain sauce through cheesecloth or very fine mesh strainer. Serve with potato pancakes and red cabbage for a traditional German dinner. Serves 10.

(*Courtesy*: Salvatore J. Campagna.)

Sweet and Sour Meatballs

❖ ❖ ❖

1 (8-ounce) can pineapple, crushed
½ cup Heinz Apple Cider Vinegar
¼ cup firmly packed brown sugar
2 tablespoons soy sauce
1 teaspoon ginger
1½ pounds lean ground beef
¾ cup dry bread crumbs
¼ cup milk
1 egg, slightly beaten
1 teaspoon salt
dash pepper
1 tablespoon vegetable oil
1 tablespoon cornstarch
1 tablespoon water

Drain pineapple, reserving liquid. Add water to reserved liquid to measure ¾ cup. Add vinegar and next 3 ingredients, set aside. Combine beef and next 5 ingredients lightly but well. Form into 30 meatballs, using a rounded tablespoon for each. Brown meatballs in oil in a large skillet; drain excess fat. Add pineapple liquid mixture. Cover; simmer 15–20 minutes or until meatballs are cooked, stirring occasionally. Stir in reserved pineapple. Combine cornstarch and water; stir into skillet. Cook until sauce is thick, stirring constantly. Makes 6 servings.

(*Courtesy:* Heinz.)

Tropical Glazed Ribs

❖ ❖ ❖

3 1½ to 4 pound lean pork baby
   back ribs
¼ cup plus 2 tablespoons Nakano
   Seasoned Rice Vinegar–Original
¼ cup unsweetened pineapple juice
   or canned papaya nectar

¼ cup lite or regular soy sauce
1 tablespoon bottled or fresh minced
   ginger
1 teaspoon bottled or fresh garlic
3 tablespoons brown sugar
½ cup pineapple or peach preserves

Place ribs in a resealable plastic bag. Combine ¼ cup vinegar, pineapple juice, soy sauce, ginger and garlic; mix well. Pour over ribs. Close bag securely; turning to coat. Marinate in refrigerator at least 4 hours or up to 24 hours before cooking. Preheat oven to 375°. Drain ribs, reserving marinade. Place ribs, meaty side up on foil-lined shallow baking sheet or jelly roll pan. Bake 30 minutes. Turn; continue to bake 15 minutes. Combine ½ cup remaining marinade (discard any remaining marinade) and brown sugar in a small saucepan. Simmer uncovered until slightly thickened and reduced to ⅓ cup, about 5 minutes. Turn ribs meaty side up; brush with brown sugar mixture. Return to oven; bake 20–25 minutes or until ribs are browned and glazed. Cool 10 minutes. Meanwhile, combine remaining 2 tablespoons vinegar with preserves; mix well. Cut ribs into individual pieces. Serve warm or at room temperature with dipping sauce. 12 servings.

(*Courtesy:* Mizkan Americas, Inc.)

Desserts

Walking on the cobblestone streets of Quebec City amid tourists from a variety of countries, I stopped at a small coffee shop and ordered a latte with a sweet fruit tart. I savored the pastry and remembered the strawberry balsamic vinegar pie I baked and froze a week before I left for my Canadian adventure. I flagged down a woman with her horse and carriage and treated myself to a ride around the city—something I've never done before, but wanted to do, sort of like adding balsamic vinegar to a fruit pie.

Surprise! Sweet foods can be good for you! Our vinegar desserts contain plenty of healthy ingredients such as yogurt, melons, and raisins. These edibles are nutritious foods—and can cure a sugar craving, too. And don't forget. Vinegar coupled with these naturally sweet treats makes dessert a healing delight.

Custard with Honey Balsamic Berries
Coconut Macaroons Dipped in White Chocolate Frosting
with Apricot Vinegar Glaze
Melon Sorbet
Pear Tart with Balsamic Fig Vinegar
Old-fashioned Raisin Pie
Strawberries with Orange and Balsamic Vinegar
Vinegar Pie

Custard with Honey Balsamic Berries

❖ ❖ ❖

1 cup half-and-half
1½ cups 2 percent organic low-fat
  milk
4–5 egg yolks
¼ cup white granulated sugar
1 teaspoon pure vanilla extract
½ cup coconut, sweetened,
  shredded (optional)
2 teaspoons nutmeg

2 cups fresh fruit (blackberries,
  blueberries, strawberries)
2 tablespoons apple cider vinegar
  (I used Honey Ridge Farms
  Balsamic Honey Vinegar)
raw sugar to taste
whipped cream, real (if preferred)
almonds, finely chopped
  (optional)

In a saucepan, heat half-and-half with milk. Do not bring to a boil. Set aside. Mix egg yolks with sugar and pour into milk, stir well. Add vanilla. Sprinkle bottom of ramekins with coconut. Pour egg mixture into 4 ramekins. Top with nutmeg and sugar. Place ramekins in a rectangular pan half-filled with water. Bake at 350 degrees for about 40 to 50 minutes till firm. Place a knife into custard and when it comes out clean, remove. Cool. In a bowl, mix fresh fruit with vinegar. Put both custard and fruit into fridge. Top with whipped cream and sprinkle almonds on top. Serves 4. (You can serve custard warm if preferred.)

Coconut Macaroons Dipped in White Chocolate Frosting with Apricot Vinegar Glaze

❖ ❖ ❖

½ cup all-purpose flour
⅛ teaspoon cream of tartar
¼ cup granulated white sugar
⅛ teaspoon salt
7 ounces sweetened condensed
  milk
1 capful each almond extract and
  pure vanilla extract

4½ to 5 cups premium sweetened
  coconut, shredded
4 egg whites
1 teaspoon orange rind
½ cup white chocolate chips or
  bar pieces

GLAZE

2 tablespoons Etruria Apricot Vinegar
2 tablespoons honey or brown sugar

In a large bowl, combine flour, cream of tartar, sugar, salt, milk, extracts, and coconut. Set aside. In a mixing bowl beat egg whites until stiff. Fold in coconut mixture. Add orange rind. Use 1/3 cup ice cream scoop or 1 teaspoon (shaped like a cone or pyramid) and place cookie dough mounds on cookie sheet lined with parchment paper. Bake at 350 degrees for approximately 15 minutes. Remove immediately. Cool.

Melt chocolate in microwave (30 seconds, watch and do not overcook). Dip bottoms or half side of each cookie into melted chocolate. Place on plate and allow to set.

For vinegar glaze: In a saucepan heat apricot vinegar and bring to boil. Turn the heat down and simmer for several minutes. Add honey or sugar. Drizzle on top of each cookie.

Makes about three dozen cookies. Store in airtight container and put in fridge or freezer. These adorable cookies with a vinegary sophistication are best fresh. Caveat: Savor in moderation due to its sugar and saturated fat.

Once I plated each cookie on the cookie sheet, I sensed this recipe was a keeper. I peeked in the oven after five minutes and the macaroons had not spread. Perfection. By 12 minutes, give or take a few, the coconut got picture-perfect toasty golden brown and kept its mound shape. Removing the macaroons from the cookie sheet was a snap—no sticking. And the first bite was heaven: crispy on the outside, moist and chewy on the inside. The frosting is sweet and tangy, thanks to the fruit-flavored vinegar. The end result: a sweet cookie to warm your home where the heart is. And I'll bet you'll convert anti-vinegar people.

Melon Sorbet

❖ ❖ ❖

2 ripe sweet melons, halved and
   deseeded
½ cup icing sugar, sifted

6 tablespoons white wine vinegar
2 egg whites, large

Scoop flesh from melons and place in a food processor with sugar
and vinegar. Blend to a puree. Place in a freezer-proof container; cover
and freeze for 4–5 hours. Whisk egg whites until stiff, then blend with
the mushy sorbet. Freeze until solid. Leave to stand at room temperature for 10–15 minutes before serving.

(*Courtesy*: The Vinegar Institute.)

Pear Tart with Balsamic Fig Vinegar

❖ ❖ ❖

A plain tart, like this one, is vibrant in earthy color. Because the
store-bought piecrust came with two, I saved one for another fruit.
These pastries boast a European flair, and can be served for breakfast,
afternoon tea, or dessert with gourmet coffee. I savored the fig treat at
night on the deck under the big, bright moon; it took me back to San
Francisco. Each bite of tart was like enjoying the exciting city lights
and enjoying the majestic mountains where I now live.

1 store-bought premium piecrust
   or make your own
2 tablespoons European-style
   butter
4 fresh pears (firm like apples
   work best), cut in quarters,
   cored, sliced in wedges

⅓ cup granulated sugar
1 teaspoon lemon rind (optional)
2 tablespoons The Olive Press Fig
   Balsamic Vinegar
2 tablespoons organic apricot
   preserves, melted
confectioners' sugar (garnish)

Line a rectangular pan with parchment paper. Unroll refrigerated
single piecrust (or use piecrust in pan). Simply shape into a rectangle

(it is very easy to do this). Fold edges so they are thick, but not perfect, to give your tart a rustic look. Sauté pears in butter. Fill piecrust with fruit slices and layer. Sprinkle with sugar, lemon rind, and vinegar. Bake at 350 degrees for 40–50 minutes till crust is golden and fruit is bubbly. Remove and spread top with preserves and sprinkle top with confectioners' sugar. Cool. Place in fridge to set overnight. Slice in nice-sized rectangles or triangles. Serve paired with all-natural vanilla ice cream, real whipped cream, or plain. Serves 8.

Old-Fashioned Raisin Pie

❖ ❖ ❖

2 cups raisins
2 cups water
½ cup packed brown sugar
2 tablespoons cornstarch
½ teaspoon cinnamon

¼ teaspoon salt
1 tablespoon vinegar
1 tablespoon butter or margarine
pastry for double 9-inch crust

Combine raisins and water; boil 5 minutes. Blend sugar, cornstarch, cinnamon, and salt. Add to raisins and cook, stirring until clear. Remove from heat. Stir in vinegar and butter. Cool slightly. Turn into pastry-lined pan. Cover with top pastry or lattice strips. Bake at 425° about 30 minutes or until golden brown. Yield: One 9-inch pie.

(*Courtesy*: Mizkan Americas, Inc.)

Strawberries with Orange and Balsamic Vinegar

❖ ❖ ❖

13 ounces fresh strawberries (pint)   1½–2 tablespoons balsamic vinegar
  washed, stemmed, sliced   1 tablespoon fructose
½ cup fresh orange juice   6 sprigs fresh mint

Slice berries into medium-sized mixing bowl. Mix together orange juice, balsamic vinegar, and fructose. Pour over berries. Gently stir berries to cover liquid. Let sit for about 1 hour. Spoon into champagne glasses or other small decorative dishes. Garnish with sprig of mint. Serves 6.

(*Courtesy:* Chef Michel Stroot of the Golden Door Spa.)

Vinegar Pie

❖ ❖ ❖

4 eggs   1 teaspoon vanilla extract
1½ cups sugar   9-inch frozen pie shell, defrosted
¼ cup butter or margarine, melted   chopped nuts (optional)
1½ tablespoons cider or white   whipped cream (optional)
  vinegar

Preheat oven to 350°. In a large mixing bowl, combine eggs, sugar, butter, vinegar, and vanilla; mix well. Pour into pie shell. Bake until firm, about 50 minutes. Cool on a rack. Serve garnished with chopped nuts or whipped cream, if desired. Yield: one 9-inch pie.

(*Courtesy:* Mizkan Americas, Inc.)

Before *You* Use
Vinegar

A FINAL DISH ON VINEGARS

Nowadays, I look back at Vinegar World and am amazed how fascinating it is in America and around the world. I cannot help but recall one early morning when I was a guest on a live radio show in the Midwest. After I was grilled on my book *The Healing Powers of Vinegar*, second edition, the host wrapped up the interview in one sentence: "Well, folks, vinegar is good for salads." I was shocked at the statement. I thought, "But what about its powers to lower the risk of developing heart disease, cancer, obesity, and home cures for a thousand and one ailments, beauty, pets, and cleaning?" My words went down the rabbit hole like in *Alice in Wonderland*. I chased a cup of joe with a large glass of water that had a splash of lemon, and a teaspoon of apple cider vinegar, and fled to the town's resort swimming pool. I knew in my heart the Vinegar World is infinite—despite feeling like I had come full circle back to when I was a kid in a world of apple cider, red wine, and white vinegars. I'm delighted to have shared the wonders of

Vinegar World, a never-ending and exciting place to me. . . . It is waiting for you. If you listen to the stories, each testimony of vinegar healing leads people to use it again and again. You, too, may experience
the good of vinegar—inside or outside your body. If you acknowledge
that an estimated 98 percent of Americans have vinegar already in
their households, it just might be worth paying attention to.

The exciting old and new ingredients in potassium-plentiful *apple
cider* and *now* antioxidant-rich *red wine vinegars* are enough to get you
started. And don't forget the variety of health benefits that are provided by *balsamic, fruit, rice* and *herbal vinegars*, too. Plus, these expert
folk remedies and vinegar recipes (and some of my personal favorites)
will keep you busy.

Keep in mind, however, if you want to prevent health ailments and
lower your risk of disease (such as alcoholism *and* cancer, in my case),
you have to learn the lessons of a healthy lifestyle (especially in the
unpredictable twenty-first century) and practice them, too. Take the
following steps:

1. Reduce the risk factor for diseases such as heart disease, stroke,
   and the most common forms of cancer by adopting a healthy
   diet, exercise, and stress-management program.

2. To combat some of the effects of air pollution and other environmental hazards, consider vitamin E and choosing foods rich
   in vitamin C, the vegetable form of vitamin A (beta-carotene),
   and a trace mineral called selenium.

3. Try to do a combination of aerobic exercise (walking, jogging,
   swimming, etc.), which is heart-healthy, and strength training
   (some type of weightlifting activity) for a minimum of three
   times a week, 20–30 minutes a day.

4. Forgo unhealthy vices and don't smoke; avoid certain foods, and
   alcohol.

5. And remember to stock your pantry full of health-boosting vinegars, garlic, onions, olive oils—plenty of fresh fruits and vegetables—and enjoy a healthy diet!

Kris Cercio, who lowered her cholesterol levels; health guru Partricia Bragg, who is living better and longer, thanks to a versatile vinegar; and me, an advocate of apple cider vinegar—as well as many others—discovered, each in our own way, that if used with a positive attitude and approach, vinegar is an amazing ancient elixir that will be around for centuries to come. You, too, can enjoy the healing powers of vinegar—nature's most remarkable remedy.

PART 9

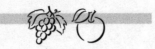

VINEGAR
RESOURCES

Where Can You Buy Vinegar?

Vinegar in hand is better than Havla to come.
—Persian Proverb

As apple cider and red wine vinegars, and other types as well, continue to be touted for their powerful health benefits, quality vinegars for the health-conscious and specialty vinegars for vinegar lovers are popping up everywhere. Currently, a wide variety of vinegars can be bought in supermarkets and health food stores, as well as through mail-order and the Internet.

Here is a list of vinegars, from organic and natural to commercial brands. If you're interested in buying any of these vinegars and can't find them locally, just contact the manufacturers directly for the locations of stores nearest you.

Bertolli
800-670-7356
www.villabertolli.com

Olive oils and vinegars.

Dove Olive Oil Co.
317 Branson Landing
Branson, MO 65616
www.doveoliveoil.com

This growing company provides oils and an impressive line of balsamic vinegars.

Gold Mine Natural Food Company
13200 Danielson Street, Suite A-1
Poway, CA 92064
www.goldminenaturalfoods.com

This company offers plant-based and organic foods. They carry a wide variety of natural, organic vinegars: apple cider, which is naturally fermented, brown rice, and ume.

HJ Heinz Company L.P.
357 6th Avenue
Pittsburgh, PA 15222
www.heinz.com

Heinz has been established since 1885 and boasts a variety of vinegars including apple cider, red wine, white distilled, and balsamic. (See Part 8 for recipes using Heinz vinegars.)

Bragg Live Foods, Inc.
Box 7
Santa Barbara, CA 93102-0007
www.bragg.com

Welcome to popular apple cider vinegars available in a variety of places, including online, grocery stores, and health food stores.

Mizkan Americas, Inc.
1661 Feehanville Drive
Suite 300
Mount Prospect, IL 60056
800-323-4358
www.mizkan.com

Mizkan is a well-established company carrying a wide variety of vinegars, including rice vinegar and specialty vinegars. (See Part 8 for recipes using Mizkan Americas products.)

Pompeian, Inc.
4201 Pulaski Highway
Baltimore, MD 21224
www.pompeian.com

Red wine varieties and balsamic vinegars. (See Part 8 of this book for recipes using their products.)

Nick Sciabica & Sons
2150 Yosemite Blvd.
Modesto, CA 95354
800-551-9612
www.sunshineinabottle.com

Sciabica specializes in cold-pressed olive oils using varieties of California olives. They also provide red wine vinegar as well as an array of balsamic vinegars. (See recipes created by Gemma Sciabica using their products.)

The Olive Press
24724 Hwy. 121 (Arnold Drive)
Sonoma, CA 95476
www.theolivepress.com

Learn about an amazing selection of olive oils and balsamic vinegars, and a variety of pantry items.

Eden Foods, Inc.
701 Tecumseh Road
Clinton, MI 49236
888-424-3336

SPECIALTY FOODS

ChefShop.com
1425 Elliott Avenue West
Seattle, WA 98119
www.ChefShop.com

ChefShop.com carries an extensive line of artisan-produced specialty foods and ingredients from around the world, including a selection of vinegars and healing oils.

King Arthur Flour
Bakery, Café, Store & School
135 US Rt. 5 South
Norwich, Vermont 05055
www.kingarthurflour.com/shop

Specialty items for all your cooking and baking needs, including herbes de provence and garlic oil.

HONEY TO PAIR WITH VINEGAR

Honey Ridge Farms
12310 NE 245th Avenue
Brush Prairie, WA 98606
www.honeyridgefarms.com

Unforgettable gourmet honey, honey crèmes (apricot, blackberry, clover, lemon, raspberry), honey vinegar, and honey grilling sauces and glazes.

INFORMATION ON VINEGAR

The Vinegar Institute
Suite 500-D
5775 Peachtree-Dunwoody Road
Atlanta, GA 30342
404-252-3663
www.versatilevinegar.org

An age-old industry association that represents vinegar manufacturers and bottlers in the United States, as well as producers in Argentina, Brazil, Canada, Germany, Panama, and Sri Lanka. Companies manufacturing and/or bottling vinegar qualify for active membership in The Institute, and suppliers of goods or services to the vinegar industry are eligible suppliers. Their job is to make sure vinegar is labeled correctly, and they test on-the-market vinegars for authenticity to protect the consumer.

Vinegar Connoisseurs International
P.O. Box 41
Roslyn, SD 57261
605-486-4536
www.vinegarman.com

Lawrence Diggs is an international consultant to vinegar makers and author of *Vinegar*. He offers a wide variety of vinegar-related website links which are fun, fascinating, and informative.

The International Vinegar Museum
502 Main Street
Roslyn, SD
Open June–September
Tuesday–Saturday
10 A.M.–6:00 P.M.

Looking for the ultimate vinegar experience? It's awaiting you, thanks to the creative Vinegar Man, at the International Vinegar Museum. See different vinegars from around the globe. Learn how paper and pottery are made from vinegar. Discover how vinegar is made in factories, villages, and homes all over the world. Buy unusual vinegars. This museum is a large brick building boasting approximately 5,000 square feet. It also has a gift shop and a vinegar-tasting bar. During the International Vinegar Festival, more exotic vinegars are brought out for people to taste.

As of this writing, I find that more manufacturers and retail outlets could be added to this list. However, because of the popularity and varied types of vinegar to choose from, it is impossible to keep up with all the new companies marketing such products.

Notes

CHAPTER 1:
THE POWER OF VINEGAR

1. Lawrence Diggs, *Vinegar* (Quiet Storm Trading Company, 1989), 249.
2. JAMA, 1998:280:1569–1575.
3. D.C. Jarvis, *Folk Medicine: A New England Almanac of Natural Health Care from a Noted Vermont Country Doctor* (Fawcett Crest, 1958), 62.
4. Dr. Paul C. Bragg and Dr. Patricia Bragg, *Apple Cider Health System* (Health Science, 1995).
5. *Williams-Sonoma Essentials Vinegars*, ed. Chuck Williams (Weldon Owen Inc., 1994), 8.
6. Maggie Oster, *Herbal Vinegar* (Storey Communications, 1994), 6.

CHAPTER 2:
A GENESIS OF SOUR WINE

1. Lawrence Diggs, *Vinegar* (Quiet Storm Trading Company, 1989), 249.
2. Op. cit., 214.
3. Ibid.

4. Emily Thacker, *The Vinegar Book* (Tresco Publishers, 1995), 4.

5. Maggie Oster, *Herbal Vinegar* (Storey Communications, 1994), 4.

6. Lawrence Diggs, *Vinegar* (Quiet Storm Trading Company, 1989), 39.

7. Ibid.

8. Maggie Oster, *Herbal Vinegar* (Storey Communications, 1994), 4.

9. Ibid.

10. Ibid.

11. Ibid.

12. Op. cit., 5.

13. Lawrence Diggs, *Vinegar* (Quiet Storm Trading Company, 1989), 214.

14. Op. cit., 214.

15. Maggie Oster, *Herbal Vinegar* (Storey Communications, 1994), 5.

16. Lawrence Diggs, *Vinegar* (Quiet Storm Trading Company, 1989), 23.

17. Op. cit., 27.

18. "Vinegar Can Be Used for What?" *Saturday Evening Post Society*, Vol. 277, No. 4, July 1, 2005, 93.

19. James O'Brien, *The Miracle of Garlic and Vinegar* (Globe Communications Corp., 1998), 58.

20. Ibid., 58, 59.

21. "Counting Her Blessing," *Town and Country*, November 2004.

CHAPTER 3:
A HISTORICAL TESTIMONY

1. Lawrence Diggs, *Vinegar* (Quiet Storm Trading Company, 1989), 250.

2. Dr. Paul C. Bragg and Dr. Patricia Bragg, *Apple Cider Vinegar: Miracle Health System* (Health Science, 1995),11.

3. Ibid.

4. Ibid.

5. D.C. Jarvis, *Folk Medicine: A New England Almanac of Natural Health Care from a Noted Vermont Country Doctor* (Fawcett Crest, 1958), 85.

6. Togo Kuroiwa, *Rice Vinegar: An Oriental Home Remedy* (Tokyo: Kenko Igakusha Co., 1977).

7. D.C. Jarvis, *Folk Medicine: A New England Almanac of Natural Health Care from a Noted Vermont Country Doctor* (Fawcett Crest, 1958), 69.

8. Op. cit., 69.

9. Dr. Paul C. Bragg and Dr. Patricia Bragg, *Apple Cider Health System* (Health Science, 1995), 8.

10. Julian Whitaker, M.D., *Health & Healing* newsletter, May 1997 (Vol. 7, No. 5).

11. Ibid.

12. Ibid.

13. Ibid.

14. Ibid.

CHAPTER 4:
WHERE ARE THE SECRET INGREDIENTS?

1. Dr. Paul C. Bragg and Dr. Patricia Bragg, *Apple Cider Health System* (Health Science, 1995), 1.

2. Product Data Sheet, Fleischmann's *Apple Cider Vinegar*; Burns Philp Food Ingredients; June 15, 1998.

3. Maggie Oster, *Herbal Vinegar* (Storey Communications, 1994).

4. D.C. Jarvis, *Folk Medicine: A New England Almanac of Natural Health Care from a Noted Vermont Country Doctor* (Fawcett Crest, 1958), 68.

5. Dr. C. Bragg and Dr. Patricia Bragg, *Apple Cider Vinegar: Miracle Health System* (Health Science, 1995), 4.

6. D.C. Jarvis, *Folk Medicine: A New England Almanac of Natural Health Care from a Noted Vermont Country Doctor* (Fawcett Crest, 1958), 48.

7. Ibid., 49.

8. Susan M. Lark, M.D., and James A. Richards, M.B.A., *The Chemistry of Success: Six Secrets of Performance* (Bay Books, 1999), 102.

Chapter 5:
Why Is Apple Cider Vinegar So Healthy?

1. Lawrence Diggs, *Vinegar* (Quiet Storm Trading Company, 1989), 248.
2. Editors of *Prevention* Magazine, *The Healing Foods Cookbook* (Rodale Press, 1991), 21.
3. "Latest News," *The Vinegar Institute*, June 2005, *http://versatile vinegar.org/june_2005.html.*
4. Earl L. Mindell, R.Ph., Ph.D. with Larry M. Johns, *Amazing Apple Cider Vinegar: The Medicinal Miracle, plus the Curative, Cleaning and Cooking Virtues from Around the World* (Keats, 1996), 18.
5. "Latest News," *The Vinegar Institute*, May 2005, *http://versatile vinegar.org/may_2005.html.*
6. *The Medical Post, Medical Bulletin,* Feb. 8, 1994.
7. "Latest News," *The Vinegar Institute*, April 12, 2005, *http://versatile vinegar.org/April* 2005.
8. *The Lancet,* March 1999.
9. "Latest News," *The Vinegar Institute*, January 2005, *http://versatile vinegar.org/january_2005.html.*
10. Cal Orey, *Doctors' Orders: What 101 Doctors Do to Stay Healthy* (Twin Streams, 2002), 56, 57.
11. C. Cortesia, et al. "Acetic Acid, the Active Component of Vinegar, Is an Effective Tuberculocidal Disinfectant." *mBio* (2014); 5 (2): eoo13–14 DOI: 10:11281mBio.00013–14.

Chapter 6:
The Red Wine Vinegar Chronicle

1. Lawrence Diggs, *Vinegar* (Quiet Storm Trading Company, 1989), 250.
2. Togo Kuoiwa, *Rice Vinegar, An Oriental Home Remedy* (Tokyo: Kenko Igakusha Co., 1977), 6, 7.

CHAPTER 7:
THE OLD AND NEW HEALTHFUL INGREDIENTS

1. Lawrence Diggs, *Vinegar* (Quiet Storm Trading Company, 1989), 250.
2. Product Data Sheet, Fleischmann's® Red Wine Vinegar, June 15, 1998.
3. M.C. Garcia-Parrilla, F.J. Heredia, and Ana M. Troncosco, *Phenolic Composition of Wine Vinegars Produced by Traditional Static Methods, Nahrung* 41 (1997, Nr. 4 S 232–235); M. C. Garcia-Parrilla, F.J. Heredia, Ana M. Troncoso, *The Influence of the Acetification Process on the Phenolic Composition of Wine Vinegars, Sciences DES* (1998, 211–221).
4. *Science,* 6/10/97; Harriet Brown, "*Cancer at the Millennium,*" *Energy Times,* May 1999.

CHAPTER 8:
TAPPING INTO THE FRENCH PARADOX

1. *France—The Good Life, Savored, Your Health,* April 18, 1995.
2. Allan Magaziner, D.O., *The Complete Idiot's Guide to Living Longer & Healthier* (Alpha Books, 1999), 56.
3. Robert Crayhon, M.S., *Robert Crayhon's Nutrition Made Simple: A Comprehensive Guide to the Latest Findings in Optimal Nutrition* (M. Evans and Company, 1994), 60.
4. Op. cit., 60–61.
5. Op. cit., 62.
6. Anne Schamberg, *Journal Sentinel Inc.,* Sun., May 7, 1995.

CHAPTER 9:
IS RED WINE VINEGAR GOOD FOR YOU?

1. Lawrence Diggs, *Vinegar* (Quiet Storm Trading Company, 1989), 250.
2. American Heart Association Journal Report: "Weekly Consumption of Wine May Cut Stroke Risk"; *Stroke: Journal of the American Heart Association,* Dec. 1998.
3. Ibid.

4. Allan Magaziner, D.O., *The Complete Idiot's Guide to Living Longer & Healthier* (Alpha Books, 1999), 54.

5. Earl Mindell, R.Ph., Ph.D., *Earl Mindell's Supplement Bible* (Fireside, 1998); 134.

6. Allan Magaziner, D.O., *The Complete Idiot's Guide to Living Longer & Healthier* (Alpha Books, 1999), 54.

CHAPTER 10:
HEALTHY RICE VINEGAR

1. Togo Kuroiwa, *Rice Vinegar: An Oriental Home Remedy* (Tokyo: Kenko Igakusha Co., 1977), 179.

2. Based on Product Data Sheet, Fleischmann's Rice Vinegar, June 15, 1998.

3. Togo Kuroiwa, *Rice Vinegar: An Oriental Home Remedy* (Tokyo: Kenko Igakusha Co., 1977), 86.

4. Op. cit.

5. Op. cit., 179.

6. Ibid.

7. Maggie Oster, *Herbal Vinegar* (Storey Communications, 1994), 12.

8. Togo Kuroiwa, *Rice Vinegar: An Oriental Home Remedy* (Tokyo: Kenko Igakusha Co., 1977), 159, 163.

CHAPTER 11:
THE BALSAMIC VINEGAR BOOM

1. Richard Simmons, "Ask Richard Simmons," *Woman's World*, June 6, 1995.

2. Lawrence Diggs.

3. Bob Rubinelli, "All About Balsamic Vinegar," Oct. 11–12, 1995.

4. Based on Product Data Sheet, Fleischmann's Balsamic Vinegar, June 15, 1998.

5. Richard Simmons, "Ask Richard Simmons," *Woman's World*, June 6, 1995.

CHAPTER 12:
HEALING HERBAL VINEGARS

1. Lawrence Diggs, *Vinegar* (Quiet Storm Trading Company, 1989), 22.
2. Ray Sahelian, M.D., *Kava: The Miracle Antianxiety Herb* (St. Martin's Paperbacks, 1998), 164.
3. Daniel B. Mowrey, Ph.D., *Herbal Tonic Therapies* (Keats Publishing, 1993), 269.
4. Op. cit., 270.
5. Jim O'Brien, "The Oregano Prescription," *Your Health*, February 1998; 55.
6. Earl Mindell, R.Ph., Ph.D., *Earl Mindell's Supplemental Bible*, (Fireside, 1998), 115.
7. Op. cit., 135.
8. Laurel Dewey, "Don't Just Look at It!" *Your Health*, Dec. 10, 1996, 80.

CHAPTER 13:
FRUIT-FLAVORED VINEGAR CRAZE

1. "Quotes by Famous People: Benjamin Franklin Quotes," *http:// www.4u.com/bfranklin/*.
2. *Journal of Neuroscience*; Research News Release by National Institutes of Health; Sept. 15, 1999.
3. A Modern Herbal Home Page, <//mgmh.html>; 1995 Electric Newt.
4. "Japanese Fad: Drinking Vinegar, "Latest News," *The Vinegar Institute*, July 2005. *http://versatilevinegar.org/latestnews.html*.
5. Akemi Nakamura, *The Japan Times*, June 11, 2005, 1.
6. Ibid., 2.
7. Budak, N. H., et al. "Functional Properties of Vinegar." *Journal of Food Science*, 79 (2014): R757-R764. doi: 10.1111/1750-3841. 12434.

CHAPTER 14:
COMBINING VINEGARS AND
GARLIC, ONIONS, AND OLIVE OIL

1. Lawrence Diggs, *Vinegar* (Quiet Storm Trading Company, 1989), 250.
2. Dr. Arnold Pike, D.C. "Garlic's Natural Medicinal Qualities" *Let's Live* (Nov. 1990).
3. James O'Brien, *Garlic and Vinegar* (Globe, 1998), 30.
4. Robert Crayhon, *Nutrition Made Simple* (M. Evans and Company, Inc., 1994), 61.
5. Nancy G. Freeman, *Bring on the Olive Oil: The Mediterranean Diet, Get Up and Go!* February 1999, 10.
6. Op. cit., 9.
7. Ibid.
8. Ibid.
9. *Circulation: Journal of the American Heart Association* (1999; 99: 779–785).

CHAPTER 15:
THE LIQUID TO HEART HEALTH

1. "Vinegar Quotes & Quotations," *http://en.thinkexist.com/quotes/with/keyword/vinegar/*.
2. Cal Orey, *Doctors' Orders: What 101 Doctors Do to Stay Healthy* (Twin Streams, 2002).
3. M.D. Espositio, et al., "Effect of a Mediterranean-Style Diet on Endothelial Dysfunction and Markers of Vascular Inflammation in the Metabolica Syndrome, *JAMA*, 2004: 292:1440–1446.
4. Joe DiAngelo, "Begin Eating European Style—The Mediterranean Diet, Celebrities Love It!" June 21, 2003, *http://www.musclebomb.com/european.html*.

Chapter 16:
Fat-Burning Vinegar

1. "Vinegar Quotes & Quotations, *http://en.thinkexist.com/quotes/with/keyword/vinegar/*.

2. Coco Masters, Alice Park, and Sora Song, "The Year in Medicine From A to Z," *Time*, December 5, 2005, 75.
3. *European Journal of Clinical Nutrition*, 2005: 59: 1266–1271.
4. Kondo, Toomoo, et al. "Vinegar Intake Reduces Body Weight, Body Fat Mass, and Serum Triglyceride Levels in Obese Japanese Subjects." *Bioscience, Biotechnology, and Biochemistry,* 73 (2009): 1837–1843.

Chapter 17:
Antiaging and Wonder Food

1. "Vinegar Quotes & Quotations," *http://en.thinkexist.com/quotes/with/keyword/vinegar/*.
2. "Life Expectancy," *Wikipedia The Free Encyclopedia*, January 6, 2006, *http://en.wikipedia.org/wiki/Life_expectancy*.
3. Sonny Fontaine, "Health Guru Gives Sun Celebs! Shapes to Brag About!" *http://www.bragg.com*.
4. "Apple Cider Vinegar"—*Women's Health & Fitness* Celebrity Scoop, The Celebrity Elixir," *http://www.bragg.com*.

CHAPTER 18:
HOME CURES

1. D.C. Jarvis, *Folk Medicine: A New England Almanac of Natural Health Care from a Noted Vermont Country Doctor* (Fawcett Crest, 1958), 9.
2. Bonnie K. McMillen, *Connections Quarterly*, Summer 1998.
3. Ibid.
4. Ibid.
5. *New York Daily News*, April 2005, *http://nydailynews.com*.
6. Mary Ann Cooper, *Natural Cures*, (Natural Health, 2005), 4
7. D.C. Jarvis, *Folk Medicine: A New England Almanac of Natural Health Care from a Noted Vermont Country Doctor* (Fawcett Crest, 1958), 86.
8. Ibid.,182.
9. George Stancliffe, "Home Remedies to Get Rid of Toenila Fungus-Now!," *http://georgestancliffe.freewebsitehosting.com*.
10. D.C. Jarvis, *Folk Medicine: A New England Alamanac of Natural Health Care from a Noted Vermont Country Doctor* (Fawcett Crest, 1958), 86.

CHAPTER 19:
VINEGARMANIA: USING VINEGAR
FOR THE HOUSEHOLD, BEAUTY, KIDS, AND PETS

1. KOBTV, November 2004, *http://www.kobtv.com*.
2. "Eco-Safety Products," April 2005, *http://news.yahoo.com*.
3. *New Zealand Herald*, March 8, 2004, *www.nzherald.co.nx*.
4. Janice Cox, *Natural Beauty for All Seasons: 250 Simple Recipes and Gift-Giving Ideas for Year-Round Beauty* (Henry Holt and Company, 1996), 55.
5. Bob Goldstein, D.V.M., and Susan Goldstein, *Love of Animals* (December 1996), 6.
6. Douglas L. Langer, D.V.M., M.S., Veterinary Medical Teaching Hospital, University of California, Davis, "Enteroliths: Do We Have a Problem in California," 1992, 3.

CHAPTER 20:
VINEGAR IS NOT FOR EVERYONE:
SOME SOUR VIEWS

1. William Shakespeare, *The Merchant of Venice* (Penguin U.S.A., 1989).
2. Susan M. Lark, M.D., and James A. Richards, M.B.A., *The Chemistry of Success: Six Secrets of Peak Performance* (Bay Books, 1999), 111.
3. Ibid.
4. Lawrence Diggs, "*Vinegar Cures a Lot of Things, But Not Everything*," excerpted from *The Vinegar Connoisseurs International Newsletter*; HealthNot Everything.html at www.vinegarman.com; 1.
5. Ibid.
6. Bill Evers, Ph.D., RD., and April Mason, Ph.D., *National Council Against Health Fraud Newsletter*, May/June 1996, Vol. 19, No. 3; *FDA Consumer*, Jan.–Feb., 1996, pp. 35–36.
7. Interstitial Cystitis Network, "Understanding Diet and IC," *ICN Handbook*, *http://www.ic-network.com/handbook/diet.html*.